S0-BFA-210

Joint Commission

Standards for Long Term Care

| 2005-2006 | SLTC |

Accreditation
Policies

Standards

Elements of
Performance

Scoring

Joint Commission Mission

The mission of the Joint Commission on Accreditation of Healthcare Organizations is to continuously improve the safety and quality of care provided to the public through the provision of health care accreditation and related services that support performance improvement in health care organizations.

© 2005 by the Joint Commission on Accreditation of Healthcare Organizations

Joint Commission Resources, Inc. (JCR), a not-for-profit affiliate of the Joint Commission on Accreditation of Healthcare Organizations (Joint Commission), has been designated by the Joint Commission to publish publications and multimedia products. JCR reproduces and distributes these materials under license from the Joint Commission.

JCR educational programs and publications support, but are separate from, the accreditation activities of the Joint Commission. Attendees at JCR educational programs and purchasers of JCR publications receive no special consideration or treatment in, or confidential information about, the accreditation process.

All rights reserved. No part of this publication may be reproduced in any form or by any means without written permission from the publisher.

Printed in the U.S.A. 5 4 3 2 1

Requests for permission to make copies of any part of this work should be mailed to:
Permissions Editor
Department of Publications
Joint Commission Resources
One Renaissance Boulevard
Oakbrook Terrace, Illinois 60181
permissions@jcrinc.com

ISBN: 0-86688-881-0
ISSN: 1096-0546

For more information about the Joint Commission on Accreditation of Healthcare Organizations, please visit http://www.jcaho.org.

Contents

Standards, Rationales, Elements of Performance, and Scoring

Section 1: Patient-Focused Functions

Section 2: Organization Functions

How to Use This Book

The "How to Use This Book" chapter is designed to help organizations understand both the purpose and the content of the *SLTC*. This chapter highlights new and updated initiatives about the evolving accreditation process and orients readers to the structure of the book.

The *2005–2006 Standards for Long Term Care (SLTC)* is designed to facilitate a long term care organization's continuous operational improvement, as well as its performance against Joint Commission long term care standards. The *SLTC* includes all the information a long term care organization needs for continuous operational improvement: standards, rationales, elements of performance (EPs), scoring, and accreditation policies and procedures. The standards are provided in a new, user-friendly format that fosters a better understanding of each standard, its rationale (when applicable), and its EPs. Additional chapters that support ongoing accreditation efforts provide guidance on how to use the standards-related information found throughout the book.

What Is the Purpose of this Book?

The *SLTC* is designed to provide long term care organizations with information about the accreditation process. The *SLTC* includes more than the latest standards and compliance information; it also includes material that supports a long term care organization's continuous operational improvement and its accreditation efforts.

The *SLTC* also provides a better understanding of the connections between safety and quality-focused standards, day-to-day activities, and the accreditation process. In essence, the book is a one-stop resource for long term care accreditation and continuous standards compliance.

To What Organizations Does This Book Apply?

This book applies to long term care organizations seeking initial or continued long term care accreditation from the Joint Commission. This scope includes the following:

- Beds licensed by the state as nursing home beds excluding intermediate care facilities specializing in care for individuals with mental retardation and other developmental disabilities
- Beds designated as long term care beds under a hospital license (excluding beds belonging to a long term acute care hospital [LTACH] and hospital swing beds)
- Beds, units, or facilities certified by Medicare or Medicaid as skilled nursing facility (SNF) beds
- Beds, units, or facilities designated as long term care by a governmental entity, such as the Veterans Administration

HB

Long term care organizations that provide care for residents with dementia, whether integrated within long term care or in a segregated special care unit, will have those services surveyed as part of that organization under the long term care standards, including those special EPs applicable to dementia care.

Many long term care facilities provide subacute care on an inpatient basis for people who have had an acute illness or injury. The standards for long term care contain additional EPs addressing subacute care. Subacute care includes the following characteristics:

- Is rendered immediately after or instead of acute hospitalization
- Treats one or more specific, active, complex, or unstable medical conditions, or administers one or more technically complex treatments
- Requires the services of an interdisciplinary team whose members are trained to assess and manage specific conditions to perform necessary procedures
- Requires frequent resident assessment and review of the clinical course and treatment plan
- Provides care at a more intensive level than that provided in a traditional nursing facility but less intensive than that provided in acute inpatient care
- Lasts for a limited time, until a condition is stabilized or until a predetermined course of treatment is completed

The types of residents who undergo subacute care include the following:

- Ventilator-dependent residents
- Closed head trauma residents, immediately after the acute phase
- Subacute rehabilitation therapy residents
- Residents requiring medically complex treatment, including wound healing, IV therapy, pain management, or AIDS treatment, for example

Subacute services may be provided in any of the organizations to which this manual applies. Organizations that provide subacute services are responsible for complying with all the standards in this manual, including those with special EPs applicable to subacute services.

What's New in the *SLTC*?

Shared Visions–New Pathways®

The Joint Commission implemented its new initiative, Shared Visions–New Pathways, in January 2004. This initiative stemmed from the Joint Commission's critical look at its services, which included significant input from health care organizations, to dramatically redesign and improve the value of the accreditation process. Shared Visions–New Pathways represents a paradigm shift away from a focus on survey preparation to one of continuous operational improvement.

Specifically, this initiative does the following:

- Focuses the survey to a greater extent on the actual delivery of care, treatment, and services
- Increases the value of and the satisfaction with accreditation among accredited long term care organizations and their staff

- Shifts the accreditation-related focus from survey preparation and scores to continuous operational improvement
- Makes the accreditation process more continuous
- Increases the public's confidence that long term care organizations continuously comply with standards that emphasize resident safety and health care quality

See "The New Joint Commission Accreditation Process" chapter for more detailed information about this initiative.

Changes to the *SLTC* are made in response to suggestions from accredited long term care organizations and relate to important issues that clearly support high-quality care, treatment, and services. Since 2002–2003, many chapters have been revised and improved to include additional information requested by customers.

The 2004 edition of the *SLTC* was valid through December 31, 2004, and is followed by the 2005–2006 edition of the *SLTC*. The one-year book for 2004 was part of a Joint Commission initiative to revise and reformat standards simultaneously across all major accreditation programs. This *2005–2006 SLTC* returns the long term care program to a two-year book cycle.

For long term care organizations needing an update from the *2002–2003 SLTC* to the *2005–2006 SLTC*, please refer to Table 1, Columns 2 and 3. Column 2 summarizes the major revisions that occurred during 2002 and 2003 for inclusion in the *2004 SLTC*. Column 3 summarizes the major revisions that occurred during 2004 for inclusion in the *2005–2006 SLTC*.

What Does This Book Include?

"The New Joint Commission Accreditation Process" chapter explains the Joint Commission's new accreditation process. This chapter includes a description of the components of the new accreditation process, a sample time line, and the new decision categories and decision rules for 2005–2006.

The "Accreditation Policies and Procedures" chapter includes current information on accreditation policies and procedures relevant to all health care organizations. This chapter, which has been updated to reflect the new accreditation process, details the types of surveys and provides in-depth discussions of, for example, the Joint Commission's Information Accuracy and Truthfulness Policy and its Public Information Policy. This chapter contains updated information about the accreditation and appeals procedures. Specific links to the "Accreditation Participation Requirements" (APR) chapter are provided to facilitate understanding of the policies that appear in both chapters.

The "Sentinel Events" chapter contains background information on the Joint Commission's Sentinel Event Policy, including the definition of a sentinel event, the goals of the Policy, which adverse events constitute sentinel events, sentinel event–related standards, definitions of what occurrences are reviewable under the Policy, and the various activities that surround the Policy.

HB

Table 1. Summary of Major Revisions to the *SLTC*

Chapter	Summary of Content Changes During 2002 and 2003	Summary of Content Changes During 2004
How to Use This Book	This chapter has been revised to include information about Shared Visions–New Pathways. It also provides a description of the reformatted standards chapters.	Updated for 2005–2006.
The New Joint Commission Accreditation Process	This **new** chapter, which replaces the "The Accreditation Decision Process and Decision Rules" chapter, details the Joint Commission's new accreditation process.	Updated for 2005–2006.
Accreditation Policies and Procedures	This chapter has been updated to reflect changes resulting from Shared Visions–New Pathways. This chapter also references the "Accreditation Participation Requirements" chapter, to facilitate understanding of the policies that appear in both chapters.	Updated for 2005–2006.
Sentinel Events	This chapter has been revised and contains extensive information on the Joint Commission's Sentinel Event Policy.	Updated for 2005–2006.
National Patient Safety Goals	N/A	This **new** chapter for 2005–2006 identifies the Joint Commission's 2005 National Patient Safety Goals and requirements for long term care. Program-specific goals have also been adopted.
Accreditation Participation Requirements	This chapter has been modified for Shared Visions–New Pathways to address the ongoing requirements for continued participation in accreditation, as well as requirements related to the Joint Commission's National Patient Safety Goals.	Updated for 2005–2006. The National Patient Safety Goalsand Requirements are no longer included in this chapter, but are their own, separate chapter.
Standards and Elements of Performance Applicability Grid	This chapter, formerly titled "Standards Applicability Grid," has been updated for 2004 and now includes EPs.	Updated for 2005–2006.

Table 1. Summary of Major Revisions to the *SLTC* *(cont.)*

Chapter	Summary of Content Changes During 2002 and 2003	Summary of Content Changes During 2004
Assessment of Residents (PE)	This chapter was **eliminated** effective January 1, 2004. Many of the requirements in this chapter have been moved to the new "Provision of Care, Treatment, and Services" chapter. See the "Crosswalks of Standards" chapter for information on where requirements from this chapter appear in the new PC chapter.	Eliminated effective January 1, 2004.
Care of Residents (TX)	This chapter was **eliminated** effective January 1, 2004. Many of the requirements in this chapter have been moved to the new "Provision of Care, Treatment, and Services" and "Medication Management" chapters. See the "Crosswalks of Standards" chapter for information on where requirements from this chapter appear in the new PC and MM chapters.	Eliminated effective January 1, 2004.
Education of Residents (PF)	This chapter was **eliminated** effective January 1, 2004. Many of the requirements in this chapter have been moved to the new "Provision of Care, Treatment, and Services" chapter. See the "Crosswalks of Standards" chapter for information on where requirements from this chapter appear in the new PC chapter.	Eliminated effective January 1, 2004.
Continuum of Care (CC)	This chapter was **eliminated** effective January 1, 2004. Many of the requirements in this chapter have been moved to the new "Provision of Care, Treatment, and Services" chapter. See the "Crosswalks of Standards" chapter for information on where requirements from this chapter appear in the new PC chapter.	Eliminated effective January 1, 2004.
Ethics, Rights, and Responsibilities (RI)	This chapter was formerly called "Patient Rights and Organization Ethics." This chapter includes reformatted standards, rationales, EPs, and scoring. For detailed information about the changes in this chapter, please see the "Crosswalks of Standards" chapter.	Updated for 2005–2006.

continued on next page

Table 1. Summary of Major Revisions to the *SLTC* (cont.)

Chapter	Summary of Content Changes During 2002 and 2003	Summary of Content Changes During 2004
Provision of Care, Treatment, and Services (PC)	This is a **new** chapter that includes requirements from the "Assessment of Residents," "Care of Resdents," "Education of Patients and Family," and "Continuum of Care" chapters. See the "Crosswalks of Standards" chapter for information on where requirements from the previous chapters appear in the PC chapter.	PC.5.10—addition of EP 4, which was inadvertently omitted from the *2004 SLTC*. PC.5.40—addition of EP 4, which was inadvertently omitted from the *2004 SLTC*. PC.8.10 was reworded.
Medication Management (MM)	This is a **new** chapter that includes requirements from the "Care of Patients" chapter. See the "Crosswalks of Standards" chapter for information on where requirements from the previous TX chapter appear in the MM chapter.	Updated for 2005–2006.
Surveillance, Prevention, and Control of Infection (IC)	This chapter includes reformatted standards, rationales, EPs, and scoring. For detailed information about the changes in this chapter, please see the "Crosswalks of Standards" chapter. This chapter has also been moved to the Resident-Focused Functions" section.	Revised chapter effective January 1, 2005.
Improving Organization Performance (PI)	This chapter includes reformatted standards, rationales, EPs, and scoring. For detailed information about the changes in this chapter, please see the "Crosswalks of Standards" chapter.	Updated for 2005–2006.
Leadership (LD)	This chapter includes reformatted standards, rationales, EPs, and scoring. For detailed information about the changes in this chapter, please see the "Crosswalks of Standards" chapter.	Updated for 2005–2006.
Management of the Environment of Care (EC)	This chapter includes reformatted standards, rationales, EPs, and scoring. For detailed information about the changes in this chapter, please see the "Crosswalks of Standards" chapter.	EC.5.20—addition of EP 5, requiring the facility to make sufficient progress toward the corrective actions described in its Statement of Conditions™ (SOC).

Table 1. Summary of Major Revisions to the *SLTC* (cont.)

Chapter	Summary of Content Changes During 2002 and 2003	Summary of Content Changes During 2004
Management of Human Resources (HR)	This chapter includes reformatted standards, rationales, EPs, and scoring. For detailed information about the changes in this chapter, please see the "Crosswalks of Standards" chapter.	Updated for 2005–2006.
Management of Information (IM)	This chapter includes reformatted standards, rationales, EPs, and scoring. For detailed information about the changes in this chapter, please see the "Crosswalks of Standards" chapter.	Updated for 2005–2006.
Medicare/ Medicaid Certification– Based LTC Accreditation Standards	This **new** chapter includes all the standards, rationales, EPs, and scoring for organizations seeking the Medicare/ Medicaid Certification–Based Long Term Care accreditation option.	Chapter revised to include some items that were inadvertently omitted in 2004: PC.5.10, EP 4 PC.13.20, EP 9 MM.2.20, EP 8, EP 9 PI.3.20 IM.3.10, EP 2 IM.6.50, EP 4
Crosswalks of Standards	*"Crosswalks of 2002–2003 Standards to 2004 Standards":* This **new** chapter includes crosswalks that identify where the 2002–2003 standards requirements appear in the reformatted standards chapters for 2004.	*"Crosswalks of 2002–2003 Standards to 2004 Standards":* This chapter includes crosswalks that identify where the 2002–2003 standards requirements appear in the reformatted standards chapters. Some standards chapters have an additional crosswalk showing changes from 2004 to 2005–2006.
Glossary	The glossary has been updated to include key terminology related to Shared Visions–New Pathways.	Updated for 2005–2006.
Index	A comprehensive, updated index appears at the end of the book.	Updated for 2005–2006.

© 2005 Joint Commission

Table 2. Scoring Category and Measure of Success (MOS) Designation Changes for 2005

This table identifies whether the scoring category and/or the measure of success (MOS) designation has changed for an element of performance (EP) for 2005. Column 1 identifies a standard and EP for which the scoring category and/or MOS has changed; if a standard and EP aren't listed, then there were no changes. Column 2 indicates what the scoring category designation was in 2004. Column 3 indicates what the scoring category designation is for 2005–2006 (that is, whether it has changed from 2004). Column 4 indicates whether an MOS designation has been added, removed, or remains for 2005–2006. If there is nothing listed in Column 4, then the EP did not require an MOS in 2004.

Standard and Element of Performance	2004 Scoring Category	2005–2006 Scoring Category	2005–2006 MOS Designation
Rights, Responsibilities, and Ethics			
RI.1.10 EP 3	B	B	Removed
RI.1.10 EP 4	A	B	Removed
RI.1.10 EP 5	C	C	Added
RI.1.10 EP 6	A	B	Removed
RI.1.10 EP 7	A	C	Remains
RI.1.20 EP 1	B	A	
RI.1.30 EP 2	A	C	Added
RI.2.10 EP 2	C	C	Added
RI.2.10 EP 3	C	C	Added
RI.2.10 EP 4	C	C	Added
RI.2.110 EP 3	A	B	
RI.2.140 EP 1	B	B	Removed
RI.2.140 EP 2	C	B	Removed
RI.2.140 EP 3	C	B	Removed
RI.2.140 EP 4	B	B	Removed
RI.2.210 EP 1	C	B	Removed
Provision of Care, Treatment, and Services			
PC.1.10 EP 1	A	B	
PC.1.10 EP 3	C	B	Removed
PC.1.10 EP 5	C	B	Removed
PC.1.10 EP 6	C	B	Removed
PC.2.20 EP 1	A	B	
PC.2.20 EP 2	A	B	
PC.2.20 EP 3	B	A	
PC.2.120 EP 8	C	A	Remains
PC.2.120 EP 9	C	A	Removed
PC.2.120 EP 11	C	A	Removed
PC.2.120 EP 12	C	A	Removed
PC.2.120 EP 13	C	A	Removed
PC.2.130 EP 3	A	A	Removed
PC.3.10 EP 2	B	B	Removed
PC.3.10 EP 4	C	B	Removed
PC.3.10 EP 5	C	B	Removed

continued on next page

Table 2. Scoring Category and Measure of Success (MOS) Designation Changes for 2005 *(continued)*

Standard and Element of Performance	2004 Scoring Category	2005–2006 Scoring Category	2005–2006 MOS Designation
PC.3.10 EP 6	A	A	Removed
PC.3.10 EP 7	A	A	Removed
PC.3.230 EP 5	B	A	Removed
PC.4.10 EP 1	C	B	Removed
PC.4.10 EP 3	C	B	Removed
PC.4.10 EP 7	C	B	Removed
PC.4.10 EP 9	B	B	Removed
PC.4.10 EP 11	C	B	Removed
PC.4.10 EP 14	C	B	Removed
PC.4.10 EP 15	C	B	Removed
PC.5.30 EP 5	B	C	Remains
PC.5.40 EP 1	C	B	Removed
PC.5.50 EP 1	C	B	Removed
PC.5.50 EP 3	C	B	Removed
PC.5.60 EP 1	B	B	Removed
PC.5.60 EP 5	C	B	Removed
PC.5.60 EP 7	B	B	Removed
PC.6.10 EP 1	C	B	Removed
PC.6.10 EP 3	C	B	Removed
PC.6.30 EP 1	C	B	Removed
PC.6.30 EP 2	C	B	Removed
PC.6.30 EP 3	C	B	Removed
PC.6.30 EP 4	C	B	Removed
PC.7.10 EP 1	C	B	Removed
PC.7.10 EP 2	B	C	Remains
PC.7.10 EP 10	B	B	Removed
PC.7.10 EP 11	B	C	Remains
PC.7.10 EP 12	A	A	Removed
PC.8.20 EP 10	C	B	Removed
PC.8.40 EP 2	B	A	Removed
PC.8.40 EP 4	B	B	Removed
PC.8.70 EP1	C	B	Removed
PC.9.10 EP10	A	A	Removed
PC.9.20 EP 1	A	B	
PC.9.20 EP 2	A	B	
PC.9.20 EP 3	A	A	Removed
PC.11.80 EP 2	B	B	Removed
PC.11.80 EP 3	A	A	Removed
PC.11.80 EP 4	A	A	Removed
PC.11.80 EP 5	A	A	Removed

HB

Table 2. Scoring Category and Measure of Success (MOS) Designation Changes for 2005 *(continued)*

Standard and Element of Performance	2004 Scoring Category	2005–2006 Scoring Category	2005–2006 MOS Designation
PC.11.80 EP 6	A	A	Removed
PC.11.90 EP 3	A	A	Removed
PC.11.90 EP 4	C	A	Removed
PC.11.90 EP 5	C	A	Removed
PC.11.90 EP 6	C	A	Removed
PC.11.90 EP 7	C	A	Removed
PC.11.90 EP 8	C	A	Removed
PC.11.90 EP 9	C	A	Removed
PC.11.90 EP 10	A	A	Removed
PC.11.90 EP 11	C	A	Removed
PC.11.90 EP 12	C	A	Removed
PC.11.90 EP 13	C	A	Removed
PC.11.90 EP 15	B	B	Removed
PC.11.90 EP 16	C	A	Removed
PC.11.90 EP 18	B	B	Removed
PC.13.10 EP 1	B	B	Removed
PC.13.20 EP 1	B	B	Removed
PC.13.20 EP 2	A	A	Removed
PC.13.20 EP 4	A	B	Removed
PC.13.20 EP 5	A	B	Removed
PC.13.20 EP 6	A	B	Removed
PC.13.20 EP 9	A	A	Removed
PC.13.20 EP 10	C	A	Removed
PC.13.20 EP 11	C	A	Removed
PC.13.20 EP 12	C	A	Removed
PC.13.30 EP 1	A	A	Removed
PC.13.40 EP 1	C	A	Removed
PC.13.40 EP 3	C	B	Removed
PC.13.40 EP 4	C	B	Removed
PC.15.10 EP 5	C	B	Removed
PC.16.10 EP 1	A	B	
PC.16.10 EP 2	B	B	Removed
PC.16.10 EP 3	B	B	Removed
PC.16.20 EP 2	B	B	Removed
PC.16.30 EP 1	A	C	Remains
PC.16.30 EP 2 (EC 1 in 2004)	A	C	Remains
PC.16.30 EP 3 (EC 1 in 2004)	A	C	Remains
PC.16.30 EP 5 (EC 2 in 2004)	B	C	Remains

continued on next page

Table 2. Scoring Category and Measure of Success (MOS) Designation Changes for 2005 *(continued)*

HB

Standard and Element of Performance	2004 Scoring Category	2005–2006 Scoring Category	2005–2006 MOS Designation
PC.16.30 EP 6 (EC 3 in 2004)	B	B	Removed
PC.16.30 EP 7 (EC 4 in 2004)	A	B	Removed
PC.16.30 EP 8 (EC 5 in 2004)	B	B	Removed
PC.16.40 EP 2	A	B	
PC.16.40 EP 3	B	C	Remains
PC.16.40 EP 4	A	A	Removed
PC.16.50 EP 1	A	B	
PC.16.50 EP 2	C	B	Removed
PC.16.50 EP 3	A	C	Remains
PC.16.50 EP 5 (EC 4 in 2004)	B	B	
PC.16.50 EP 6 (EC 5 in 2004)	A	B	Removed
PC.16.60 EP 3	C	B	Removed
PC.16.60 EP 4	C	B	Removed
Medication Management			
MM.1.10 EP 1	A	B	
MM.1.10 EP 2	B	A	
MM.2.10 EP 2	B	A	
MM.2.10 EP 4	B	B	Removed
MM.2.10 EP 5	B	B	Removed
MM.2.10 EP 6	A	B	
MM.2.20 EP 2	B	A	
MM.2.20 EP 3	B	A	Removed
MM.2.20 EP 4	B	A	Removed
MM.2.20 EP 5	B	A	Removed
MM.2.20 EP 6	B	B	Removed
MM.2.20 EP 7	B	A	Removed
MM.2.20 EP 9	A	A	Added
MM.2.30 EP 4	C	A	Remains
MM.2.30 EP 7	C	B	Removed
MM.4.10 EP 1	B	C	Remains
MM.4.10 EP 5	B	B	Removed
MM.4.10 EP 6	B	B	Removed
MM.4.20 EP 1	B	B	Removed
MM.4.20 EP 2	B	C	Remains
MM.4.20 EP 3	B	C	Remains
MM.4.20 EP 4	B	C	Remains
MM.4.30 EP 1	B	B	Removed

HB

Table 2. Scoring Category and Measure of Success (MOS) Designation Changes for 2005 *(continued)*

Standard and Element of Performance	2004 Scoring Category	2005–2006 Scoring Category	2005–2006 MOS Designation
MM.4.30 EP 2	B	B	Removed
MM.4.30 EP 3	B	A	Removed
MM.4.30 EP 4	B	A	Removed
MM.4.40 EP 1	B	B	Removed
MM.4.40 EP 2	B	B	Removed
MM.4.40 EP 3	B	C	Remains
MM.4.40 EP 4	B	C	Remains
MM.4.40 EP 5	B	B	Removed
MM.4.70 EP 1	A	A	Removed
MM.4.70 EP 2	A	A	Removed
MM.4.70 EP 3	A	A	Removed
MM.4.80 EP 4	B	C	Remains
MM.7.10 EP 1	B	A	
MM.7.20 EP 4	B	B	Removed
MM.7.40 EP 1	B	B	Removed
MM.8.10 EP 1	B	B	Removed
MM.8.10 EP 2	B	B	Removed
MM.8.10 EP 3	B	B	Removed
MM.8.10 EP 4	B	B	Removed
MM.8.10 EP 5	B	B	Removed
MM.8.10 EP 6	B	B	Removed
Surveillance, Prevention, and Control of Infection			
IC.4.10 EP 2	C	B	Removed
IC.4.10 EP 3	C	B	Removed
IC.4.10 EP 6	C	C	Added
IC.4.10 EP 7	C	C	Added
IC.7.10 EP 1	B	A	
Improving Organization Performance			
PI.1.10 EP 1	B	B	Removed
PI.1.10 EP 2	B	A	Removed
PI.1.10 EP 3	B	B	Removed
PI.1.10 EP 4	A	A	Removed
PI.1.10 EP 5	A	A	Removed
PI.1.10 EP 6	A	A	Removed
PI.1.10 EP 8	A	A	Removed
PI.1.10 EP 13	B	B	Removed
PI.1.10 EP 14	B	B	Removed
PI.1.10 EP 15	B	B	Removed
PI.1.10 EP 16	B	B	Removed
PI.1.10 EP 17	B	B	Removed

continued on next page

Table 2. Scoring Category and Measure of Success (MOS) Designation Changes for 2005 *(continued)*

Standard and Element of Performance	2004 Scoring Category	2005–2006 Scoring Category	2005–2006 MOS Designation
PI.2.10 EP 1	B	B	Removed
PI.2.10 EP 2	B	B	Removed
PI.2.10 EP 3	B	B	Removed
PI.2.10 EP 4	B	B	Removed
PI.2.10 EP 5	B	B	Removed
PI.2.20 EP 1	B	B	Removed
PI.2.20 EP 2	B	B	Removed
PI.2.20 EP 3	B	B	Removed
PI.2.20 EP 4	A	A	Removed
PI.2.20 EP 5	A	A	Removed
PI.2.20 EP 6	A	A	Removed
PI.2.20 EP 9	A	A	Removed
PI.2.20 EP 10	A	A	Removed
PI.2.30 EP 2	A	A	Removed
PI.2.30 EP 3	B	B	Removed
PI.2.30 EP 4	B	B	Removed
PI.2.30 EP 5	B	B	Removed
PI.3.10 EP 1	B	B	Removed
PI.3.10 EP 2	B	B	Removed
PI.3.10 EP 3	B	B	Removed
PI.3.10 EP 4	B	B	Removed
PI.3.10 EP 5	B	B	Removed
PI.3.20EP 4	B	B	Removed
PI.3.20 EP 5	B	B	Removed
PI.3.20 EP 6	B	B	Removed
PI.3.20 EP 7	B	B	Removed
PI.3.20 EP 8	B	B	Removed
PI.3.20 EP 9	B	B	Removed
Leadership			
LD.1.10 EP 3	A	A	Removed
LD.1.20 EP 1	A	A	Removed
LD.1.20 EP 2	A	A	Removed
LD.1.20 EP 3	B	B	Removed
LD.1.20 EP 4	A	A	Removed
LD.1.20 EP 5	A	A	Removed
LD.1.20 EP 6	B	B	Removed
LD.2.10 EP 2	A	A	Removed
LD.2.10 EP 3	A	A	Removed
LD.2.10 EP 4	B	B	Removed
LD.2.20 EP 1	B	B	Removed

HB

Table 2. Scoring Category and Measure of Success (MOS) Designation Changes for 2005 *(continued)*

Standard and Element of Performance	2004 Scoring Category	2005–2006 Scoring Category	2005–2006 MOS Designation
LD.2.20 EP 2	B	B	Removed
LD.2.20 EP 5	B	B	Removed
LD.2.30 EP 1	A	A	Removed
LD.2.30 EP 2	A	A	Removed
LD.2.30 EP 3	A	A	Removed
LD.2.40 EP 1	A	A	Removed
LD.2.40 EP 2	A	A	Removed
LD.2.40 EP 3	B	B	Removed
LD.2.40 EP 4	B	B	Removed
LD.2.40 EP 5	B	B	Removed
LD.2.40 EP 6	B	B	Removed
LD.3.20 EP 1	C	B	Removed
LD.3.20 EP 2	B	B	Removed
LD.3.50 EP 1	B	A	
LD.3.50 EP 2	B	A	Removed
LD.3.50 EP 4	B	A	
LD.3.50 EP 5	A	B	
LD.3.50 EP 6	B	B	Removed
LD.3.50 EP 7	B	A	
LD.3.60 EP 1	C	B	Removed
LD.3.60 EP 2	C	B	Removed
LD.3.60 EP 3	C	B	Removed
LD.3.70 EP 1	B	B	Removed
LD.3.80 EP 1	C	B	Removed
LD.3.80 EP 2	C	B	Removed
LD.3.80 EP 3	C	B	Removed
LD.3.80 EP 4	C	B	Removed
LD.3.90 EP 1	B	B	Removed
LD.3.120 EP 1	B	B	Removed
LD.3.120 EP 2	C	B	Removed
LD.3.130 EP 1	A	A	Removed
LD.3.130 EP 2	B	B	Removed
LD.3.130 EP 3	C	C	Removed
LD.4.20 EP 1	B	B	Removed
LD.4.20 EP 2	B	B	Removed
LD.4.20 EP 3	B	B	Removed
LD.4.20 EP 4	B	B	Removed
LD.4.20 EP 5	B	B	Removed
LD.4.20 EP 6	B	B	Removed
LD.4.50 EP 3	C	B	

continued on next page

Table 2. Scoring Category and Measure of Success (MOS) Designation Changes for 2005 *(continued)*

Standard and Element of Performance	2004 Scoring Category	2005–2006 Scoring Category	2005–2006 MOS Designation
LD.4.60 EP 4	A	B	
LD.4.70 EP 1	C	B	
LD.4.70 EP 2	C	B	
LD.4.70 EP 3	C	B	
Management of the Environment of Care			
EC.1.10 EP 4	B	B	Removed
EC.1.10 EP 6	C	C	Added
EC.1.10 EP 9	C	B	Removed
EC.1.20 EP 2	A	C	Remains
EC.1.20 EP 3 (EP 4 in 2004)	C	C	Added
EC.1.30 EP 4	C	B	Removed
EC.1.30 EP 6	C	B	Removed
EC.1.30 EP 7	C	B	Removed
EC.2.10 EP 3	B	B	Removed
EC.2.10 EP 5	C	B	Removed
EC.2.10 EP 7	A	B	
EC.2.10 EP 9	C	B	
EC.3.10 EP 2	C	B	Removed
EC.3.10 EP 7	C	B	Removed
EC.3.10 EP 9	A	B	
EC.3.10 EP 10	C	A	Removed
EC.3.10 EP 11	C	C	Remains
EC.3.10 EP 12	C	C	Remains
EC.3.10 EP 13	C	B	Removed
EC.4.20 EP 2	C	A	
EC.5.10 EP 2	C	B	Removed
EC.5.10 EP 3	C	B	Removed
EC.5.10 EP 5	C	B	
EC.5.30 EP 4	C	C	Added
EC.5.30 EP 5	C	B	Removed
EC.5.40 EP 3	A	A	Removed
EC.5.40 EP 9	A	A	Removed
EC.5.40 EP 10	A	A	Removed
EC.5.50 EP 3	A	A	Removed
EC.7.10 EP 8	C	B	
EC.7.10 EP 11	C	B	
EC.7.10 EP 12	B	A	
EC.7.10 EP 13	C	B	
EC.7.10 EP 15 (EP 14 in 2004)	C	B	Removed

HB

Table 2. Scoring Category and Measure of Success (MOS) Designation Changes for 2005 *(continued)*

Standard and Element of Performance	2004 Scoring Category	2005–2006 Scoring Category	2005–2006 MOS Designation
EC.7.10 EP 16 (EP 15 in 2004)	A	A	Removed
EC.7.20 EP 2	C	C	Added
EC.7.20 EP 4	C	C	Added
EC.7.50 EP 1	A	A	Removed
EC.7.50 EP 2	A	A	Removed
EC.7.50 EP 3	A	A	Removed
EC.8.10 EP 2	C	B	
EC.8.10 EP 3	C	B	
EC.8.10 EP 5	C	B	
EC.8.10 EP 7	C	B	
EC.8.10 EP 11	A	A	Removed
EC.8.10 EP 12 (EP 11 IN 2004)	A	A	Removed
EC.8.10 EP 15	B	C	
EC.8.10 EP 16	B	C	
EC.8.20 EP 1	C	C	Added
EC.8.20 EP 6 (EP 5 IN 2004)	C	C	Added
EC.8.30 EP 1	C	B	
EC.8.30 EP 2	C	B	Removed
EC.8.30 EP 3	C	B	
EC.8.30 EP 4	C	B	Removed
EC.9.10 EP 1	B	B	Removed
EC.9.10 EP 2	B	B	Removed
EC.9.10 EP 3	A	B	
EC.9.10 EP 10 (EP 9 in 2004)	C	B	Removed
EC.9.20 EP 1	C	B	Removed
EC.9.20 EP 3	C	B	Removed
EC.9.20 EP 4	C	B	Removed
EC.9.20 EP 5	C	B	Removed
EC.9.20 EP 6	C	B	Removed
EC.9.20 EP 8	C	A	Removed
EC.9.20 EP 9	C	B	Removed
EC.9.30 EP 1	C	B	Removed
EC.9.30 EP 2	C	B	Removed
EC.9.30 EP 3	C	B	Removed
EC.9.30 EP 4	C	B	Removed
EC.9.30 EP 5	C	B	Removed
Management of Human Resources			
HR.1.10 EP 1	B	B	Removed

continued on next page

Table 2. Scoring Category and Measure of Success (MOS) Designation Changes for 2005 *(continued)*

HB

Standard and Element of Performance	2004 Scoring Category	2005–2006 Scoring Category	2005–2006 MOS Designation
HR.1.10 EP 2	A	A	Removed
HR.1.10 EP 3	A	A	Removed
HR.1.10 EP 4	A	A	Removed
HR.1.20 EP 1	B	B	Removed
HR.1.20 EP 18	A	A	Removed
HR.1.20 EP 19	A	A	Removed
HR.1.30 EP 1	B	A	Removed
HR.1.30 EP 4	B	B	Removed
HR.1.30 EP 5	B	B	Removed
HR.1.30 EP 6	B	B	Removed
HR.1.30 EP 7	B	B	Removed
HR.1.30 EP 8	A	A	Removed
HR.2.30 EP 1	C	B	Removed
HR.2.30 EP 10	B	B	Removed
HR.3.10 EP 1	A	B	Removed
HR.3.10 EP 2	A	B	Removed
HR.3.10 EP 3	A	B	Removed
HR.3.10 EP 4	A	B	Removed
HR.3.10 EP 5	A	B	Removed
HR.3.10 EP 6	B	B	Removed
HR.3.10 EP 7	A	B	Removed
HR.3.10 EP 9 (EP 8 IN 2004)	C	C	Remains
HR.3.10 EP 10 (EP 9 IN 2004)	B	B	Removed
HR.4.10 EP 10	A	B	Removed
HR.4.10 EP 11	A	A	Removed
HR.4.10 EP 12	A	A	Removed
HR.4.10 EP 13	B	B	Removed
HR.4.10 EP 14	A	A	Removed
HR.4.10 EP 16	B	B	Removed
HR.4.10 EP 17	A	A	Removed
HR.4.10 EP 18	A	A	Removed
HR.4.20 EP 1	A	B	Removed
HR.4.20 EP 2	A	C	Remains
HR.4.20 EP 3	A	A	Removed
HR.4.30 EP 1	A	B	Removed
HR.4.30 EP 2	A	A	Removed
HR.4.30 EP 3	A	A	Removed
HR.4.30 EP 4	B	A	Removed
HR.4.30 EP 5	A	A	Removed
HR.4.30 EP 6	A	A	Removed

HB

Table 2. Scoring Category and Measure of Success (MOS) Designation Changes for 2005 *(continued)*

Standard and Element of Performance	2004 Scoring Category	2005–2006 Scoring Category	2005–2006 MOS Designation
HR.4.40 EP 2	A	B	
HR.4.40 EP 3	A	B	
HR.4.40 EP 4	A	B	
HR.4.40 EP 5	A	B	
HR.4.50 EP 1	A	A	Removed
HR.4.50 EP 3	A	A	Removed
Management of Information			
IM.1.10 EP 1	C	B	
IM.1.10 EP 2	C	B	
IM.2.10 EP 1	B	B	Removed
IM.2.10 EP 2	B	B	Removed
IM.2.10 EP 3	C	B	Removed
IM.2.10 EP 4	C	B	Removed
IM.2.10 EP 6	C	B	Removed
IM.2.10 EP 8	C	B	Removed
IM.2.20 EP 2	B	B	Removed
IM.2.20 EP 7	C	B	Removed
IM.3.10 EP 2	A	A	Added
IM.3.10 EP 5	B	A	
IM.4.10 EP 6 (EP 2 IN 2004)	B	B	
IM.4.10 EP 7 (EP 3 IN 2004)	B	B	
IM.5.10 EP 2	A	B	
IM.5.10 EP 3	A	B	
IM.6.10 EP 8	A	B	
IM.6.10 EP 12 (EP 11 in 2004)	C	B	Removed
IM.6.10 EP 13 (EP 11 in 2004)	C	B	Removed
IM.6.10 EP 14 (EP 12 in 2004)	B	B	
IM.6.10 EP 15 (EP 12 in 2004)	B	A	
IM.6.10 EP 16 (EP 12 in 2004)	B	A	
IM.6.10 EP 17 (EP 13 in 2004)	A	A	
IM.6.10 EP 19 (EP 15 in 2004)	A	A	Removed
IM.6.50 EP 3	C	A	Removed
IM.6.50 EP 4	B	A	Removed

© Joint Commission 2005

The new "National Patient Safety Goals" chapter details the Joint Commission's 2005 National Patient Safety Goals for long term care.

The "Accreditation Participation Requirements" chapter addresses the ongoing requirements for continued participation in the accreditation process and includes requirements related to the integration of the Periodic Performance Review (PPR) in the accreditation process. These requirements are scorable.

The central portion of the book is divided into sections—"Resident-Focused Functions" and "Organization Functions." The first two sections contain the nine functional chapters of the safety- and quality-focused standards, rationales, EPs, and scoring that apply to long term care organizations. The third section lists the standards used in the Medicare/Medicaid Certification–Based Long Term Care Accreditation.

Section 1 includes resident functions directly related to the provision of care, treatment, and services. Resident-focused standards appear in the following four functional chapters:
1. "Ethics, Rights, and Responsibilities" (RI)
2. "Provision of Care, Treatment, and Services" (PC), a new chapter including requirements from the former "Assessment of Residents" (PE), "Care and Treatment of Residents" (TX), "Education of Residents" (PF), and "Continuum of Care" (CC) chapters
3. "Medication Management" (MM), a new chapter including medication requirements that previously appeared in the "Care and Treatment of Residents" (TX) chapter
4. "Surveillance, Prevention, and Control of Infection" (IC), which has been moved from the "Organization Functions" section because of its direct relationship to resident care, treatment, and services

Section 2 contains organization functions that, although not directly experienced by the resident, are vital to the organization's ability to provide high-quality care, treatment, and services. Organization standards appear in the following five functional chapters:
1. "Improving Organization Performance" (PI)
2. "Leadership" (LD)
3. "Management of the Environment of Care" (EC)
4. "Management of Human Resources" (HR)
5. "Management of Information" (IM)

Immediately following the functional chapters is the new "Medicare/Medicaid Certification–Based LTC Accreditation Standards" chapter, which pulls from the functional chapters the standards, rationales, and EPs for the Medicare/Medicaid Certification–Based LTC Accreditation Standards option.

The "Crosswalks of Standards" chapter provides crosswalks that identify where the 2004 standards requirements appear in the reformatted standards chapters for 2005–2006. The crosswalks list the 2004 standards and the corresponding reformatted standards, if applicable, and identify where the 2004 standards requirements appear in the reformatted standards.

The glossary provides definitions of many terms used throughout the book. In addition, a comprehensive index appears at the end of the book.

HB

What Do the Reformatted Functional Chapters Include?

One goal of the Shared Visions–New Pathways initiative is to ensure and enhance the relevance of the Joint Commission standards to critical resident safety and health care quality issues.

Through the Standards Review Task Force, the Joint Commission has streamlined standards and reduced documentation burdens to do the following:
- Ensure the relevance of standards to safety and quality
- Reduce redundancy
- Improve the clarity of standards
- Reduce the associated paperwork and the documentation of compliance burden

As a result of this review, the standards are displayed in a new format, which includes the following:
- Each chapter has an "Overview" section that provides background and explanatory information.
- Standards are statements that define the performance expectations and/or structures or processes that must be in place for an organization to provide safe, high-quality care, treatment, and services.

Accreditation decisions are based on simple counts of the standards that are determined to be not compliant.
- A rationale is background, justification, or additional information about a standard. A rationale is included for those standards needing additional text describing the purpose of the standard. In some cases, the rationale for a standard is self-evident. Therefore, not every standard has a written rationale.
- Elements of performance (EPs) are statements that detail the specific performance expectations and/or structures or processes that must be in place for an organization to provide high-quality care, treatment, and services.

Note: *For more information about how to score each EP, please refer to the "Understanding the Parts of This Chapter" section at the beginning of each functional chapter.*

What Are Some Tips for Success?

The following tips are intended as helpful suggestions for using this book to successfully achieve continuous compliance with the standards:
- Make the *SLTC* available to staff by keeping a complete copy or multiple copies of the book in a resource center. Let staff and others know that the book is available and how they can access it.
- Read all parts of each chapter in this book.

- Keep a record of calls to the Joint Commission's Standards Interpretation Group (630/792-5900), including both questions and answers, for future reference and to avoid duplicate calls by other staff members.
- Focus on the concepts described and the points made in all standards and EPs. Concentrate on incorporating the frameworks and concepts of standards and EPs into day-to-day work, rather than on viewing the concepts as rules that must be followed just for Joint Commission survey purposes.
- Keep up with *SLTC* changes as they occur instead of waiting until your survey is near. Read *Joint Commission Perspectives*®, the official monthly Joint Commission newsletter, to find new scoring, standard interpretations, and other useful information as the year progresses.
- View changes to requirements under the "JCAHO Requirements" section on the *Perspectives* page of the JCR Web site for free access to standards and policy revisions and requirements that are specific to your organization. Look for the "Joint Commission Requirement" page at http://www.jcrinc.com/subscribers/perspectives.asp?durki+2815&site=10&return=27.
- Check the Joint Commission's Web site (*www.jcaho.org*) for any revisions to long term care standards.
- Go to http://www.jcaho.org/accredited+organizations/standards+faqs.htm for Standards Frequently Asked Questions. You can also use the online form for submitting standards questions to the Joint Commission at http://www.jcaho.org/onlineform/onlineform.asp.
- Keep a year's track record of evidence of implementation on hand. Data from the preceding 12 months will be reviewed and assessed during the onsite accreditation survey.
- Develop a team responsible for creating innovative ways to achieve and maintain continuous operational improvement and standards compliance, such as the following:
  - ○ Question of the week or month
  - ○ Standards-related posters
  - ○ Column in a weekly all-staff newsletter

Where Should I Go if I Still Have Questions?

If you still have questions about how to use this book, *see* Table 3 (page HB-22), "Whom Do I Call?" which includes Joint Commission staff to whom specific questions can be directed.

HB

Table 3. Whom Do I Call?

The following is a list of information resources at the Joint Commission and Joint Commission Resources.

The Joint Commission's **main** telephone number is **630/792-5000**. The Joint Commission's business hours are 8:30 A.M. to 5:00 P.M. Central Standard Time, Monday through Friday.

Written correspondence should be sent to:
Joint Commission on Accreditation of Healthcare Organizations
One Renaissance Boulevard
Oakbrook Terrace, IL 60181
ATTN: _____
[Area Indicated (such as Account Representative or Accreditation Operations)]

The Joint Commission's **main fax number** is **630/792-5005**. If you experience difficulties in transmission, please call 630/792-5541.

The **Customer Service** telephone number is **630/792-5800**. Joint Commission customer service representatives are available from 8:00 A.M. to 5:00 P.M. Central Standard Time, Monday through Friday. Call Joint Commission's Customer Service with questions about:
- General information on Joint Commission services, mission, or history
- How to apply for a survey for the first time
- Ernest A. Codman Award program and applications
- Your organization's accreditation status or history
- Obtaining a list of accredited organizations
- Checking the current accreditation status of an organization
- Quality reports
- Help in accessing information on the Joint Commission's Web site

Call your **account representative** at **630/792-3007** for information about long term care or with questions about the following:
- Application for accreditation for long term care
- Scheduling of surveys
- Survey agenda or survey process
- Status of a survey report
- Content of a survey report
- Focused surveys

Call the **Standards Interpretation Group** at **630/792-5900** for information and questions about:
- Interpretation of long term care standards
- How to comply with long term care standards
- Credentialing

Organizations seeking accreditation or wanting to learn more about the process should **call Business Development** at the appropriate number listed below:
- Ambulatory Care   x5286 or x5290
- Assisted Living   x5722 or x5720
- Behavioral Health Care   x5771 or x5790
- Critical Access Hospitals   x5822 or x5810

continued on next page

Table 3. Whom Do I Call? *(cont.)*

- Disease-Specific Care   x5291 or x5256
- Health Care Networks, including
  Managed Care Organizations,
  Preferred Provider Organizations,
  and Integrated Delivery Systems   x5291 or x5293
- Home Care or Hospice   x5771 or x5742
- Hospital   x5810 or x5811
- Laboratory   x5286 or x5287
- Long Term Care   x5286 or x5722
- Office-Based Surgery   x5286 or x5259

The Joint Commission's **Web site** address is http://www.jcaho.org. For an extensive e-mail or telephone list of contacts, click **"Contact Us"** located near the top of the Joint Commission's home page. Throughout the online directory you will see e-mail addresses listed in parentheses. In general, e-mail addresses consist of the first letter of the person's first name and the entire last name @jcaho.org. In most cases, to reach the appropriate person and department by telephone, dial 630/792- and the extension number listed.

Joint Commission Resources' **main** telephone number is **630/268-7400.** Joint Commission Resources' business hours are 8:30 A.M. to 5:00 P.M. Central Standard Time, Monday through Friday. Visit the **Web site** at http://www.jcrinc.com for information, questions, or to order the following:

- Continuous service readiness
- Custom education
- Domestic consulting services
- Educational seminars
- International accreditation services
- Publications

Joint Commission Resources' **Customer Service** telephone number for publications orders and education program registrations is **877/223-6866.** Customer service representatives are available from 8:00 A.M. to 8:00 P.M. Central Standard Time, Monday through Friday. Call Customer Service for the following:

- Obtaining a free catalog for Joint Commission Resources publications or education
- Orders for Joint Commission Resources publications and registration for education seminars
- Multimedia education products
- Publications or education related to specific care programs (such as Disease Management)
- Call **630/792-5429** with requests for permission to reprint any Joint Commission Resources publication

Call the **Joint Commission Satellite Network (JCSN)** at **800/711-6549** for information and questions about how to sign up for the series of education programs broadcast across the United States.

HB

The New Joint Commission Accreditation Process

Overview

The Joint Commission's new accreditation process focuses on systems critical to the safety and the quality of care, treatment, and services. It represents a shift from a focus on survey preparation to a focus on continuous operational improvement by encouraging long term care organizations to incorporate the standards as a guide for routine operations.

Under this new accreditation process, the survey is the on-site evaluation piece of a continuous process. The new accreditation process encourages long term care organizations to continuously use the standards to achieve and maintain excellent operational systems. Initiatives like the Periodic Performance Review (PPR) (discussed on page ACC-5) and the sharing of Priority Focus Process (PFP) information (discussed on page ACC-6) will facilitate this.

This chapter explains the following:
- Implementation and time line
- Revised standards and scoring format
- Periodic Performance Review
- Priority Focus Process
- Priority focus areas
- Clinical/service groups
- Tracer methodology and changes in the on-site survey process
- Evidence of Standards Compliance and measures of success

Implementation and Time Line

The time line in Figure 1 on page ACC-2 shows how components of the new accreditation process play out across a time continuum. The graphic displays the three-year accreditation cycle in terms of how it is experienced by a long term care organization from its full on-site survey in July 2002 to its next full on-site survey in July 2005.*

---

* Organizations that were surveyed in July 2002 were the first to submit their PPR at the midpoint in their accreditation cycle. These organizations will undergo another full on-site survey in July 2005.

ACC

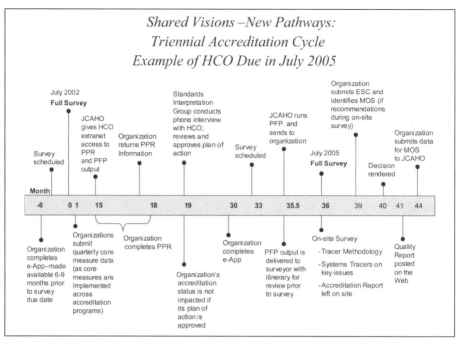

Figure 1. *This time line depicts the events experienced by an organization through a three-year accreditation cycle from 6 months before one survey (–6) to 39 months later, or 3 months after its next full survey. Joint Commission events appear above the time line and health care organization (HCO) events appear below the time line.** *

Key Milestones in the Time Line[†]

- Approximately 15 months after your last on-site survey, the Joint Commission will electronically send PPR access,[‡] the output of the PFP (*see* pages ACC-5–ACC-8 for more information), and instructions to your long term care organization on how to proceed.

- Your long term care organization has three months to complete its PPR, during which time staff will evaluate compliance with standards using elements of performance (EPs) (*see* the section "Revised Standards and Scoring Format" on pages ACC-4–ACC-5 for more information). For standards identified as not compliant,

---

* In 2004, the Joint Commission continued to conduct voluntary unannounced surveys on a limited basis, opening the option to all types of accredited organizations, and will transition to a completely unannounced survey process in 2006. *See* page APP-5 of the "Accreditation Policies and Procedures" chapter for more information on random unannounced surveys.

† The Joint Commission will be transitioning to a completely unannounced survey process in 2006. These key milestones will all still be a part of the accreditation process, and their time lines will be adjusted to fit into an unannounced survey model.

‡ **Note:** *Beginning in 2005, you will have continual access to the continuous PPR tool, but you will receive access to the official PPR tool for submission at the 15- through 18-month point in your accreditation cycle. There will be an annual update to the continuous PPR beginning in 2006. See pages APR-9–APR-11 for more information on the PPR options.*

your long term care organization will develop a plan of action with measures of success (MOS), if required. At the 18-month point in the accreditation cycle, you will submit (via a secure extranet Web space) your PPR containing plan(s) of action to the Joint Commission.

- Approximately 30 days after your plan of action has been submitted, Joint Commission staff will review plans of action over the telephone* and indicate whether the corrective actions, MOS, and the time frames are acceptable. Your accreditation decision is not affected if you conduct a PPR.
- Nine months before your next triennial on-site survey, your long term care organization will complete an electronic application (e-App) for accreditation.
- Two weeks before your survey, Joint Commission will provide the most current output of the PFP for your long term care organization. (For more information on this process, please see the PFP component on page ACC-6.) The surveyor(s) scheduled to conduct your survey will also receive the PFP output for your long term care organization. This information will help the surveyor(s) develop a survey process that focuses on issues that are unique to your long term care organization.
- The triennial on-site survey occurs. The surveyor(s) will visit various units/programs or services using tracer methodology. (For more information on this process, please see the "Tracer Methodology" component on pages ACC-18–ACC-20.) During the survey, the surveyor(s) will also look for evidence that your plan of action from the PPR has been implemented.
- After evaluating your long term care organization's performance, the survey team will review the results of its individual findings. Before the closing conference, the survey team will enter its findings into laptop computers, thus producing a report of survey findings. After the report has been rendered, the team leader will meet with your long term care organization's chief executive officer (CEO) to provide him or her with a copy of the report. It is up to the CEO to decide whether the report will be distributed at the exit conference; however, the survey team will use the contents of the report during its exit conference. (For more information on this process, please *see* the "Accreditation Policies and Procedures" chapter on page APP-1.)
- Approximately 48 hours after your survey has taken place, the Joint Commission will post your report of survey findings on a secure automated area of the extranet site that is password protected for each organization. If the surveyor(s) find requirements for improvement in your long term care organization, you have 90 days (45 days beginning July 1, 2005) following the posting of your organization's Accreditation Report on the Jayco® extranet to submit an Evidence of Standards Compliance (ESC). During the 90-day/45-day period, your long term care organization's prior accreditation decision will remain in effect.
- If, at the end of the 90-day/45-day period, your long term care organization successfully addresses its requirements for improvement, it will be moved to an accreditation decision of "Accredited." After the 90-day/45-day time frame, either the ESC report is received and approved or your long term care organization is moved to an accreditation decision of "Provisional Accreditation." Your Quality Report will be made available to the public on Joint Commission's Quality Check®.

---

* Joint Commission staff will phone your organization to set up a time for this telephone call.

Revised Standards and Scoring Format

ACC

As part of the Shared Visions–New Pathways® initiative, the Joint Commission conducted a major review of the standards. During this process, all standards were reviewed and subsequently streamlined to enhance the focus on key quality and safety issues. The revisions achieve the following:

- Reduce redundancy
- Improve the clarity of standards language
- Reduce the associated paperwork and documentation of compliance burden

The standards chapters have been reformatted significantly. Please refer to the section "Understanding the Parts of This Chapter" at the beginning of each functional chapter and to page HB-20 in the "How to Use This Book" chapter for a detailed explanation.

For a complete crosswalk of standards from the *2002–2003 SLTC* to the *2005–2006 SLTC*, please *see* the "Crosswalks of Standards" chapter.

Scoring was also revised. The revised framework provides for the scoring of the standards as compliant or not compliant. The accreditation decision will be based on a simple count of the standards that are judged not compliant. The EPs for each standard will be scored on the following scale:

0	Insufficient compliance
1	Partial compliance
2	Satisfactory compliance
NA	Not applicable

The determination as to whether a long term care organization is compliant with a given standard is based on the scoring of that standard's EPs. An EP is a specific performance expectation related to a standard that details the specific structures or processes that must be in place for a long term care organization to provide quality care, treatment, and services.

Two components are scored for each EP: (1) compliance with the requirement itself **and** (2) compliance with the track record* for that requirement. Scoring has been simplified, and track record achievements (which have always been part of the scoring) have been appropriately modified.

To determine your compliance with an EP, first look at the EP scoring category listed immediately preceding the scoring scale in the margin next to the EP. There are three scoring categories: A, B, and C. For more information on scoring, please refer to the "Understanding the Parts of This Chapter" at the beginning of each standards chapter as well as the "How to Use This Book" chapter.

In addition to the requirements specifically stated in the EPs, EPs are also scored in accordance with the following track record achievements:

---

* **Track record** The amount of time that an organization has been in compliance with a standard, EP, or other requirement.

Score	Initial Survey*	Full Survey
2	4 months or more	12 months or more
1	2 to 3 months	6 to 11 months
0	Fewer than 2 months	Fewer than 6 months

ACC

If during an on-site survey, your organization has been found to be not compliant with one or more standards, you must submit an Evidence of Standards Compliance (ESC)[†] for each standard that is not compliant. The ESC must address compliance at the EP level; when an EP within a noncompliant standard requires a measure of success (MOS),[‡] your organization must demonstrate achievement with the MOS when completing the ESC.[§]

See the "Understanding the Parts of this Chapter" section at the beginning of each functional chapter for detailed information on sample sizes.

After you have evaluated and scored each EP for a particular standard, use these simple rules to determine your compliance with the standard itself:
● Your organization is not in compliance (that is, not compliant) with the standard if any EP is scored 0.
● Otherwise, your organization is in compliance with a standard if more than 65% of its EPs are scored 2.

Revised Accreditation Process

Presurvey Activities
Periodic Performance Review

The Joint Commission's new accreditation process is designed to shift the focus from survey preparation and passing the triennial exam to continuous standards compliance and operational improvement in the provision of safe, high-quality care, treatment, and services. One component of the accreditation process that supports this paradigm shift is the Periodic Performance Review (PPR), a compliance assessment at the midpoint of your organization's accreditation cycle. The

---

* **Initial survey** An accreditation survey of a health care organization not previously accredited by the Joint Commission, or an accreditation survey of an organization performed without reference to any prior survey findings.

[†] **Evidence of Standards Compliance (ESC)** A report submitted by a surveyed organization within 45 days (90 days between January 1, 2004, and June 30, 2005) of its survey, which details the action(s) that it took to bring itself into compliance with a standard or clarifies why the organization believes it was in compliance with the standard for which it received a requirement for improvement. An ESC must address compliance at the element of performance (EP) level and include a measure of success (MOS) (*see* definition) for all appropriate EP corrections.

[‡] **Measure of Success (MOS)** A numerical or quantifiable measure usually related to an audit that determines whether an action was effective and sustained, due four months after Evidence of Standards Compliance (ESC) (*see* definition) approval.

[§] **Note:** *Not every EP requires an MOS. EPs that do require an MOS are clearly marked in the standards chapters in this manual. Organizations are required to demonstrate achievement with an MOS only for EPs within a not compliant standard that require an MOS. Organizations* do not *need to demonstrate achievement with an MOS for any EP within a compliant standard.*

ACC

PPR is an Accreditation Participation Requirement (APR) for ambulatory care, behavioral health care, home care, hospitals, and long term care organizations.

The PPR helps your organization review applicable standards, assess compliance, develop and implement plans of action, and identify measures by which you will gauge your success in carrying out those plans. By participating in the PPR, your organization will be better able to incorporate Joint Commission standards into routine operations, which in turn will help to ensure the provision of safe, high-quality care on an ongoing basis.

Beginning January 1, 2005, your organization will have continuous access to the PPR tool through the password-protected Jayco extranet site. At the 15-month point of the accreditation cycle, your organization will be notified that it must submit to the Joint Commission (no later than the 18-month point of your accreditation cycle) your selection and completion of the full PPR, option 1, option 2, or option 3. Table 1 outlines some of the activities in each of these options.

Plans of Action

A plan of action is a detailed description of how a long term care organization plans to bring into compliance any standard identified as not compliant in the PPR. (Plans of action are not required for standards where some EPs are marked "partial compliance" but where the standard does not meet the level of not compliant.) The plan of action should include the planned action to be taken and target dates. If the EP has an MOS, you must also describe the MOS or how you plan to gauge your successful implementation of your plans of action.

The PPR will only affect an organization's accreditation decision if the organization fails to participate in the PPR process, whether the full or one of the three options, or if through the PPR process, an immediate threat to life situation* is identified.

If you need more information while completing your PPR, please contact your account representative.

Priority Focus Process

An important component of the Joint Commission's accreditation process is the Priority Focus Process (PFP), which guides surveyors in planning and conducting your on-site survey. The PFP uses an automated tool, which takes available data from a variety of sources—including e-Apps for accreditation, previous survey findings, complaint data, ORYX core measure data (for hospitals only), and publicly available external data (such as MedPAR or OASIS)—and integrates them to identify clinical/service groups (CSGs) and priority focus areas (PFAs) for your organization. The PFP converts this data into information that focuses survey activities, increases consistency in the accreditation process, and customizes the accreditation process to make it specific to your long term care organization.

Surveyors will receive enhanced information and insight about a long term care organization before the on-site survey. The PFP integrates various presurvey data

---

* *See* page APP-29 of this book for more information.

Table 1. Current PPR Options

Full PPR

- Organization uses the automated PPR tool to assess and score compliance with elements of performance (EPs) for each applicable standard
- Organization creates a plan of action* addressing each EP scored partial or insufficient compliance within any standards found not compliant
- Organization identifies a measure of success (MOS),† if required, for each EP scored partial or insufficient compliance within any standards scored not compliant
- Organization submits PPR data to the Joint Commission
- Organization and the Joint Commission's Standards Interpretation Group (SIG) hold a conference call within 30 days after PPR submission to discuss standards scored not compliant, plan(s) of action, and MOS
- SIG reviews and approves plan(s) of action during conference call
- Surveyors review any required MOS at triennial survey

Option 1

- Organization uses PPR tool to affirm that, for substantive reasons, legal counsel advises organization not to participate in the full PPR
- Organizations cannot use PPR tool to score compliance, but can print and view standards and EPs to conduct an assessment on paper
- Organization affirms that it has completed an assessment of its compliance with applicable EPs and developed plans of action and MOS, as necessary, but does not submit data to Joint Commission
- Organization can submit standards-related issues in the PPR tool for telephone discussion with SIG, if desired, and receive design approval
- Surveyors review any required MOS at triennial survey

continued on next page

(listed below) on each long term care organization and recommends the PFAs and CSGs for the on-site survey. This information will guide tracer activities. (*See* pages ACC-18–ACC-20 for more information on the tracer methodology.) However, the PFP does not preclude any area from being surveyed.

From these sources, the PFP identifies PFAs for each long term care organization on which surveyors initially will focus during the first part of the on-site survey. Surveyors will use the PFP in the following ways:

---

* A plan of action details the action(s) an organization will take to come into compliance with each standard identified as not compliant.

† An MOS is a numerical or quantifiable measure, usually related to an audit that determines whether an action was effective and sustained.

ACC

Table 1. Current PPR Options *(continued)*

Option 2

- Organization uses PPR tool to affirm that, for substantive reasons, legal counsel advises organization not to participate in full PPR
- Decision triggers scheduling of on-site survey at the midpoint of accreditation cycle
- Survey will be approximately one-third the length of the triennial survey; a fee will be charged
- Survey will be conducted primarily using tracer methodology and Priority Focus Process (PFP) output; all standards are subject to review
- Surveyor leaves written report of findings with organization
- Organization creates a plan of action and any required MOS for each standard scored not compliant and submits data to the Joint Commission via the PPR tool within 30 days of survey
- Organization and SIG hold a conference call to discuss any standards scored not compliant, plan(s) of action, and MOS
- SIG reviews and approves plan(s) of action during conference call
- Surveyors will review any required MOS at triennial survey

Option 3

- Organization must attest that after careful consideration with legal counsel, it has decided not to participate in the full PPR and instead intends to undergo a limited survey at the midpoint in its accreditation cycle
- Organization is subject to an on-site survey (like option 2)
- Survey will be approximately one-third the length of the triennial survey; a fee will be charged
- Survey will be conducted primarily using tracer methodology and PFP output; all standards are subject to review
- Unlike option 2, however, option 3 stipulates that no report of findings will be submitted to the Joint Commission and that the surveyor delivers the results orally at the closing conference of the on-site survey
- Additionally, there is no review of the PPR survey findings during the organization's next triennial survey
- Following the survey, the organization may elect to participate in a conference call to discuss standards-related issues with Joint Commission staff. At the time of the organization's triennial survey, the surveyors will receive no information relating to the organization's option 3 survey findings

- Two weeks before the triennial survey, the surveyor(s) assigned to your long term care organization will have access to your long term care organization's PFP information via the surveyor extranet
- Surveyors will review the PFP information for long term care organization–specific PFAs as well as for long term care organization–specific CSGs

- As part of the planning process, surveyors will begin to assess and plan their tracer activities
- During the on-site survey, the surveyors will use the long term care organization's active resident list to select tracer residents

The PFP will also be used for a long term care organization undergoing its initial survey. The only difference with this type of long term care organization (versus a long term care organization that has already gone through a survey) is in the available data inputs that feed the PFP. Long term care organizations undergoing an initial survey will not have previous requirements for improvement (referred to as "Type I Recommendations" before January 1, 2004) or ORYX data available to feed into the PFP. For initial surveys, the Joint Commission will only be able to feed e-App data, external data (as applicable), and OQM data into the PFP.

After these data are transformed to become the PFP information, the process for initial surveys is no different from any other type of survey. The data will be aggregated in the same manner to determine the PFAs and CSGs for the long term care organization.

Priority Focus Areas

PFAs are processes, systems, or structures in a health care organization that significantly impact safety and/or the quality of care provided. The list of PFAs was developed from information provided by the Joint Commission Office of Quality Monitoring, expert literature, and expert opinions. The Joint Commission categorized the different processes, systems, and structures leading to improved health care in 14 PFAs. The PFAs evolved from this process of identifying common patterns useful toward building positive health care outcomes and safe, high-quality health care.

The PFAs provide a consistent yet customized approach to providing an initial focus for the on-site survey process, and they may assist the health care organization at the time of its PPR.

The PFAs are the following:
- Assessment and Care/Services
- Communication
- Credentialed Practitioners
- Equipment Use
- Infection Control
- Information Management
- Medication Management
- Organizational Structure
- Orientation & Training
- Patient Safety
- Physical Environment
- Quality Improvement Expertise/Activities
- Rights & Ethics
- Staffing

ACC

PFAs guide the surveyor throughout a portion of the survey—namely, the tracer portion. Outside of formal conferences/interviews, much of the survey will consist of reviewing systems issues in the form of tracer methodology (for more information, please see the "Tracer Methodology" section on page ACC-18). The CSGs affect tracer selection more than the PFAs do. When a resident is selected for a tracer activity, the surveyor will put more focus on the prioritized list of PFAs for your long term care organization.

Definitions for each PFA follow.

Assessment and Care/Services Assessment and Care/Services for residents comprise the execution of a series of processes including, as relevant: assessment; planning care, treatment, and/or services; provision of care; ongoing reassessment of care; and discharge planning, referral for continuing care, or discontinuation of services. Assessment and Care/Services are fluid in nature to accommodate a resident's needs while in a care setting. While some elements of Assessment and Care/Services might occur only once, other aspects might be repeated or revisited as the resident's needs or care delivery priorities change. Successful implementation of improvements in Assessment and Care/Services relies on the full support of leadership.

Subprocesses of Assessment and Care/Services include:
- Assessment
- Reassessment
- Planning care, treatment, and/or services
- Provision of care, treatment, and services
- Discharge planning or discontinuation of services

Communication Communication is the process by which information is exchanged between individuals, departments, or organizations. Effective Communication successfully permeates every aspect of a health care organization, from the provision of care to performance improvement, resulting in a marked improvement in the quality of care delivery and functioning.

Subprocesses of Communication include:
- Provider and/or staff-resident communication
- Resident and family education
- Staff communication and collaboration
- Information dissemination
- Multidisciplinary teamwork

Credentialed Practitioners Credentialed Practitioners are health care professionals whose qualifications to provide resident care services have been verified and assessed, resulting in the granting of clinical privileges. They typically are not employed staff at the health care organization. The category varies from organization to organization and from state to state. It includes licensed independent practitioners and, in some settings, nurse practitioners, advanced practice registered nurses, and physician assistants who are permitted to provide resident care services under the direction of a sponsoring physician. Licensed independent practitioners are permitted by law and the health care organization to provide care and services without clinical supervision or direction within the scope of their license and consistent with individually granted clinical privileges.

Equipment Use Equipment Use incorporates the selection, delivery, setup, and maintenance of equipment and supplies to meet resident and staff needs. It generally includes movable equipment, as well as management of supplies that staff members use (for example, gloves, syringes). (Equipment Use does not include fixed equipment such as built-in oxygen and gas lines and central air conditioning systems; this is included in the Physical Environment focus area.) Equipment Use includes planning and selecting; maintaining, testing, and inspecting; educating and providing instructions; delivery and setup; and risk prevention related to equipment and/or supplies.

Subprocesses of Equipment Use include:
- Selection
- Maintenance strategies
- Periodic evaluation
- Orientation and training

Infection Control Infection Control includes the surveillance/identification, prevention, and control of infections among residents, employees, physicians, and other licensed independent practitioners, contract service workers, volunteers, students, and visitors. This is a systemwide, integrated process that is applied to all programs, services, and settings.

Subprocesses of Infection Control include:
- Surveillance/identification
- Prevention and control
- Reporting
- Measurement

Information Management Information Management is the interdisciplinary field concerning the timely and accurate creation, collection, storage, retrieval, transmission, analysis, control, dissemination, and use of data or information, both within an organization and externally, as allowed by law and regulation. In addition to written and verbal information, supporting information technology and information services are also included in Information Management.

Subprocesses of Information Management include:
- Planning
- Procurement
- Implementation
- Collection
- Recording
- Protection
- Aggregation
- Interpretation
- Storage and retrieval

- Data integrity
- Information dissemination

ACC

Medication Management Medication Management encompasses the systems and processes an organization uses to provide medication to individuals served by the organization. This is usually a multidisciplinary, coordinated effort of health care staff, implementing, evaluating, and constantly improving the processes of selecting, procuring, storing, ordering, transcribing, preparing, dispensing, administering (including self-administering), and monitoring the effects of medications throughout the residents' continuum of care. In addition, Medication Management involves educating residents and, as appropriate, their families, about the medication, its administration and use, and potential side effects.

Subprocesses of Medication Management include:
- Selection
- Procurement
- Storage
- Prescribing or ordering
- Preparing
- Dispensing
- Administration
- Monitoring

Organizational Structure The Organizational Structure is the framework for an organization to carry out its vision and mission. The implementation is accomplished through corporate bylaws and governing body polices, organization management, compliance, planning, integration and coordination, and performance improvement. Included are the organization's governance, business ethics, contracted organizations, and management requirements.

Subprocesses of Organizational Structure include:
- Management requirements
- Corporate by-laws and governing body plans
- Organization management
- Compliance
- Planning
- Business ethics
- Contracted services

Orientation & Training Orientation is the process of educating newly hired staff in health care organizations to organizationwide, departmental, and job-specific competencies before they provide resident care services. *Newly hired staff* includes, but is not limited to, regular staff employees, contracted staff, agency (temporary) staff, float staff, volunteer staff, students, housekeeping, and maintenance staff.

Training refers to the development and implementation of programs that foster staff development and continued learning, address skill deficiencies, and thereby help to ensure staff retention. More specifically, it entails providing opportunities for staff to develop enhanced skills related to revised processes that may have been addressed during orientation, new resident care techniques, or expanded job responsibilities. Whereas Orientation is a one-time process, Training is a continuous one.

Subprocesses of Orientation & Training include:
- Organizationwide orientation
- Departmental orientation
- Job-specific orientation
- Training and continuing or ongoing education

Patient Safety Effective Patient Safety entails proactively identifying the potential and actual risks to safety, identifying the underlying cause(s) of the potential risks, and making the necessary improvements so that risk is reduced. It also entails establishing processes to respond to sentinel events, identifying cause through root cause analysis, and making necessary improvements. This involves a systems-based approach that examines all activities within an organization that contribute to the maintenance and improvement of resident safety, such as performance improvement and risk management to ensure the activities work together, not independently, to improve care and safety. The systems-based approach is driven by organization leadership; anchored in the organization's mission, vision, and strategic plan; endorsed and actively supported by medical staff and nursing leadership; implemented by directors; integrated and coordinated throughout the organization's staff; and continuously re-engineered using proven, proactive performance improvement modalities. In addition, effective reduction of errors and other factors that contribute to unintended adverse outcomes in an organization requires an environment in which residents, their families, and organization staff and leaders can identify and manage actual and potential risks to safety.

Subprocesses of Patient Safety include:
- Planning and designing services
- Directing services
- Integrating and coordinating services
- Error reduction and prevention
- The use of sentinel event alerts
- National Patient Safety Goals
- Clinical practice guidelines
- Active resident involvement in care

Physical Environment The Physical Environment refers to a safe, accessible, functional, supportive, and effective Physical Environment for residents, staff members, workers, and other individuals, by managing physical design; construction and redesign; maintenance and testing; planning and improvement; and risk prevention, defined in terms of utilities, fire protection, security, privacy, storage, and hazardous materials and waste. The Physical Environment might include the home in the case of home care and foster care.

Subprocesses of Physical Environment include:
- Physical design
- Construction and redesign
- Maintenance and testing
- Planning and improvement
- Risk prevention

ACC

Quality Improvement Expertise/Activities Quality Improvement identifies the collaborative and interdisciplinary approach to the continuous study and improvement of the processes of providing health care services to meet the needs of consumers and others. Quality Improvement depends on understanding and revising processes on the basis of data and knowledge about the processes themselves. Quality Improvement involves identifying, measuring, implementing, monitoring, analyzing, planning, and maintaining processes to ensure they function effectively. Examples of Quality Improvement Activities include designing a new service, flowcharting a clinical process, collecting and analyzing data about performance measures or resident outcomes, comparing the organization's performance to that of other organizations, selecting areas for priority attention, and experimenting with new ways of carrying out a function.

Subprocesses of Quality Improvement Expertise/Activities include:
- Identifying issues and establishing priorities
- Developing measures
- Collecting data to evaluate status on outcomes, processes, or structures
- Analyzing and interpreting data
- Making and implementing recommendations
- Monitoring and sustaining performance improvement

Rights & Ethics Rights & Ethics include resident rights and organizational ethics as they pertain to resident care. Rights & Ethics addresses issues such as resident privacy, confidentiality and protection of health information, advance directives (as appropriate), organ procurement, use of restraints, informed consent for various procedures, and the right to participate in care decisions.

Subprocesses of Rights & Ethics include:
- Resident rights
- Organizational ethics pertaining to resident care
- Organizational responsibility
- Consideration of resident
- Care sensitivity
- Informing residents and/or family

Staffing Effective Staffing entails providing the optimal number of competent personnel with the appropriate skill mix to meet the needs of a health care organization's residents based on that organization's mission, values, and vision. As such, it involves defining competencies and expectations for all staff (the competency of licensed independent practitioners and medical staff are addressed in the Credentialed Practitioners priority focus area for all accreditation programs); Staffing includes assessing those defined competencies and allocating human resources necessary for resident safety and improved resident outcomes.

Subprocesses of Staffing include:
- Competency
- Skill mix
- Number of staff

ACC

Clinical/Service Groups CSGs categorize residents and/or services into distinct populations for which data can be collected. The Joint Commission created the list of CSGs based on data gathered from e-Apps from each accreditation program and on publicly available data from external sources. The list then underwent a thorough review to make sure that all categories were actually representative of populations served or services provided by the organizations surveyed by the individual accreditation programs. Joint Commission surveyors use a long term care organization's CSGs combined with other long term care organization-specific data to get a better understanding of the long term care organization's systems and the residents it serves. Tracer residents are selected according to CSGs.

CSGs for Long Term Care:
- LTC—Hospital operated
- LTC—Freestanding
- Residents needing subacute care
- Dementia care
- Geriatric psychiatric care
- Pediatric care
- Rehabilitation services
- Skilled nursing care/complex medical care
- Transitional care unit
- Traumatic brain injury services
- Ventilator services

Additional CSGs based on Centers for Medicare & Medicaid Services' Nursing Home Compare Data:
- Residents having delirium
- Residents having infections
- Residents having loss of ability in activities of daily living
- Residents having mobility concerns
- Residents having pressure ulcers
- Residents needing pain control
- Residents needing physical restraints

On-Site Survey Activities
Survey Agenda
The on-site survey process shifts the focus from survey preparation and scores to continuous operational improvement in support of safe, high-quality care, treatment, and services.

The survey agenda will include the following elements (in no particular order):*

- *Opening Conference and Orientation to the Organization.* The opening session will be an opportunity for introductions and for an orientation to the structure and content of the survey. At this time, your long term care organization will briefly explain its structures, mission, vision, and relationship with the community.
- *Surveyor Planning Session.* During this session, the surveyor(s) will review data and information about the long term care organization, including plans of action generated from the PPR, and plan the survey agenda. The surveyor(s) will also select initial tracer residents.
- *Leadership Session.* Surveyors will discuss the following with leaders:
  - ○ Information gathering and baseline assessment of leadership-level, system issues—system standards, management oversight and direction, and other leadership responsibilities
  - ○ Leadership's approach to the PPR and methods used to address areas needing improvement
  - ○ Ongoing initiatives to improve delivery of health care
  - ○ Safety program and National Patient Safety Goals
  - ○ Oversight by trustees or board
- *Individual Tracer Activity.* During the tracer activity, the surveyor will do the following:
  - ○ Follow the course of a type of care, treatment, and service provided to the resident by the long term care organization
  - ○ Assess the interrelationships among disciplines and departments (where applicable) and the important functions in the care, treatment, and services provided
  - ○ Evaluate the performance of processes relevant to the care, treatment, and service needs of the resident, with particular focus on the integration and coordination of distinct, but related, processes
  - ○ Identify vulnerabilities in the care processes
- *Special Issue Resolution.* This session provides an opportunity for surveyors to follow up on potential findings that could not be resolved in other survey activities.
- *Daily Briefing.* During the daily briefing, the surveyor will do the following:
  - ○ Facilitate leadership's understanding of the survey process and the findings that contribute to the accreditation decision
  - ○ Report on findings from the previous day's survey activities
  - ○ Emphasize patterns or trends of significant concern that could lead to non-compliance determinations
  - ○ Highlight any positive findings or exemplary performance
  - ○ Allow the long term care organization to provide information that may have been missed during the previous survey day
  - ○ Review the agenda for the survey day ahead and make any necessary adjustments based on long term care organization needs or the need for more intensive assessment of an issue

---

* Please *see* the *Survey Activity Guide*, available by calling your Account Representative, for more detailed information on the survey process.

- *Competence Assessment Process.* This process will help the long term care organization and the surveyor to do the following:
  - ○ Identify the competence-assessment, process-related strengths and vulnerabilities of staff and, as applicable, licensed independent practitioners
  - ○ Begin the assessment or determine the degree of compliance with relevant standards
  - ○ Identify human resources issues requiring further exploration
- *Environment of Care Session.* This session will help the long term care organization and the surveyor do the following:
  - ○ Identify vulnerabilities and strengths in processes
  - ○ Begin to identify or determine the action(s) necessary to address any identified vulnerabilities
  - ○ Begin the assessment or determine the long term care organization's actual degree of compliance with relevant standards
  - ○ Identify Environment of Care (EC) processes requiring further evaluation of implementation
  - ○ Identify issues requiring further exploration
- *System Tracer Sessions.* System tracers are interactive sessions with surveyors and long term care organization staff that explore the performance of important resident-related functions that cross the long term care organization. Surveyors and long term care organization staff address critical risk points and provide education during the system tracer sessions. The following are the system tracers:
  - ○ Medication Management
  - ○ Infection Control
  - ○ Data Use
- *CEO Exit Briefing and Organization Exit Conference.* During this conference, the surveyor(s) will do the following:
  - ○ Report the outcome of the survey and present the Accreditation Report if desired by the CEO or administrator
  - ○ Review the issues of standards compliance that have been identified during the survey
  - ○ Allow the long term care organization a final on-site opportunity to question the survey findings or provide additional material regarding standards compliance
  - ○ Gain agreement between the surveyor(s) and the long term care organization regarding the survey findings, when possible
  - ○ Review required follow-up actions, as applicable
- *Credentialing and Privileging.* During this session, the surveyor(s) will discuss organization-specific issues related to the following:
  - ○ The process the organization uses to collect relevant data for decisions for appointment
  - ○ Consistent implementation of the credentialing and privileging process for licensed independent practitioners and other professionals
  - ○ Processes for granting, and appropriate delineation of, privileges
  - ○ Whether practitioners practice within the limited scope of delineated privileges

○ Linkage of results of peer review and focused monitoring to the credentialing and privileging process

○ Identification of potential concerns in the credentialing, privileging, and appointment process

ACC

- *Life Safety Code® (LSC) * Building Tour.* This session will help the organization and surveyor do the following:
    ○ Identify areas of concern in the organization's processes for designing buildings to *LSC* requirements
    ○ Identify areas of concern in the organization's processes for maintaining buildings to *LSC* requirements
    ○ Identify areas of concern in the organization's processes for identifying and resolving *LSC* problems
    ○ Determine the organization's degree of compliance with relevant *LSC* requirements
    ○ Identify or determine the action(s) necessary to address any identified *LSC* problems
- *Surveyor Team Meeting.* On surveys being conducted by more than one surveyor, scheduled team meetings provide an opportunity for surveyors to share information and observations, plan for upcoming survey activities, and plan for communication and coordination with the organization.
- *Surveyor Report Preparation.* The surveyor(s) will use this time to compile, analyze, and organize the data he or she has collected throughout the survey into a report reflecting the organization's compliance with standards.

Tracer Methodology
Individual Tracer Activity

The tracer methodology is the cornerstone of the new survey process. The individual tracer activity is an evaluation method conducted during an on-site survey designed to trace the care experiences that a resident had while at the long term care organization. The tracer methodology is a way to analyze an organization's systems of providing care, treatment, and services using actual care recipients as the framework for assessing standards compliance. Surveyors will use the following general criteria to select initial individual tracers:

- Residents in top CSGs and PFAs for that organization
- Residents who cross programs, for example, long term care residents who present at a hospital or some residents received from a hospital in complex organizations
- Residents related to system tracer topics (*see* the section "System Tracer Activity" on page ACC-19), such as infection control or medication management
- Residents receiving complex services, such as surgery or treatment in an intensive care unit[†]

---

* *LIfe Safety Code®* is a registered trademark of the National Fire Protection Association, Quincy, MA.

[†] Please *see* the *Survey Activity Guide,* available by calling your Account Representative, for more detailed information on other program-specific criteria for tracer selection.

The typical residents selected for initial tracer activity will be those identified in the long term care organization's PFP information as listed in the CSGs. Based on identified PFAs and CSGs, the surveyor will identify resident tracers and follow specific residents through the long term care organization's processes. A surveyor will not only examine the individual components of a system but will also evaluate how the components of a system interact with each other. In other words, a surveyor will look at the care, treatment, and services provided by each department and service, as well as how departments and services work together. Surveyors may start where the resident is currently located. They then can move to where the resident first entered the organization's systems, an area of care provided to the resident that may be a priority for that organization, or to any areas in which the resident received care, treatment, or services. The order will vary. Along the way, surveyors will speak with health care staff members who actually provided the care to that tracer resident—or, if that staff member is not available, will speak with another staff member who provides the same type of care. Based on the surveyor's findings, he or she may select similar residents to trace. The tracer methodology permits surveyors to "pull the threads" if there is a reason to believe that an issue needs further exploration.

System Tracer Activity

System tracers differ from individual tracers in that during individual tracers, the surveyor follows a specific resident through his or her course of care, evaluating all aspects of care. System tracers follow the flow of one specific system or process across the organization. During the system tracer sessions, surveyors evaluate the system/process, including the integration of related processes and the coordination and communication among disciplines and departments in those processes.

A system tracer includes an interactive session (involving a surveyor and relevant staff members). Points of discussion in the interactive session include the following:
- The flow of the process across the organization, including identification and management of risk points, integration of key activities, and communication among staff/units involved in the process
- Strengths in the process and possible actions to be taken in areas needing improvement
- Issues requiring further exploration in other survey activities
- A baseline assessment of standards compliance
- Education by the surveyor, as appropriate

The three topics evaluated with system tracers are data use, infection control, and medication management, although the number of system tracers varies based on survey length.

Data Use. The data use system tracer focuses on how the organization collects, analyzes, interprets, and uses data to improve resident safety and care.

Infection Control. The infection control system tracer explores the organization's infection control processes. The goals of this session are to assess your organization's compliance with the relevant infection control standards, identify infection control issues that require further exploration, and determine actions that may be necessary to address any identified risks and improve resident safety.

ACC

Medication Management. The medication management system tracer explores the organization's medication management processes, while focusing on subprocesses and potential risk points (such as hand-off points). This tracer activity helps the surveyors evaluate the continuity of medication management from procurement of medications through the monitoring of their effects on residents.

The Role of Staff in Tracer Methodology

To help the surveyor or survey team in the tracer methodology, staff will be instructed to provide the surveyor or survey team with a list of active residents including the residents' names, current locations in the long term care organization, and diagnoses, as appropriate. Surveyors may request assistance from long term care organization staff for selection of appropriate tracer residents. As surveyors move around a long term care organization, they will ask to speak with the staff members who have been involved in the tracer resident's care, treatment, and services. If those staff members are not available, they will ask to speak to another staff member who would perform the same function(s) as the member who has cared for or is caring for the tracer resident. Although it is preferable to speak with the direct caregiver, it is not mandatory since the questions that will be asked are questions that any caregiver should be able to answer in providing care to the resident being traced.

Accreditation Policies and Procedures

Overview

This chapter provides information on the Joint Commission's accreditation policies and procedures relevant to all health care organizations interested in Joint Commission accreditation, whether they are applying for the first time or on a renewal basis. These policies and procedures apply to all organizations either currently accredited by, or seeking accreditation by, the Joint Commission.

This chapter includes information about the continuous accreditation process and specific components that occur at various stages, including information long term care organizations need to know about the Periodic Performance Review (PPR), the on-site survey, and the Evidence of Standards Compliance (ESC) process. The time line on page ACC-2 of "The New Joint Commission Accreditation Process" chapter identifies all the stages of the continuous accreditation process and their timing in that process.

The chapter is organized into major sections reflecting the elements of the accreditation process. You will be able to locate the policies and procedures applicable to your organization according to where your organization is in the accreditation process or cycle. An organization must follow the policies and procedures described in this chapter to participate and continue to participate in the accreditation process. Failure to follow the policies and procedures described in this chapter can result in denial or withdrawal of accreditation.

Note: *The "Accreditation Participation Requirements" chapter includes specific requirements for accreditation participation. The requirements are existing policies within this "Accreditation Policies and Procedures" chapter and are currently effective for accreditation purposes. Cross-references to the Accreditation Participation Requirements (APRs) can be found in the applicable sections of this chapter.*

General Information

This section provides information relevant to an organization either applying for initial Joint Commission accreditation or seeking continued accreditation. Because this material is revised on a regular basis, all organizations are encouraged to review it.

Organizations Eligible for Accreditation
General Eligibility Requirements

Any health care organization may apply for Joint Commission accreditation under the standards in this book* if all the following requirements are met:

- The organization is in the United States or its territories or, if outside the United States, is operated by the U.S. government, under a charter of the U.S. Congress, meeting the following criteria:
  - The nature of the health care practices in the applicant organization is compatible with that of Joint Commission standards and their elements of performance (EPs).
  - With the use of interpreters provided by the organization, as necessary, the surveyor(s) can effectively communicate with substantially all the organization's management and clinical personnel and at least half of the organization's residents, and can understand medical records and documents that relate to the organization's performance
  - United States citizens make up at least 10% of the organization's resident population

    or

    A United States government agency contracts with the organization to provide services to United States citizens

    or

    United States citizens preferentially use the organization in that country
- The organization assesses and improves the quality of its services. This process includes a review of care by clinicians, when appropriate.
- The organization identifies the services it provides, indicating which services it provides directly, under contract, or through some other arrangement.
- The organization provides services addressed by the Joint Commission's standards.

Scope of Accreditation Surveys
General Survey Categories

The Joint Commission surveys and accredits health care organizations using standards from one or more of the following manuals:

- *Accreditation Manual for Assisted Living*
- *Accreditation Manual for Critical Access Hospitals*
- *Accreditation Manual for Office-Based Surgery Practices*
- *Accreditation Manual for Preferred Provider Organizations*
- *Comprehensive Accreditation Manual for Ambulatory Care*
- *Comprehensive Accreditation Manual for Behavioral Health Care*
- *Comprehensive Accreditation Manual for Home Care* (includes standards for home health, personal/support care, hospice, home medical equipment, and pharmacies)
- *Comprehensive Accreditation Manual for Hospitals: The Official Handbook*

---

* The Joint Commission will work with the organization to determine which standards from other accreditation publications are applicable.

- *Comprehensive Accreditation Manual for Integrated Delivery Systems*
- *Comprehensive Accreditation Manual for Long Term Care* (includes standards for subacute care programs)
- *Comprehensive Accreditation Manual for Laboratory and Point-of-Care Testing*
- *Comprehensive Accreditation Manual for Managed Care Organizations*

In addition to standards, the Joint Commission also surveys organizations using the standards' EPs, performance measurement data (when applicable), and APRs, including the Joint Commission National Patient Safety Goals. Used in conjunction with the standards, these items help assess an organization's performance.

Tailored Survey Policy

The Joint Commission survey, assuming satisfactory compliance, provides one accreditation award for all the organization's services, programs, and related organizations. Another service, program, or related entity (that is, component), whether providing services or through a contractual arrangement, will be included in the survey of the applicant organization under the following circumstances:

- There are Joint Commission standards applicable to the component
- The component is overseen and managed by the applicant organization through organizational and functional integration

Note: *Any service, program, or related entity that is a component of an accreditation-eligible organization may independently seek accreditation if it can meet Joint Commission survey-eligibility requirements.*

Organizational and functional integration refers to the degree to which the component is overseen and managed by the applicant organization. An *applicant organization* refers both to an organization seeking accreditation and to an organization that is currently accredited. A *component* is a service, program, or related entity that delivers care or services and is eligible for survey under one of the Joint Commission's accreditation programs. These include the following:

- General, psychiatric, pediatric, critical access, surgical specialty, and rehabilitation hospitals
- Home care organizations, including those that provide home health services, personal care and support services, home infusion and other pharmacy services, long term care pharmacies and infusion centers, durable medical equipment services, and hospice services
- Nursing homes and other long term care facilities, including subacute care programs and dementia programs
- Assisted living residences that provide or coordinate personal services, 24-hour supervision and assistance (scheduled and unscheduled) activities, and health-related services
- Behavioral health care organizations, including those that provide mental health services, substance abuse treatment services, foster care services, and services for persons with developmental disabilities of various ages in various organized service settings

- Ambulatory care providers, including outpatient surgery facilities and office-based surgery, rehabilitation centers, sleep labs, imaging centers, group practices, and others
- Clinical laboratories

Organizational integration exists when the applicant organization's governing body, either directly or ultimately, controls budgetary and resource allocation decisions for the component or, where individual corporate entities are involved, there is greater than 50% common governing board membership for the applicant organization as well as on the board of the component.

Functional integration exists when the entity meets at least three of the following eight criteria:
1. The applicant organization and the component do the following:
   - Use the same process for determining membership of licensed independent practitioners in practitioner panels or medical or professional staff and/or
   - Have a common organized medical or professional staff for the applicant organization and the component
2. The applicant organization's human resources function hires and assigns staff at the component and has the authority to do the following:
   - Terminate staff at the component
   - Transfer or rotate staff between the applicant organization and the component
   - Conduct performance appraisals of the staff who work in the component
3. The applicant organization's policies and procedures are applicable to the component with few or no exceptions
4. The applicant organization manages significant operations of the component; that is, the component has little or no management authority or autonomy independent of the applicant organization
5. The component's resident records are integrated in the applicant organization's resident record system
6. The applicant organization applies its performance improvement program to the component and has authority to implement actions intended to improve performance at the component
7. The applicant organization bills for services provided by the component under the name of the applicant organization
8. The applicant organization and/or the component portrays to the public that the component is part of the organization through the use of common names or logos; references on letterheads, brochures, telephone-book listings, or Web sites; or representations in other published materials

The Joint Commission evaluates all health care services provided by the organization for which the Joint Commission has standards and makes one accreditation decision and survey report. An organization must be prepared to provide evidence of its compliance with each applicable standard. To gain accreditation, an organization must demonstrate overall compliance with the standards and their EPs.

Complex Organization Survey Process

The complex organization survey process is applied to organizations that are governed by the Tailored Survey Policy (*see* pages APP-3–APP-4). The Joint Commission will conduct a complex organization survey based on the services provided by the organization, as reported in its application for accreditation. Because a complex organization survey process will involve standards in more than one of the manuals listed in this chapter, the Joint Commission provides the organization with a copy of each of the manuals to be used in the survey before it is conducted.

Organizations that have acquired a new component will be given a 12-month grace period from the time the component is acquired before the performance of that component will be factored into the organization's overall accreditation decision. The newly acquired component will usually be surveyed within six months of its acquisition as an extension survey; however, the accreditation decision rendered from the extension survey will be in effect only for the component for 12 months following the acquisition before impacting the organization's overall accreditation decision.

Contracted Services

The Joint Commission evaluates the organization's assessment of the quality of services provided under contractual arrangements. The Joint Commission reserves the right to evaluate, as part of its survey, services provided by another organization or provider. It may survey performance issues between the contracted organization and the applicant organization, regardless of the accreditation decision of the contracted organization. The Joint Commission also surveys services provided on-site under contract.

Unannounced Surveys

Historically, the Joint Commission's regular, triennial surveys have been conducted in an announced fashion. Beginning in 2004 and through 2005, the Joint Commission will conduct unannounced triennial surveys on an optional and limited basis. The Joint Commission plans to transition to all unannounced surveys by 2006.

For organizations that elect to undergo an unannounced survey in 2004 or 2005, the following policies are applicable:

- The survey can be scheduled anywhere between January and December in the year that the organization is due for survey
- The organization will be invoiced immediately after the survey
- The organization will be removed from the pool of organizations eligible for a random unannounced survey throughout its accreditation cycle
- Because the date of an organization's survey cannot be announced and, therefore, a Public Information Interview (PII) will most often not be able to be scheduled during the organization's survey, the PII policy no longer applies. In place of the PII policy, the organization is required to fulfill the new APR for continuous public involvement. This APR is effective in 2006 for all programs and immediately for the organizations that voluntarily undergo unannounced surveys. Through this APR, the organization will be required to demonstrate how it com-

municates with its public to provide information on how an individual can contact the Joint Commission with any resident safety or quality-of-care concerns.

All other policies and procedures in this chapter will apply to organizations undergoing an unannounced regular survey.

Multiorganization Option

The Joint Commission offers multiorganization systems that own or lease at least two organizations the option of a modified survey process. This option has the following three components:

1. A corporate orientation
2. A consecutive survey of participating organizations with the same survey team leader
3. A corporate summation

A system may choose to have either a corporate orientation, a corporate summation, or both. The orientation session provides an opportunity for corporate staff to orient the survey team to the structure and practices of the system. The survey team will also survey centralized corporate services, documentation, and policies and procedures applicable to Joint Commission standards. The corporate summation provides an overall analysis of the system's strengths and weaknesses. It also provides consultation and education related to accreditation survey findings across the system. There is one fee for both the corporate orientation and corporate summation.

Continuity in the composition of the survey team will be maintained by the survey team leader(s). The remaining members of the survey team will rotate in and out of the system's scheduled route. The survey team leader will compile the information necessary to support the corporate summation.

To allow for consecutive surveys of a system's participating organizations, the Joint Commission can advance or extend the survey due dates of participating organizations by up to six months. Any participating organization that requires an extension of the due date greater than six months must undergo an extension survey. Successful completion of the extension survey will extend the organization's accreditation survey due date for up to one year from its original survey due date.

Through the multiorganization option, the Joint Commission accredits the individual health care organizations that are part of a multiorganization system, not the system itself. Therefore, each organization within a system will receive its own accreditation decision and report. The findings and decision for one organization within a system will have no bearing on those of another organization within the system.

Early Survey Policy

The sidebar on page APP-9 highlights Early Survey Policy Options 1 and 2 described in the following sections. An organization wishing to be accredited for the first time by the Joint Commission may choose one of two Early Survey Policy Options. Under both Option 1 and Option 2, organizations are required to undergo two surveys. However, the nature of the surveys and potential outcomes differ. The first survey under Option 1 is a more limited survey, while the first survey under Option 2 is a full accreditation survey. The Public Information Policy (pages APP-12–APP-16) applies to both Option 1 and Option 2.

Early Survey Policy Option 1 (Preliminary Accreditation)

A. Eligibility. This option is available to any organization that is currently not accredited except an organization that has been denied accreditation. Organizations must declare during the application process that they wish to be surveyed under this option.

B. The First Survey. When an organization chooses Option 1, the Joint Commission will conduct two on-site surveys. The Joint Commission can conduct the first survey as early as two months before the organization begins operating, provided the organization meets the following criteria:

- It is licensed or has a provisional license, according to applicable law and regulation
- The building in which the services will be offered or from which the services will be coordinated is identified, constructed, and equipped to support such services
- It has identified its chief executive officer or administrator, its director of clinical or medical services, and its nurse executive, if applicable
- It has identified the date it will begin operations

Generally, the first survey uses a limited set of standards and assesses only the organization's physical facilities, policies and procedures, plans, and related structural considerations. For this reason, the Early Survey Policy Option 1 has not been recognized by the Centers for Medicare & Medicaid Services (CMS) to meet the requirements for Medicare certification.

C. Preliminary Accreditation. The Joint Commission grants Preliminary Accreditation to an organization in satisfactory compliance with a subset of the standards and their EPs assessed in the first survey under Option 1. An organization not in satisfactory compliance must reapply and begin the accreditation process again. An organization that meets the decision rules for Conditional Accreditation will also be granted a Preliminary Accreditation decision.

The Preliminary Accreditation decision will include assignment of an additional survey against the full set of applicable standards within six months of the first survey. The survey will assess evidence of compliance with the standards for at least four months.

For an organization operating when the survey is conducted, the effective date for its Preliminary Accreditation decision is the day after the survey is conducted. For an organization not in operation, the effective date is the day after it begins operating. If the organization is not in operation at the time of survey, the organization must confirm in writing the date it begins operating.

A Preliminary Accreditation decision remains until the organization has completed a second, full survey or until the Joint Commission has withdrawn the Preliminary

Accreditation. The Joint Commission may withdraw Preliminary Accreditation in the following situations:

- When an organization that was not providing services at the time of the first survey does not begin services when expected
- If an organization does not meet the survey eligibility criteria (*see* page APP-2) or
- If an organization fails to accept the date of the second survey
- If an organization is found not in satisfactory compliance with the applicable standards and their EPs

In these cases, the organization must begin the accreditation process again.

D. The Second Survey. The second survey is a full accreditation survey. The Joint Commission conducts this survey at the following times:

- Approximately six months after the first survey
- At least four months after the organization has begun operating

The organization's accreditation status, based on survey results, will change to one of the following:

- Accredited
- Provisional Accreditation
- Conditional Accreditation
- Preliminary Denial of Accreditation
- Denial of Accreditation

The effective date of the accreditation decision is the day after the second survey. The organization's three-year accreditation cycle begins the day after the second survey is conducted, unless the Joint Commission reaches a decision to deny accreditation. Submission of ESC may be required based on the survey findings of the second survey under this option.

Early Survey Policy Option 2

A. Eligibility. Option 2 is available only to an organization that has the following:

- Never been surveyed by the Joint Commission or has been unaccredited by the Joint Commission for the previous two years
- Been in actual operation for at least one month
- Cared for at least 10 residents by the time of the first survey with at least one resident in active treatment at the time of survey
- Not been denied participation in the Medicare program as a result of a survey conducted by or action taken by CMS or the state on behalf of CMS

B. The First Survey. When an organization chooses Early Survey Policy Option 2, the Joint Commission will conduct an initial full accreditation survey. If the organization demonstrates satisfactory compliance with standards and EPs in the first survey, it will be granted an Accredited decision,* including a requirement for a second survey to assess that the track record of compliance is sufficient. This accreditation decision reflects the preliminary nature of the assessed performance. The effective date of the accreditation decision is the day after the first survey.

---

* Effective immediately.

Early Survey Policy Options

Early Survey Policy Option 1
First Survey
- Conducted up to two months before opening if the following criteria are met:
  - ○ Licensed
  - ○ Building identified, constructed, and equipped
  - ○ CEO or administrator, director of clinical or medical services (medical director) identified
  - ○ Identified opening date
- Limited set of standards (physical plant, policies and procedures)
- Outcome: Preliminary Accreditation

Second Survey
- Six months after first survey
- Full survey
- Outcome: Change in Preliminary Accreditation decision to Accreditation, Provisional Accreditation, Conditional Accreditation, or Preliminary Denial of Accreditation. The effective date of the accreditation decision is the day after the *second* survey.

Early Survey Policy Option 2
First Survey
- Conducted when an organization
  - ○ Has been in operation (licensed) at least one month
  - ○ Has cared for at least 10 residents
  - ○ Has one resident in active treatment at time of survey
- Full survey; no track record
- Outcome: Accredited, Conditional Accreditation, or Preliminary Denial of Accreditation

Second Survey
- A full, follow-up survey four months after first survey
- Addresses track record and standards compliance issues
- Outcome: Accredited or Provisional Accreditation, Conditional Accreditation, or Preliminary Denial of Accreditation. The effective date of the accreditation decision is the day after the *first* survey.

Note: *For all surveys, the organization will incur a fee. Contact the Department of Planning and Financial Affairs at 630/792-5115 for more information.*

C. The Second Survey. The organization will undergo a full follow-up survey in four months to address track record achievements that could not be assessed during the first survey due to the limited time of operation. The full scope of applicable standards will be reviewed with particular attention being paid to the issue of sustained performance since the first survey. Organizations surveyed under the Early Survey Policy will also be required to complete an ESC after the first and second surveys, as appropriate.

Initial Surveys

Organizations that are seeking Joint Commission accreditation for the first time or have been unaccredited by the Joint Commission during the previous six months are eligible for an initial survey. The full scope of applicable standards will be reviewed during the survey. The scoring of the standards will be based on a 4-month track record of compliance (prior to survey), rather than the 12-month track record of compliance required for triennial surveys.

Information Accuracy and Truthfulness Policy

The accuracy and veracity of relevant information, whether actually used in the accreditation process or not, are essential to the integrity of the Joint Commission's accreditation process. Information provided at any time by the organization must be accurate and truthful.* Such information can be obtained in the following ways:

APP

- Be provided verbally or in writing
- Be obtained through direct observation or interview by Joint Commission surveyors
- Be derived from documents supplied by the organization to the Joint Commission including, but not limited to, an organization's root cause analysis in response to a sentinel event, an organization's request for accreditation, or a plan of correction submitted as part of the Conditional Accreditation process
- Involve data or documents transmitted electronically to the Joint Commission, including, but not limited to, data or documents provided as part of the electronic application (e-App) process
  or
- Involve an attestation that an organization has not knowingly used Joint Commission full-time, part-time, or intermittent surveyors to provide any accreditation-related consulting services after January 1, 2004. Examples of such services include, but are not limited to, the following:
  - Helping an organization to meet Joint Commission standards
  - Helping an organization in the PPR process
  - Conducting mock surveys for an organization
    or
  - Providing consultation to an organization to address Priority Focus Process (PFP) information

Falsification, as the term is used in this policy, applies to both commissions and omissions in sharing information with the Joint Commission.

Policy Requirements

The Joint Commission's Information Accuracy and Truthfulness Policy includes the following:

1. An organization must never provide the Joint Commission with falsified information relevant to the accreditation process. The Joint Commission construes any efforts to do so as a violation of the organization's obligation to engage in the accreditation process in good faith.
2. *Falsification* is defined for this policy as the fabrication, in whole or in part, and through commission or omission, of any information provided by an applicant or accredited organization to the Joint Commission. This includes, but is not limited to, any redrafting, reformatting, or content deletion of documents.
3. The organization may submit additional material that summarizes or otherwise explains original information submitted to the Joint Commission. These materials must be properly identified, dated, and accompanied by the original documents.

---

* *See* APR 10 on page APR-7 in the "Accreditation Participation Requirements" chapter.

4. As part of the application for the accreditation process and annually thereafter, each organization will be required to attest to its compliance with the requirements of this policy. Such certification should be signed by the director and/or manager, the chairperson of the governing body, and the chief of the medical staff (or leader of the professional staff).

5. The Joint Commission conducts an evaluation when it has cause to believe that an accredited organization might have provided falsified information to the Joint Commission relevant to the accreditation process. Except as otherwise authorized by the president of the Joint Commission, the evaluation includes an unannounced on-site survey. This survey uses special protocols designed to address the alleged information falsification. It assesses the degree of actual organization compliance with the standards and their EPs that are the subject of the allegation, if appropriate.

6. The Joint Commission immediately takes action to deny accreditation or remove the accreditation award from an accredited organization whenever the Joint Commission is reasonably persuaded that the organization has provided falsified information. If nonmanagerial employees or contractors have undertaken the falsification and the organization's leadership takes no immediate action upon becoming aware of the falsification, or at least one individual in a supervisory or managerial position directs or participates in the falsification, the Joint Commission acts to declare Preliminary Denial of Accreditation or to remove the accreditation award from an accredited organization.

7. The Joint Commission notifies responsible federal and state government agencies of any organization subject to such action.

8. If an organization is denied accreditation because it provided falsified information, the Joint Commission prohibits it from participating in the accreditation process for a period of one year. The president of the Joint Commission, for good cause only, may waive all or a portion of this waiting period.

Good Faith Participation in Accreditation

The Joint Commission requires each organization seeking accreditation or reaccreditation to engage in the accreditation process in good faith. The Joint Commission may deny accreditation to any organization failing to participate in good faith in the accreditation process.

Certain categories of issues interfering with good faith participation can be described as follows:

- *Deceiving the Joint Commission.* Compliance with the Information Accuracy and Truthfulness Policy requires a commitment on the part of the accredited organization not to deceive the Joint Commission in any aspect of the accreditation process. The Joint Commission believes that appropriate preparation for an accreditation survey is a fully acceptable and positive practice, which helps improve the quality and safety of individual care. It is rare that such preparation could overstep the bounds of good faith activity to reach the level of deception. For example, to hire additional caregiving staff shortly before a survey for the express purpose of their presence during the survey, with the intent to terminate the employment of such caregivers promptly after the survey, is an act of such deception.

- *Deceiving the Public.* Accredited organizations are not acting in good faith if they mislead the public about the meaning and limitations of accreditation. Also, accredited organizations must not inaccurately suggest to the public that their accreditation award applies to any unaccredited affiliated or otherwise related activities.
- *Reprisals.* The Joint Commission invites open communication from any accredited organization's staff and recipients of care and services about any standards compliance or other issues relating to the accreditation process. An organization's good faith participation in the accreditation process would be questioned if the organization does the following:
  - ○ Attempts to discourage such communication, for example, by taking disciplinary steps against an employee solely because that employee provides information to the Joint Commission
  - ○ Threatens those who communicate with the Joint Commission with a defamation lawsuit based solely on what was said to the Joint Commission or
  - ○ Allows the treatment or access to services of any individual or staff to be adversely impacted by his or her or a family member's communication with the Joint Commission
- *Standards Compliance.* If an organization's conduct reflects a lack of commitment to standards compliance, issues of good faith may be raised. For example, an intentional refusal to attempt to comply with a standard could suggest a cavalier view of the accreditation process.

The Good Faith Participation requirement applies continuously throughout the accreditation cycle.

Public Information Policy*

The Joint Commission is committed to making relevant and accurate information about surveyed health care organizations available to interested parties. Information regarding a health care
organization's quality and safety of care helps organizations improve their services. This information can also help educate consumers and health care purchasers in making informed choices about health care. At the same time, it is important that confidentiality be maintained for certain information to encourage candor in the accreditation process.

Quality Reports

The Quality Report provides summary information about the provision of quality and safety at an accredited organization. Quality Reports are created at the organization level and are designed to provide national and state information that can be compared against other accredited organizations and nonaccredited organizations.

Joint Commission Quality Reports for each accredited organization include the following information:

---

* This policy meets the requirements of the Health Insurance Portability and Accountability Act of 1996.

APP

- The date of the most recent triennial survey
- The accreditation decision based on the most recent triennial survey
- An organization's current accreditation decision
- The current decision of any component or program whose accreditation decision is different from that of the organization as a whole
- The date of the most recent evaluation activity for the organization, if any
- Standards areas with requirements for improvement
- Subsequent satisfaction of requirements for improvement and the date(s) of resolution for specific standards areas
- Subsequent new requirements for improvement and the date(s) assigned
- Services included in the accreditation survey
- Joint Commission policies or rules that lead to a Preliminary Denial of Accreditation or Denial of Accreditation
- Disease-specific care certification(s) and the effective date of each certification
- The receipt of Special Quality Recognition Awards, as recognized by the Joint Commission's Board of Commissioners (for example, the Ernest A. Codman Award, Magnet Status)
- Achievement of National Patient Safety Goals
- Performance against National Quality Improvement Goals
- Performance in relation to Patient Experience of Care Measures

Each accredited organization is afforded the opportunity to prepare a commentary of up to two pages regarding its Quality Report. The commentary accompanies any organization Quality Reports distributed by the Joint Commission, whether via hard copy or the Joint Commission's Web site.

Each Quality Report released by the Joint Commission also includes appropriate background information.

The Joint Commission may also make available information contained in Quality Reports to other third-party providers of information. An organization's Quality Report may be obtained via the Customer Service Department or through Quality Check®, a directory on the Joint Commission's Web site (http://www.jcaho.org).

Performance measurement data is included in Quality Reports when all the following conditions are met:
- Accredited organizations are reporting data on standardized core measures.
- Performance measurement data have been integrated into the accreditation process.
- Sufficient data to assure statistical significance are available.
- Appropriate reporting formats have been developed and approved by the Board of Commissioners.

In addition, released data must satisfy the following requirement:
- The data are accompanied by an explanation of the following:
  - Source or derivation
  - Accuracy, reliability, and validity
  - Appropriate uses
  - Limitations and potential misuses

Information That Is Publicly Disclosed on Request

In addition to information provided in Quality Reports, the following information may be obtained by writing or calling the Joint Commission:

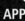

- The organization's accreditation history
- Survey fees paid by an accredited organization
- The organization's scheduled survey date(s) after the organization has been notified of the dates
- Applicable standards used for an accreditation survey
- For a complex survey, the organizational component(s) contributing to a Conditional Accreditation or Denial of Accreditation decision
- Requirements for improvement for which the Joint Commission had no or insufficient evidence of resolution when an organization withdrew from accreditation
- The standards areas for which the Joint Commission had no or insufficient evidence of resolution of requirements for improvement when an organization withdrew from accreditation
- As applicable, confirmation of the occurrence of a sentinel event at an accredited organization and the Joint Commission's intent to apply its Sentinel Event Policy to this occurrence

Release of Complaint-Related Information on Request

The Joint Commission addresses all complaints that pertain to resident safety or quality-of-care issues within the scope of Joint Commission standards. Complaints may be forwarded by CMS or other federal or state agencies having oversight responsibilities for health care organizations, or may be received directly from consumers, payers, or health care professionals.

The Joint Commission has a toll-free hotline to provide residents, their families, caregivers, and others with an opportunity to share concerns regarding quality-of-care issues at accredited health care organizations. The toll-free number is 800/994-6610 and is available 24 hours a day, seven days a week; however, staff members are available weekdays between 8:30 A.M. and 5:00 P.M. central standard time to answer calls.

Upon request from any party, the Joint Commission releases the following aggregate information relating to complaints about an accredited organization for the three-year period prior to receipt of the request:

- The number of standards-related written complaints filed against an accredited organization that have met criteria for review
- The applicable standards areas involved in a specific complaint review
- The standards areas in which requirements for improvement were issued as a result of complaint evaluation activities
- When an unannounced or unscheduled survey is based on information derived from a complaint or public sources, the standards areas related to the complaint

The Joint Commission also provides the following information as appropriate to complainants regarding their complaints:

- Any determination that the complaint is not related to Joint Commission standards

- If the complaint is related to standards, the course of action to be taken regarding the complaint
- Whether the Joint Commission has decided to take action regarding an organization's accreditation decision following completion of the complaint investigation
- Any change in an organization's accreditation decision following completion of the complaint investigation

Release of Aggregate Performance Data

The Joint Commission reserves the right to publish or release aggregate performance data.

Data Release to Government Agencies*

The Joint Commission makes available to federal, state, local, or other government certification or licensing agencies specific accreditation-related information under the following circumstances:

- When the Joint Commission identifies a serious situation in an organization that might jeopardize the health or safety of residents or the public and immediately takes action to deny accreditation
- Upon request, when the request involves otherwise publicly available information

Additional information is made available when an organization is certified for participation in a federal or state program or licensed to operate by a state agency on the basis of its accreditation. The Joint Commission so advises the organization's chief executive officer and provides timely notice to local, state, and federal authorities having jurisdiction. The information available to government agencies includes the following:

- The official accreditation decision and any subsequent change in this decision or any designation, such as Accreditation Watch
- Complaint information requested by CMS or state agencies in accordance with deemed status or other recognition requirements, including the following:
  - Action taken on the complaint
  - The standards area(s) in which a requirement for improvement was issued as a result of the complaint evaluation
  - The status of the case
- Specific information when an organization is assigned a Conditional Accreditation, Preliminary Denial of Accreditation, or Denial of Accreditation decision, which includes the following:
  - All final requirements for improvement

_____

* Section 92, PL 96-499, the Omnibus Budget Reconciliation Act of 1980, requires that Medicare providers include, in all their contracts for services costing $10,000 or more in any 12-month period, a clause allowing the Secretary of the U.S. Department of Health and Human Services (DHHS), the U.S. Comptroller General, or their representatives to examine the contract and the contractor's books and records. The Joint Commission herein stipulates that if its charges to any such provider amount to $10,000 or more in any 12-month period, the contract or any agreement on which such charges are based and any of the Joint Commission's books, documents, and records that might be necessary to verify the extent and nature of Joint Commission costs will be available to the Secretary of DHHS, the Comptroller General, or any of their duly authorized representatives for four years after the survey. The same conditions apply to any related subcontracts the Joint Commission has if the payments under such subcontracts amount to $10,000 or more in any 12-month period.

○ A statement, if any, from the organization regarding its views on the validity of the Joint Commission survey findings

○ A copy of the approved plan of correction and the results of the plan of correction follow-up survey

- Notification of upcoming triennial or focused surveys and retrospective dates of other surveys conducted, such as random unannounced, other announced, or unannounced for-cause surveys. A copy of the Accreditation Report is included for the following:

○ CMS upon request respecting deemed status determinations

○ State agencies that have entered into specific information-sharing agreements that permit provider-authorized release of such reports to the state agency

Joint Commission Right to Clarify

The Joint Commission reserves the right to clarify information, even if the information involved is otherwise considered confidential, when an organization disseminates inaccurate information regarding its accreditation.

Confidential Information

The Joint Commission keeps confidential the following information received or developed during the accreditation process:

- The Accreditation Report unless its submission is required by a government agency *(see* "Data Release to Government Agencies" on pages APP-15–APP-16)
- Information learned from the organization before, during, or following the accreditation survey, which is used to determine compliance with specific accreditation standards
- An organization's root cause analysis and related action plan prepared in response to a sentinel event or in response to other circumstances specified by the Joint Commission
- All other materials that might contribute to the accreditation decision
- Written staff analyses and Accreditation Committee minutes and agenda materials
- The algorithms used in the PFP
- The PFP information used in an organization's survey
- An organization's PPR and related plan of action and measures of success (MOS)

This policy applies to all organizations with an accreditation history, subject to any requirements of any applicable laws.

Survey Fees

The Joint Commission determines survey fees annually as needed to meet the cost of its operations. Surveyed organizations are charged for all surveys with the exception of random unannounced surveys. The Joint Commission bases an organization's survey fees on several factors, including the volume and type of services provided, and the sites to be included in the organization's accreditation. Contact the Pricing Unit at the Joint Commission at 630/792-5115 for a fee schedule or more information on survey fees.

The survey fee is not finalized until the Joint Commission has received and reviewed the organization's application. The Joint Commission sends an invoice when it schedules an organization for survey. It asks the organization to pay the fees according to specified terms. The Joint Commission charges an organization the fee rate in effect at the time of survey. For an initial survey, an organization must send a nonrefundable processing fee with the application for accreditation (e-App). The Joint Commission credits this payment toward the organization's total fee.

APP

The Joint Commission offers organizations two payment options. An organization can do one of the following:

- Pay the full survey fee upon receipt of the invoice, which is sent approximately 30 calendar days before the survey is scheduled
- Pay 50% of the fee upon receipt of the invoice and the remaining 50% within 60 calendar days after completion of the survey

An organization *that did not pay* its survey fee in full prior to issuance of the accreditation decision and report must remit the outstanding balance within 60 calendar days from receipt of the report. Failure to provide timely payment can result in the loss of accreditation. The Joint Commission notifies an organization with significant standards compliance problems of either a Conditional Accreditation or a Preliminary Denial of Accreditation decision as soon as possible, whether or not payment has been received.

Organizations participating in optional, voluntary, unannounced triennial surveys in 2004 and 2005 will be invoiced after their survey takes place.

Before the Survey

This section provides information on the steps leading to a full accreditation survey. These include the application process, the assignment of an account representative, the PPR process, the PFP, survey scheduling, the assignment of a survey team, policies regarding survey scheduling, postponements and delays, the notification of the public about a forthcoming Joint Commission survey, and the conduct of a PII. The accreditation time line included on page ACC-2 is also a good reference for viewing the accreditation process as a whole. In accordance with the requirements of the Health Insurance Portability and Accountability Act of 1996 (HIPAA), a health care organization and the Joint Commission must have a signed Business Associate agreement before the organization's survey can begin.

An Organization's Extranet Site

A key feature of the Shared Visions–New Pathways® initiative is increased use of technology in the accreditation process. The use of technology better enables the Joint Commission and accredited organizations to communicate accreditation-related information in a more efficient and timely manner.

To fully use technology in the accreditation process, each organization will have a secured Web site on the Joint Commission's extranet. Access to the site can only be accomplished through the use of the organization's password. This site will permit organizations to complete their e-App and PPR electronically. In addition, approximately 48 hours following an organization's survey, the organization's Accreditation Report and its ESC report will be posted on the organization's Web site. Only the accredited organization will have access to this site when it is ready for the organization to complete.

Periodic Performance Review

The PPR process is a key component in a more continuous accreditation process. It is designed to help organizations incorporate Joint Commission standards as part of routine operations and ongoing quality improvement efforts. As such, organizations will have access to their PPR tool on a continuous basis throughout their accreditation cycle. The PPR tool will permit organizations to evaluate compliance with all applicable Joint Commission standards and EPs. However, approximately 15 months into the accreditation cycle, the Joint Commission will notify that the organization needs to complete its PPR and submit it to the Joint Commission by the 18th month in the accreditation cycle.* For every not compliant standard, the organization must identify a plan of action at the EP level identifying how it plans to come into compliance with the requirement(s). This plan must include an MOS, if applicable, for each EP within a standard identified as not compliant that requires an MOS (not all EPs require an MOS, and organizations need to demonstrate achievement with an MOS only for an EP that's within a not compliant standard that requires an MOS). The MOS is a numerical or other quantitative measure usually related to an audit that can help determine whether a planned action was effective and sustained.

The evaluation and plan of action must be completed electronically on the organization's secure site on the Joint Commission's extranet and transmitted to the Joint Commission within three months. Following receipt of the evaluation and plan of action, staff from the Joint Commission's Standards Interpretation Group will schedule a telephone call with the organization to discuss and agree upon an acceptable plan of action. The time line for the PPR is such that the organization should have sufficient time (at least 6 months) to implement the actions identified in the plan of action and demonstrate a 12-month track record prior to the organization's regular on-site survey. (The PPR process will not be applicable to organizations undergoing an initial survey.) Beginning in 2006, organizations will be required to submit to the Joint Commission an update to their PPR on an annual basis. (*See* APR chapter, pages APR-9–APR-11, for the full text of the PPR and its options.)

Application for Accreditation

An organization begins the accreditation process by completing an application. An electronic version of the application for accreditation can be completed via the organization's extranet site. When an organization is due to complete its application, the Joint Commission will electronically notify the organization about how to access its application electronically. Likewise, when an organization notifies the

---

* Beginning in 2005, organizations will have continual access to the continuous PPR tool. There will be an annual update to the continuous PPR beginning in 2006. *See* pages APR-9–APR-11 for more information on the PPR.

Joint Commission that it wishes to become accredited, the Joint Commission will provide the organization with information explaining how to access and complete its application on its extranet site.

Organizations using this e-App will type data directly in the application and, when complete, will submit the application to the Joint Commission electronically. The application provides essential information about an organization, including owner- ship, demographics, and types and volume of services provided.

APP

The application does the following:
● Describes the organization seeking accreditation
● Requires the organization to provide the Joint Commission with all official records and reports of public or publicly recognized licensing (for example, a state license), examining, reviewing, or planning bodies*
● Authorizes the Joint Commission to obtain any records and reports not pos- sessed by the organization
● When accepted, establishes the terms of the relationship between the organiza- tion and the Joint Commission

Organizations choosing not to complete an application via the extranet site may request a print copy of the application by contacting their account representative. If you do not know who your account representative is, please call 630/792-3007.

Except for unannounced surveys, the Joint Commission will notify the organization of the scheduled survey at least four weeks before the survey date. For information on receiving applications for resurvey, see "Continuing Accreditation" on page APP-36.

Accuracy of the Application Information
The Joint Commission schedules surveys based on information provided in the organization's e-App. With the information provided, the Joint Commission deter- mines the number of days required for a survey and the composition of the survey team.

Inaccurate or incomplete information in the e-App might necessitate an additional survey, which could delay the Joint Commission's survey report and accreditation decision. The organization might also incur additional survey charges.

Handling Changes Affecting the Application Information†
At any time during the accreditation process, if an organization undergoes a change that modifies the information reported in its e-App, the organization must notify the Joint Commission in writing within 30 calendar days after such change is made. Information that must be reported includes the following:
● A change in ownership
● A change in location
● A significant increase or decrease in the volume of services

---

* *See* APR 1 on page APR-2 in the "Accreditation Participation Requirements" chapter.

† *See* APR 2 on page APR-2 in the "Accreditation Participation Requirements" chapter.

- The addition of a new type of health service or site of care
- The acquisition of a new component
- The deletion of an existing health service or site of care
  or
- The deletion of an existing component

The Joint Commission may schedule an additional survey for a later date if its surveyor or survey team arrives at the organization and discovers that a change was not reported. The Joint Commission may also survey any unreported services and sites addressed by its standards. The Joint Commission will make the final accreditation decision for the organization only after surveying all or an appropriate sample of all services and sites provided by the organization for which the Joint Commission has standards. Information reported in the e-App is subject to the Joint Commission's policy on information accuracy and truthfulness (*see* pages APP-10–APP-12).

Role of the Account Representative

The Joint Commission assigns an account representative to each organization after receipt of the e-App. This person serves as the primary contact between the organization and the Joint Commission. He or she coordinates survey planning and covers policies, procedures, accreditation issues or services, and inquiries throughout the accreditation process. If your organization does not know who your account representative is, please call 630/792-3007.

Survey Scheduling and Postponements

Note: *This section is not applicable to organizations that choose to have their survey conducted unannounced.*

Schedules for Surveys

The Joint Commission schedules surveys systematically and efficiently to keep survey fees to a minimum. Resurveys are scheduled within 45 calendar days before or after the organization's triennial due date. An organization's first full accreditation survey, an initial survey, must be scheduled within six months from the time the Joint Commission receives the organization's application.

Survey Postponement Policy

A postponement is an organization's request to alter an already scheduled survey date. An organization should direct a request for a postponement to its account representative. A request to postpone a survey may be granted if one or more of the following criteria are met:

- A natural disaster or other major unforeseen event has occurred that has totally or substantially disrupted operations
- The organization is involved in a major strike, has ceased admitting residents, and is transferring residents to other facilities or organizations

- Residents and/or the organization is being moved to a new building on the day or days of the survey
  or
- The Joint Commission has provided fewer than four weeks advance notice to the organization (by telephone or in writing) of the survey date(s)

Note: *If a survey postponement is requested because of a natural disaster, strike, or movement to a new building, an on-site extension survey might be required if the organization is continuing to provide resident care services.*

APP

An organization undergoing its first Joint Commission survey will be asked to specify on its application the month in which it wishes to be surveyed. Following the scheduling of the survey, the organization will be permitted to postpone its survey only if it meets the above criteria.

Fees for Postponements

In rare circumstances, the Joint Commission may, at its discretion, approve a request to postpone a survey for an organization not meeting any of the preceding criteria. In such cases, the organization may be charged a fee to defray costs and may be required to undergo an extension survey. Please contact your account representative or the Pricing Unit at 630/792-5115.

Timeliness of Application and Deposits

The Joint Commission requires an organization to submit a new e-App if the organization does not accept a scheduled survey within six months. This ensures that the organization's information is current.

A nonrefundable, nontransferable survey deposit is required for initial surveys only. The Joint Commission applies the deposit to the organization's survey fee if a survey is conducted.

Forfeiture of Survey Deposit

An organization scheduled for an initial survey will forfeit its survey deposit if its survey is not conducted within six months of submission of its application. The organization must then reapply and submit a new survey deposit to begin the accreditation process again.

The Survey Agenda

The Joint Commission's account representative works with the organization to develop a tentative survey agenda based on survey task assignments required as part of the survey. A generic agenda template will be sent to all organizations with a similar number of required survey days and similar survey teams. The draft of the tentative agenda is reviewed and revisions made, as appropriate.

Notifying the Public About a Joint Commission Survey

The Joint Commission evaluates all relevant information about an organization's compliance with applicable standards and intent statements. It therefore requires an organization to inform the public of a scheduled full survey and invite them to provide the surveyor or survey team with relevant information.* The organization must provide an opportunity for members of the public to participate in a PII during a full survey, including the second survey under Early Survey Policy Option 1 and both surveys under Early Survey Policy Option 2 (*see* pages APP-6–APP-9). A full survey refers to the survey of all components of an organization under all applicable standards and intent statements. The public includes, but is not limited to the following:

- Residents and their families
- Resident advocates and advocacy groups
- Members of the community for whom services are provided
- Staff

Public Posting

The organization is responsible for making the PII process widely known and effective as a source of compliance information in the accreditation process. The Joint Commission requires an organization scheduled for full survey to post or make announcements of the following:

- The survey date
- The opportunity for a PII
- How to request an interview

In the event that all organization components are not surveyed at the same time, the requirement to announce the upcoming full survey applies at the time the primary program is surveyed. For example, if an organization with ambulatory, long term care, and home care components is scheduled for a tailored survey in which the organization is the primary program and each component's survey is scheduled for a different date, the notice of survey is to be posted consistent with the organization's survey dates.

To maximize participation, postings or announcements must be made throughout the organization, including components being surveyed at a different time, in a form consistent with one provided by the Joint Commission. *See* Figure 1, page APP-23, for an example of a Public Notice form. This example may be used by the organization, or the organization may design its own Public Notice form that conveys the same information as this example. An organization should post notices in staff eating areas, break rooms, on bulletin boards near major entrances, and in treatment areas. In addition, the organization must provide each staff person with a written announcement of the survey if such postings are not likely to be seen by all staff.

---

* *See* APR 8 on page APR-5 in the "Accreditation Participation Requirements" chapter.

PUBLIC NOTICE

The Joint Commission on Accreditation of Healthcare Organizations will conduct an accreditation survey of _____ on _____.

               (Insert the name of your organization)   *(Insert your survey dates)*

The purpose of the survey will be to evaluate the organization's compliance with nationally established Joint Commission standards. The survey results will be used to determine whether, and the conditions under which, accreditation should be awarded the organization.

Joint Commission standards deal with organization quality, safety-of-care issues, and the safety of the environment in which care is provided. Anyone believing that he or she has pertinent and valid information about such matters may request a public information interview with the Joint Commission's field representatives at the time of the survey. Information presented at the interview will be carefully evaluated for relevance to the accreditation process. Requests for a public information interview must be made in writing and should be sent to the Joint Commission no later than five working days before the survey begins. The request must also indicate the nature of the information to be provided at the interview. Such requests should be addressed to

Division of Accreditation Operations
Office of Quality Monitoring
Joint Commission on Accreditation of Healthcare Organizations
One Renaissance Boulevard
Oakbrook Terrace, IL 60181

Or
Faxed to 630/792-5636

Or
E-mailed to complaint@jcaho.org

The Joint Commission's Office of Quality Monitoring will acknowledge in writing or by telephone requests received 10 days before the survey begins. An Account Representative will contact the individual requesting the public information interview prior to survey, indicating the location, date, and time of the interview and the name of the surveyor who will conduct the interview.

This notice is posted in accordance with the Joint Commission's requirements and may not be removed before the survey is complete.

Date Posted: _____

Figure 1. *This is a sample Public Notice form.*

Advance Notice

The Joint Commission requires an organization scheduled for survey to post public notices at least 30 calendar days before the scheduled date. An organization receiving the scheduled date fewer than 30 calendar days before the survey date should post public notices promptly. Notices must remain posted until the survey is completed.

Informing the Public to Notify the Joint Commission Regarding Safety and Quality-of-Care Concerns

The organization must take reasonable steps to inform its community of the opportunity for PIIs during the full survey at least 30 calendar days before the survey. Steps include the following:

APP

- Informing all advocacy groups (such as organized resident groups and unions) that have substantively communicated with the organization in the previous 12 months
- Reaching other members of the community through means such as a public service announcement on radio or television, a classified advertisement in a local newspaper, postings on the organization's Web site, or a notice in a community newsletter or other publication*
- Informing individuals who inquire about the survey of the survey date(s) and opportunity to participate

An organization opting to have its survey conducted on an unannounced basis will not be required to comply with the requirements of this policy. Rather, the organization will be required, by a new APR, to demonstrate how it informs its public(s) that they should notify the Joint Commission if they have issues concerning safety and quality of care in that organization on a continuous basis. The organization can demonstrate its compliance with this APR by distributing information about the Joint Commission, including contact information in published materials such as admission brochures, and/or posting this information on the organization's Web site.

Compliance with the Public Information Interview Policy

The surveyor(s) reviews the organization's compliance with the policy outlined in the preceding section. The team indicates at the exit conference whether it believes the organization has complied with the policy and reports on this to the Joint Commission. Failure to comply with the PII policy ordinarily results in a recommendation, which needs to be addressed as part of the ESC process (*see* "Accreditation Decisions" on page APP-31). As a result, the Joint Commission may also conduct a postsurvey PII at the organization's expense, if requested.

In addition, the surveyor(s) conducting a postsurvey PII also conducts whatever follow-up survey he or she (they) believes appropriate in view of the information obtained during the PII. An organization's subsequent failure to comply with the Joint Commission's PII policy can result in loss or denial of its accreditation.

Conduct of the Public Information Interview
Handling Requests†

Individuals requesting a PII are to forward their requests and the nature of the information they will provide in writing to the Joint Commission. The organization must explain this process in its communications. To ensure participation, individuals are

---

* *See* APR 8 on page APR-5 in the "Accreditation Participation Requirements" chapter.

† This type of notification must be published or broadcast at least once.

encouraged to forward written requests as soon as possible, and no later than five calendar days before the scheduled survey.

Sometimes an individual may make a written request for a PII directly to the organization. When this occurs, the organization must promptly forward it to the Office of Quality Monitoring at the Joint Commission. An organization receiving *oral requests* should instruct individuals to make the request in writing and mail it to the Joint Commission. The organization should provide individuals needing assistance in doing this with the necessary support.

APP

Scheduling Interviews

The organization must provide potential PII participants with sufficient advance notice. The Joint Commission acknowledges all PII requests to the individual participants. Prior to the survey, the Joint Commission schedules a time-limited PII to be conducted during the survey. The Joint Commission is responsible for notifying the individuals requesting PIIs of the interview's exact date, time, and place. The organization must try to alleviate any potential concerns about reprisals to individuals who participate in the interview process.

Interview Eligibility

Individuals whose written requests arrive late or who simply appear at the stated time, requesting the opportunity to be heard without a prior written request, are heard by a Joint Commission surveyor if time permits. Otherwise, the surveyor informs them that it is not possible to honor their requests and then offers them the opportunity to provide a subsequent written statement.

Individuals contacting the Joint Commission and stating an interest in supplying information anonymously are informed that they may provide written complaints through the Joint Commission's Office of Quality Monitoring at 800/994-6610. The Joint Commission will maintain confidentiality, as requested.

The Interview Process

The Joint Commission's survey team conducts the PII. A representative of the organization may attend, unless the individual requesting the PII asks that no representative from the organization be present. The Joint Commission will honor such requests. The interview will be conducted on the organization's premises, whether a representative from the organization is present or not.

The organization is expected to provide reasonable accommodations for all PIIs.

An interview consists of the orderly receipt of information, orally or in writing, within a set time limit. The interview is not a debate between an organization's representative and an interviewee. Surveyors may, however, ask clarifying questions.

In addition, surveyors will not debate with or convey conclusions to any interviewee. Rather, the Joint Commission considers the information gathered in the interview by the surveyor along with the surveyor's findings and recommendations during the survey process.

The On-Site Survey

This section includes information relevant to an organization that has applied for an accreditation survey and is ready for the survey process. It provides an overview of the survey process, including use of the PFP.

Priority Focus Process

APP

The PFP guides the overall survey process, including planning and the on-site survey, by providing enhanced insight into and information about each organization before its survey. This focuses survey activities on organization-specific issues that are most relevant to safety and quality of care (referred to as priority focus areas [PFAs]). The PFP can be considered as a process for standardizing the PFAs for review during survey.

As part of the PFP, an automated tool called the Priority Focus Tool (PFT) takes data gathered before the survey about an organization and, through the use of algorithms or sets of rules, transforms the data into information that guides the survey process. Examples of sources for the data may include but are not limited to the following:

- Data from an organization's application
- Complaint and sentinel event information
- Performance measurement data, when applicable
- An organization's previous survey results
- Data collected from external sources, such as the Nursing Home Compare section of the Medicare Web site

For additional information on the PFP process, *see* "The New Joint Commission Accreditation Process" chapter.

The Survey Process in Brief

Overview

During an accreditation survey, the Joint Commission evaluates an organization's performance of functions and processes aimed at continuously improving resident outcomes. The survey process focuses on assessing performance of important resident-centered and organization functions that support the safety and quality of resident care and may include the conduct of a PII. This assessment is accomplished through evaluating an organization's compliance with the applicable standards in this manual based on the following:

- Tracing the care delivered to residents
- Verbal and written information provided to the Joint Commission
- On-site observations and interviews by Joint Commission surveyors
- Documents provided by the organization

In addition, throughout the survey, MOS identified by an organization as part of its PPR process will be validated.

The Joint Commission's accreditation process seeks to help organizations identify and correct problems and improve the safety and quality of care and services provided. In addition to evaluating continuous compliance with standards and their EPs, significant time is spent on education.

The Joint Commission began conducting surveys on an unannounced basis in 2004 for organizations that volunteered. Unannounced surveys will be optional and conducted on a limited basis throughout 2005. Beginning in 2006, all accreditation resurveys will be unannounced. Initial surveys will remain announced.

Surveys are designed to be individualized to each organization, to be consistent, and to support the organization's efforts to improve performance. The length of the survey is determined by the Joint Commission based on information supplied in the application describing organization size and scope of services. In addition, Joint Commission surveyors may conduct some survey activities during evening, night, and weekend shifts (off-shift) for full surveys of three or more days and a sample of two-day surveys in health care organizations that provide 24-hour care. These off-shift visits will not occur before the opening conference at the start of the survey.

Survey Agenda

The survey agenda will contain the following elements:

Opening Conference. The opening session of the survey process will be an opportunity for organization leaders and key staff to meet with the surveyor(s) and make any last-minute adjustments to the survey schedule or elements.

Leadership Conference. During the conference, surveyors will discuss with leaders (including nursing, performance improvement, and safety leadership) their roles in performance improvement and other key issues of organization operations, such as resident safety, review of National Patient Safety Goals, and PFP output related to clinical/service groups (CSGs) and clinical focus areas. Some organizations might experience two Leadership Conferences, as necessary.

Validating the Organization's Implementation of Its Plan of Action Generated as Part of the PPR Process. The organization will have already submitted this plan to the Joint Commission for review and approval as part of the PPR process and will have worked with Joint Commission Standards Interpretation Group staff on areas for improvement. As part of conducting an organization's full survey, surveyors will review MOS information and verify that the organization has implemented the plan of action.

Visits to Care and Service Areas Guided by the PFP Using the Tracer Methodology. These two elements of the Joint Commission's survey process, PFP and tracer, allow surveyors to analyze the functioning of organization systems.

Tracer Methodology. One element driving this revised accreditation process is analysis of the organization's systems of providing care and services using actual residents as the framework for assessing compliance with selected standards. This process, called tracer methodology, works with PFP to trace residents, using PFAs as a starting point, within the health care organization's systems. For more information on tracer methodology, *see* "The New Joint Commission Accreditation Process" chapter.

Systems Tracer Session. During this session, high-priority safety and quality-of-care issues on a systemwide basis will be evaluated throughout the organization.

Daily Briefings. During this session, organization staff will be briefed on the previous day's survey findings and any significant patterns or trends that are becoming evident in the survey.

APP

Closing Conference. The closing or exit conference will be devoted to a discussion of the surveyor's findings. At the completion of the survey, the surveyors will provide the organization's accreditation report before leaving the organization.

Survey Team Composition

Accreditation surveys may be conducted by a survey team rather than an individual surveyor. The composition of an organization's survey team is also based on the information provided in its e-App. In most instances, an organization survey team is composed of one to five surveyors, including physicians, nurses, administrators, or other specialties as needed. All surveyors assess and provide consultation regarding all functions addressed by the standards.

In addition, depending on the organization's service configuration, additional surveyors may be assigned to survey specialized areas, such as long term care, home care, and behavioral health care. The findings of additional surveyors are integrated into the organization's accreditation decision and survey report.

Survey Team Leadership

If more than one surveyor is required, one of the surveyors on each organization survey team is designated as the team leader. The team leader is responsible for integration, coordination, and communication of on-site survey activities. In addition to direct participation as an active member of the survey team, the team leader serves as the primary point of on-site contact between the organization and the Joint Commission. Among other responsibilities, the team leader leads the opening conference and the daily and exit briefings.

Scoring Compliance and Track Record Achievements

Accredited organizations are expected to remain in continuous compliance with the standards and their EPs throughout their accreditation cycle. Standards will be judged "compliant" or "not compliant." EPs will be scored on the following scale:

0	Insufficient compliance
1	Partial compliance
2	Satisfactory compliance
NA	Not applicable

For a complete discussion on the scoring methodology, see "The New Joint Commission Accreditation Process" chapter.

For practical purposes in conducting the survey, surveyors will ordinarily limit their evaluation of the organization's track record of compliance, which is 12 months for a triennial survey and 4 months prior to an initial survey.

Surveyors may evaluate compliance over a shorter or longer time frame depending on circumstances encountered during the survey. For example, the required time frame for full compliance with applicable standards and EPs for new services will not exceed the time the service has been in operation. In another example, certain activities that are conducted infrequently, such as biennial credentialing, might require evaluation over a longer interval to ensure an adequate sample size for valid assessment. For a triennial survey, an organization's track record will generally impact the scoring of standards according to the following:

Score 0   Fewer than 6 consecutive months before survey
Score 1   6 to 11 consecutive months before survey
Score 2   12 consecutive months before survey

During initial surveys, an organization's track record will generally impact the scoring of standards according to the following:

Score 0   Fewer than 2 consecutive months before survey
Score 1   2 to 3 consecutive months before survey
Score 2   4 consecutive months before survey

Feedback Sessions

Final scores about compliance are not reached until all required resident care settings have been visited and all survey activities have been conducted. However, surveyors will communicate their observations at daily briefings, as requested by the organization. If the organization has additional information that would demonstrate compliance with a standard that the surveyor has indicated might be a recommendation, the organization should supply that information to the surveyor(s) as soon as possible.

Final On-Site Survey Activities

At the leadership closing conference, the survey team will present survey findings and a written Accreditation Report.

Immediate Threat to Life

The Joint Commission may consider for accreditation purposes a surveyor's finding that some aspect of an organization's operation is having or might have a serious, adverse effect on resident health or safety, and that immediate action must be taken.

In these cases, surveyors will notify the organization's chief executive officer and the Joint Commission's headquarters staff immediately if they identify any condition they believe poses a serious threat to public or resident health and safety. The president of the Joint Commission, or if the president is unavailable his or her designee, can then issue an expedited Preliminary Denial of Accreditation decision based on such notification. He or she will promptly inform the organization's chief executive officer and appropriate governmental authorities of this decision and the findings that led to this action. The Accreditation Committee of the Board of Commissioners will confirm or reverse the decision at its next meeting. The Accreditation Committee may take into consideration an organization's corrective actions or responses to a serious threat situation. The organization can provide information to demonstrate that the serious threat-to-life situation has been corrected prior to the Accreditation Committee's consideration of the Preliminary Denial of Accreditation decision.

In these situations, the corrective action will be considered when a single issue leads to the adverse finding and the organization demonstrates that it did the following:

- Took immediate action to completely remedy the situation
- Prepared a thorough and credible root cause analysis
- Adopted systems changes to prevent a future recurrence of the problem

Accreditation Reports

Following evaluation of the organization's performance of functions and processes, the survey team reviews the results of integrated individual findings. Then, with the use of laptop-based decision support software, the team produces the organization's Accreditation Report. The team leader meets with the organization's chief executive officer prior to the closing conference and provides him or her with a copy of the report. The CEO determines whether the preliminary report is distributed at the closing conference. The survey team uses the report contents in making its closing conference presentations.

Within approximately 48 hours of a survey, the organization's report of survey findings will be posted on the organization's secured extranet site. The report will include, as appropriate, an organization's strengths, requirements for improvement, and supplemental findings.

If an organization does not receive any recommendations, then the organization's accreditation decision will be rendered at the same time that the organization's Accreditation Report is available and will be effective the day after the completion of the survey. If an organization receives requirements for improvement, then the organization's accreditation decision will be rendered following the submission of an ESC report. The ESC report is due within 90 calendar days following the survey; however, the organization's accreditation decision will be retroactive to the day after the last day of the survey.* For organizations that receive a notification that they will be recommended for either Conditional Accreditation or Preliminary Denial of Accreditation, their accreditation decisions will be rendered by the Joint Commission's Accreditation Committee. (*See* the "Evidence of Standards Compliance" section below.)

After the Survey

This section includes information relevant to an organization that recently has participated in an accreditation survey. Material includes information on the ESC process, the MOS process, the types of accreditation decisions, how to request review of Preliminary Denial of Accreditation decisions, how to appeal Denial of Accreditation decisions, and how to use and display an accreditation award.

---

* Beginning July 1, 2005, the ESC report will be due within 45 days of survey.

APP

Evidence of Standards Compliance Process

For every requirement for improvement cited in an organization's Accreditation Report, the organization must submit an ESC report. The ESC report will be available for completion on the organization's extranet site at the same time the organization's Accreditation Report is posted, which is approximately 48 hours after the organization's survey.

APP

The ESC report must detail the action(s) that the organization took to bring itself into compliance with a standard or clarify why the organization believes that it is in compliance with the standard in which it received a requirement for improvement. An ESC report must address compliance at the EP level and include an MOS, if applicable. An MOS is a numerical or quantifiable measure usually related to an audit that will determine if an action is effective and sustained. (*See* "Measure[s] of Success Report" below.)

The ESC report is due within 90 calendar days* after an organization's survey. Following submission of the report, an organization will receive an accreditation decision. If an organization implements actions to address its requirements for improvement, the organization's accreditation decision will be "Accredited." If an organization's ESC report does not address its requirements for improvement, then the organization's accreditation decision will be "Provisional Accreditation."

Conditional Accreditation, Preliminary Denial of Accreditation, and the ESC Report

If an organization is notified that a recommendation will be made to the Joint Commission's Accreditation Committee for either Conditional Accreditation or Preliminary Denial of Accreditation, the organization will have an opportunity to provide information to clarify any of the recommendations cited in its Accreditation Report through its ESC report. This information will be provided to the Accreditation Committee.

Measure(s) of Success Report

An organization will be required to submit an MOS report within four months of submitting an acceptable ESC report. The MOS report will demonstrate whether each MOS identified in the organization's ESC report was reached.

Accreditation Decisions

An organization's accreditation decision becomes official following submission of its ESC report, which is retroactive to the day after the last day of the survey, or, in the case of Conditional Accreditation or Preliminary Denial of Accreditation, on the date the Accreditation Committee makes a decision. When an organization's accreditation decision becomes official, it is publicly disclosable. There are six possible accreditation decisions, as follows:

1. Accredited
2. Provisional Accreditation

---

* 45 days beginning July 1, 2005.

3. Conditional Accreditation
4. Preliminary Denial of Accreditation
5. Denial of Accreditation
6. Preliminary Accreditation

Table 1 (page APP-33) provides a description of each category and the conditions that lead to it.

APP

An organization's request to withdraw from the accreditation process after undergoing survey and before a final decision has been made does not terminate the decision-making process. The Joint Commission will issue a final accreditation decision.

Review and Appeal of Preliminary Denial of Accreditation or Denial of Accreditation Decisions

The appeal procedures are set forth in the "Review and Appeal Procedures" section of this chapter on pages APP-40–APP-50. Two additional procedures specific to Preliminary Denial of Accreditation and Denial of Accreditation decisions are listed here.

When an organization receives written notice from the Joint Commission that a recommendation of Preliminary Denial of Accreditation is proposed for submission to the Accreditation Committee, the organization has 10 business days from receipt of that notification to submit to the Joint Commission an ESC report, clarifying information that demonstrates that it was in fact in compliance with one or more standards in question at the time of survey. If, after Joint Commission review of any submitted materials, the Preliminary Denial of Accreditation recommendation stands, the organization will have five business days from receipt of notification to submit a written response directly to the Accreditation Committee.

Weighted Decision Rules

Recently, the Joint Commission has reevaluated how a complex organization's overall accreditation decision should be impacted by a component's decision involving threats to resident safety, instances in which inaccurate information is provided to the Joint Commission, or violation of other APRs.

As such, the Joint Commission has revised the weighted decision rules so that, when a secondary component of a complex organization meets the rules of Conditional Accreditation or Preliminary Denial of Accreditation as a consequence of invoking the Immediate Threat to Life Policy or not complying with the Information Accuracy and Truthfulness Policy or APRs, that accreditation decision would apply equally to the component and the complex organization of which the component is a part. *See* Table 2 on page APP-35 for more information on the weighted decision rules.

Table 1. Types of Joint Commission Accreditation Decisions

The Joint Commission has six accreditation decision categories. Each decision and the conditions that lead to it are described below.

APP

Accreditation Decision Category	Conditions That Lead to This Type of Decision
Accredited	The organization is in compliance with all standards at the time of the on-site survey or has successfully addressed all requirements for improvement in an ESC report within 90 days following the survey (45 days beginning July 1, 2005).
Provisional Accreditation	The organization fails to successfully address all requirements for improvement in an ESC report within 90 days following the survey (45 days beginning July 1, 2005).
Conditional Accreditation	The organization is not in substantial compliance with the standards, as usually evidenced by a count of the number of standards identified as not compliant at the time of survey, which is between two and three standard deviations above the mean number of noncompliant standards for organizations in that accreditation program. The organization must remedy identified problem areas through preparation and submission of an ESC report and subsequently undergo an on-site, follow-up survey.
Preliminary Denial of Accreditation	There is justification to deny accreditation to the organization as usually evidenced by a count of the number of noncompliant standards at the time of survey, which is at least three standard deviations above the mean number of standards identified as not compliant for organizations in that accreditation program. The decision is subject to appeal prior to the determination to deny accreditation; the appeal process may also result in a decision other than Denial of Accreditation.

continued on next page

Table 1. Types of Joint Commission Accreditation Decisions *(continued)*

Denial of Accreditation	The organization has been denied accreditation. All review and appeal opportunities have been exhausted.
Preliminary Accreditation	The organization demonstrates compliance with selected standards in the first of two surveys conducted under Early Survey Policy Option 1.

APP

Award Display and Use

The Joint Commission provides each accredited organization with one certificate of accreditation per site. There is no charge for the initial certificate(s). Additional certificates may be purchased. Such requests should be sent to the Certificate Coordinator, Division of Accreditation Operations at the Joint Commission.

The certificate and all copies remain the Joint Commission's property. They must be returned if either of the following situations occur:
- The organization is issued a new certificate reflecting a name change
- The organization's accreditation status is changed, withdrawn, or denied, for any reason

An organization accredited by the Joint Commission must be accurate in describing to the public the nature and meaning of its accreditation and its award.* When an organization receives an accreditation award, the Joint Commission sends the organization guidelines for characterizing the accreditation award.

Accreditation award certificates will include language about educating residents and their families on how to contact the Joint Commission.

An organization may not engage in any false or misleading advertising of the accreditation award. Any such advertising may be grounds to deny accreditation. For example, an organization may not represent its accreditation as being awarded by any of the Joint Commission's corporate members. These include the American College of Physicians, the American College of Surgeons, the American Dental Association, the American Hospital Association, and the American Medical Association. The Joint Commission has permission to reprint the seals of its corporate members on the certificates of accreditation. However, these seals must not be reproduced or displayed separately from the certificate.

Any organization that materially misleads the public about any matter relating to its accreditation must undertake corrective advertising of a degree acceptable to the

---

* *See* APR 11 on page APR-8 in the "Accreditation Participation Requirements" chapter.

Table 2. Weighted Decision Rules

Primary Program

One program in a complex organization is to be identified as "primary" (this is not a change from the previous rule).

If the primary program meets a rule for Provisional Accreditation, Conditional Accreditation, or Preliminary Denial of Accreditation, the overall decision for the organization will be Provisional Accreditation, Conditional Accreditation, or Preliminary Denial of Accreditation, respectively.

Secondary Programs

If one of the secondary programs meets a rule for Preliminary Denial of Accreditation, the overall decision for the organization will be Conditional Accreditation.

If one of the secondary programs meets a rule for Conditional Accreditation, the overall decision for the organization will be Provisional Accreditation.

If two or more of the secondary programs meet rules for Preliminary Denial of Accreditation, the overall decision for the organization will be Preliminary Denial of Accreditation.

If two or more of the secondary programs meet rules for Conditional Accreditation, the overall decision for the organization will be Conditional Accreditation.

If the primary or any secondary program meets a rule for Provisional Accreditation, the overall decision for the organization will be Provisional Accreditation.

Joint Commission in the same medium in which the misrepresentation occurred. If an organization fails to undertake the required corrective advertising following the communication of false or misleading advertising about its accreditation status, the organization may be subject to loss of accreditation.

The Joint Commission's logo is a registered trademark. An accredited organization may use the logo if it follows the following guidelines:
- The logo must remain in the same proportional relationship as provided and should not be displayed any larger than an organization's own logo
- The logo's format cannot be changed, the name cannot be separated from the symbol, and it must be printed in the original color
- Graphic devices such as seals, other words, or slogans cannot be added to the logo except for the words "Accredited by"

These guidelines apply to logo use on all print materials, Internet Web pages, and promotional items, such as coffee mugs, T-shirts, and notepads. Contact the Department of Communications at the Joint Commission at 630/792-5631 for questions about using the Joint Commission logo.

Before the Next Survey

This section provides information relevant to organizations between Joint Commission surveys. Material includes the duration of an accreditation award; the process for continuing accreditation; how to notify the Joint Commission in the event of organizational changes including the opening or closing of a unit or services, addition or deletion of components, leadership changes, mergers, consolidations, and acquisitions; and unscheduled and unannounced for-cause surveys.

APP

Reentering the Accreditation Process

For a previously accredited organization to be designated as "new" and be subject to only a 4 month track record period for demonstrating standards compliance, it must not have participated in the accreditation process during the previous 6 months. If an organization is *reentering* the accreditation process before 6 months have passed, it must demonstrate a continuing 12-month track record of compliance with the standards.

Duration of Accreditation Award

An accreditation award is continuous until the organization has its next full survey, which is usually around three years unless revoked for cause or as otherwise outlined in this chapter. Accreditation is effective on the first day after the Joint Commission completes the organization's survey. An organization may request a full accreditation survey more frequently than once every three years. The Joint Commission will, at its discretion and in accordance with its mission, determine whether to honor the request. Such requests should be sent to the organization's account representative.

Continuous Compliance

The Joint Commission expects an accredited organization to be in continuous compliance with all applicable standards and EPs. It may ask an organization to supply, in writing, information about compliance with standards. It may also survey an organization at any time with or without notice in response to complaints, media coverage, or other information that raises questions about the adequacy of resident health and safety protections (*see* "Unscheduled and Unannounced For-Cause Surveys" on pages APP-39–APP-40). The Joint Commission might also conduct a survey if an organization fails to respond to a request for more information.

An organization's failure to permit a survey can be viewed by the Joint Commission as the organization no longer wanting to participate in the accreditation process. Therefore, the Joint Commission will begin proceedings to deny accreditation to the organization.*

Continuing Accreditation

The Joint Commission does not automatically renew an organization's accreditation. An organization seeking to continue its accreditation must reapply for accredi-

---

* *See* APR 3 on pages APR-2–APR-3 in the "Accreditation Participation Requirements" chapter.

tation, undergo a full accreditation survey, and be found in compliance with the standards and intent statements.

Accreditation Renewal Process

The Joint Commission will notify an organization approximately six to nine months before the organization's triennial accreditation due date that it needs to complete an application for a resurvey and provide information about how the application can be accessed, completed, and transmitted to the Joint Commission electronically via the organization's extranet site. The organization should call 630/792-5800 if it has not received such a notification four months before its accreditation due date.

APP

Note: *Effective January 1, 2006, all triennial surveys will be conducted on an unannounced basis. As such the accreditation renewal process will change. Please consult future issues of* Joint Commission Perspectives® *or the 2006 update to this manual for more information on the anticipated changes.*

Generally, the Joint Commission conducts a triennial survey in the time period between 45 calendar days before the organization's three-year survey due date and 45 calendar days after the due date. The Joint Commission notifies the organization of the survey date at least four weeks before the survey. If there are any specific dates within the 45 calendar days before and after the due date range that would conflict with other organization activities, the organization should identify those dates in the application as dates to avoid.

Accreditation Decision During Triennial Survey

An organization's previous accreditation decision remains in effect until a decision is made either to accredit or to preliminarily deny accreditation to the organization.

Notification of Changes Made Between Surveys

Accreditation is neither automatically transferred nor continued if significant changes occur within the organization. When significant changes occur, the organization must notify the Joint Commission in writing not more than 30 calendar days after such change is made. The organization must also notify the Joint Commission in writing if it opens or closes any units or services.

When an organization offers at least 25% of its services at a new location or in a significantly altered physical plant, the organization must also fill out and submit to the Joint Commission Part 2: Basic Building Information of the Statement of Conditions™ (SOC) Compliance Document, Part 3E or 3F of the Statement of Fire Safety (SFS), and Part 4: Plan for Improvement, should *Life Safety Code*®* deficiencies be present. (For a copy of the SOC, visit the Joint Commission's Web site at http://www.jcaho.org, select Accredited Organizations, then your accreditation program, then Standards, and then Statement of Conditions™.) Failure to provide timely notification to the Joint Commission of these changes may result in the loss of accreditation.

---

* *Life Safety Code*® is a registered trademark of the National Fire Protection Association, Quincy, MA.

Mergers, Consolidations, and Acquisitions

In the case of a merger, consolidation, or acquisition, the Joint Commission may decide that the organization responsible for services must have a survey. Barring exceptional circumstances, the Joint Commission continues the accreditation of the organization undergoing the kind of changes described previously until it determines whether an extension survey is necessary.

APP

Note: *When an accredited organization acquires another organization and an extension survey is conducted, the survey findings resulting from the extension survey would be maintained separately from, and would not be reflected in, the accreditation decision of the acquiring organization for 12 months following the acquisition. After the 12-month period, any outstanding standards compliance problems in the acquired component(s) would be reflected in the accreditation decision of the acquiring organization.*

Extension Surveys

An extension survey is conducted at an accredited organization or at a site that is owned and operated by the organization if the accredited organization's current accreditation is not due to expire for at least nine months and when at least one of the following conditions is met. The results of an extension survey can affect the organization's accreditation decision.

An extension survey of the organization might be necessary if the organization has done one of the following:
- Instituted a new service or program for which the Joint Commission has standards
- Changed ownership and there are a significant number of changes in the management and clinical staff or operating policies and procedures
- Offered at least 25% of its services at a new location or in a significantly altered physical plant
- Expanded its capacity to provide services by 25% or more as measured by resident volume, pieces of equipment, or other relevant measures
- Provided a more intensive level of service
  or
- Merged with, consolidated with, or acquired an unaccredited site, service, or program for which there are applicable Joint Commission standards and EPs

An extension survey can also occur in the following situations:
- The Joint Commission grants an organization's request to continue its current accreditation beyond the conclusion of the three-year cycle*
  or
- An organization has merged with, consolidated with, or acquired an accredited organization whose accreditation expiration date is within three months of the merger, consolidation, or acquisition, while its own accreditation expiration date is at least nine months away.

---

* Such requests are granted only for unusual or compelling reasons.

Unscheduled and Unannounced For-Cause Surveys

The Joint Commission may perform either an unscheduled survey or an unannounced survey when it becomes aware of potentially serious standards compliance or resident care or safety issues, or it has other valid reasons for surveying in an accredited organization.*

Note: *The for-cause unscheduled or unannounced surveys should not be confused with regular unannounced surveys, as described on page APP-5.*

Either type of survey can take place at any point in an organization's three-year accreditation cycle. The Joint Commission usually provides the organization with 24 to 48 hours advance notice of an unscheduled survey. No preliminary report is generated after an unscheduled survey whether announced or unannounced.

Note: *Organizations are charged for these surveys, regardless of the outcome. The cost of the survey can be obtained by calling the Pricing Unit at 630/792-5115. However, organizations are not charged for random unannounced surveys. (For additional information on random unannounced surveys, see below.)*

No advance notice is provided for unannounced surveys. Reasons for unannounced surveys include occurrence of any event or series of events in an accredited organization that creates one of the following significant situations:

- Concern that a continuing threat might exist to the safety or care of residents, or that the safety or care of residents is at risk
  or
- Indication that the organization is not or has not been in compliance with the Joint Commission's Information Accuracy and Truthfulness Policy

Such a survey can either include all the organization's services or only those areas where a serious concern may exist.

Results of any unannounced or unscheduled surveys can generate follow-up activities and can affect an organization's current accreditation decision. The Joint Commission may deny accreditation if the organization does not allow the Joint Commission to conduct unscheduled or unannounced surveys.

Random Unannounced Surveys

The Joint Commission also conducts unannounced surveys on a 5% random sample of accredited organizations. The survey is generally conducted 9–30 months following the accreditation date (that is, the date after the last day of the full survey). An organization will receive no advance notice of the random unannounced survey. One surveyor conducts each survey for one day. Organizations are not charged for random unannounced surveys.

Note: *As part of the move toward all accreditation surveys being conducted on an unannounced basis in 2006, the Joint Commission will no longer conduct random unannounced surveys after January 1, 2006.*

---

* *See* APR 3 on pages APR-2–APR-3 in the "Accreditation Participation Requirements" chapter.

During the random unannounced survey, the surveyor assesses both *fixed* and *variable* components, or performance areas. Fixed components are identified each year for organizations based on the highest PFAs and selected National Patient Safety Goals. Fixed components are identified based on the degree of actual or perceived risk to the care of residents posed by noncompliance with standards related to these elements. Fixed components for each accreditation program are published in *Perspectives* and are listed on the Joint Commission Web site. Variable components are identified through the PFP. Presurvey information run through the PFP identifies prioritized organization-specific PFAs to be evaluated. (*See* the "Priority Focus Process" section of this chapter [page APP-26] for more on presurvey information.) The surveyor may also expand the scope of the random unannounced survey based on findings at the time of the survey.

No random unannounced surveys will be conducted at an organization undergoing an unannounced triennial survey.

Review and Appeal Procedures

After any Preliminary Denial of Accreditation decision, the organization has the right to make a detailed presentation before a Review Hearing Panel. The Accreditation Committee will then review the findings of the Review Hearing Panel and either deny accreditation to the organization or select an appropriate alternative accreditation decision. The organization may appeal any decision of the Accreditation Committee to deny accreditation before the decision becomes the final decision of the Joint Commission.

The following outline details review and appeal procedures:

I. **Evaluation by Joint Commission Staff**
   A. **Review and Determination by Joint Commission Staff.** Following a triennial or other survey activity, the Joint Commission staff shall review survey findings, survey documents, and any other relevant materials or information received from any source. Except as provided in paragraphs I.B, I.C, and I.D, Joint Commission staff shall, in accordance with decision rules approved by the Accreditation Committee of the Board of Commissioners, do the following:
   1. Determine or recommend to the Accreditation Committee that the organization be accredited, as described in paragraph VII of these procedures
      or
   2. Recommend to the Accreditation Committee that the organization be conditionally accredited
      or
   3. Determine that the organization be conditionally accredited, if the organization does not submit ESC in accordance with paragraph I.B.I.a or I.B.I.b
      or

4. Recommend to the Accreditation Committee that the organization be preliminarily denied accreditation

   or

5. Defer consideration while additional information regarding the organization's compliance status is reviewed by Joint Commission staff

   or

6. Determine or recommend to the Accreditation Committee that the organization be preliminarily accredited in accordance with the Early Survey Policy set forth on pages APP-6–APP-9

   or

7. Recommend to the Accreditation Committee that the organization be initially denied Preliminary Accreditation in accordance with the Early Survey Policy set forth on pages APP-6–APP-9

B. Determination to Recommend Conditional Accreditation Based on Full Triennial Surveys.

1. Notification to Organization of Areas of Noncompliance with Standards. In the case of full triennial surveys, if the Joint Commission staff, based on survey findings, survey documents, and any other relevant materials or information received from any source, determines to recommend that the organization be conditionally accredited, it will outline its findings and determination. The organization may do the following:

   a. Accept the findings and determination of the staff through submission of the ESC report.

      or

   b. Submit to the Joint Commission, through an ESC report, any clarification of its compliance with Joint Commission standards at the time of the survey that is not reflected in the Accreditation Report, along with an explanation of why such documentation was not available for review at the time of the survey.

2. Consideration of the Organization's Response. Joint Commission staff shall review the organization's submission of any additional information and shall, in accordance with decision rules approved by the Accreditation Committee, do the following:

   a. Recommend to the Accreditation Committee that the organization be conditionally accredited

      or

   b. Recommend to the Accreditation Committee that the organization be preliminarily denied accreditation

      or

   c. Recommend to the Accreditation Committee that the organization be accredited, as described in paragraph VII of these procedures

APP

C. **Determination to Recommend That Accreditation Be Preliminarily Denied Based on Full Triennial or Other Survey Activity.**

1. Notification to Organization of Areas of Noncompliance with Standards. In the case of full triennial surveys, if the Joint Commission staff, based on survey findings, survey documents, and any other relevant materials or information received from any source, determines, in accordance with decision rules approved by the Accreditation Committee, to recommend to the Accreditation Committee that the organization be preliminarily denied accreditation, it will outline its findings and determination. The organization may do the following:

    a. Accept the findings and determination of the staff through submission of the ESC report.

    or

    b. Submit to the Joint Commission through the ESC report any clarification of its compliance with Joint Commission standards at the time of the survey that is not reflected in the Accreditation Report, along with an explanation of why such information was not available for review at the time of the survey.

2. Consideration of the Organization's Response. Joint Commission staff members shall review the organization's submission of any additional information and shall, in accordance with decision rules approved by the Accreditation Committee, do the following:

    a. Recommend to the Accreditation Committee that the organization be conditionally accredited

    or

    b. Recommend to the Accreditation Committee that the organization be preliminarily denied accreditation

    or

    c. Recommend to the Accreditation Committee that the organization be accredited, as described in paragraph VII of these procedures.

D. **Decisions by the President of the Joint Commission.** Notwithstanding anything outlined in paragraphs I.A–I.C.1 of these procedures to the contrary, if the findings of any survey identify any condition that poses a threat to public or resident safety, the president of the Joint Commission, or if the president is not available, a vice president of the Joint Commission designated by the president to do so, may promptly decide that the organization be immediately placed in Preliminary Denial of Accreditation. This action and the findings that led to this action shall be reported by telephone and in writing to the organization's chief executive officer and in writing to the authorities having jurisdiction. The president's or his or her designee's decision shall be promptly reviewed by the Accreditation Committee in accordance with paragraph II of these procedures.

II. Review by the Accreditation Committee

A. Scope of Review. The Accreditation Committee shall consider the Joint Commission president's, or the president's designee's, decision and the Joint Commission staff's report and recommendation and may review the survey findings, survey documents, and any other relevant materials or information received from any source, including any additional information supplied by the organization in response to this information or, in the case of a Preliminary Denial of Accreditation decision by the president or his or her designee, information supplied by the organization regarding corrective actions taken in response to the identification of a serious threat to resident or public health or safety.

B. Decision. Following such consideration, the Accreditation Committee shall do the following:
1. Or accredit the organization, as described in paragraph VII of these procedures.
2. Or conditionally accredit the organization.
3. Or preliminarily deny accreditation to the organization or confirm a decision by the president or his or her designee to preliminarily deny accreditation.
4. Or defer consideration while additional information regarding the organization's compliance status is gathered and reviewed by Joint Commission staff.
5. Or order a resurvey or partial resurvey of the organization and an evaluation of the results, to the extent appropriate, by the Joint Commission staff. Thereafter, Joint Commission staff shall transmit the report and recommendation to the Accreditation Committee for action, as provided in paragraph II.C of these procedures.
6. Or preliminarily accredit the organization.
7. Or initially deny Preliminary Accreditation to those organizations that apply for Early Survey Policy Option 1.

C. Deferred Consideration. When the Accreditation Committee defers consideration pursuant to paragraph II.B.4 or II.B.5 of these procedures, Joint Commission staff shall review and report to the Accreditation Committee concerning the organization's compliance decision. The Accreditation Committee may order any resurvey or partial resurvey necessary to reach such a decision. Following such consideration and review, the Accreditation Committee shall do the following:
1. Accredit the organization, as described in paragraph VII of these procedures.
2. Or conditionally accredit the organization.
3. Or preliminarily deny accreditation or confirm a decision of the president or his or her designee to preliminarily deny accreditation to the organization.
4. Or defer consideration while additional information regarding the organization's compliance status is gathered and reviewed by the Joint Commission staff.

APP

5. Or order an additional resurvey or partial resurvey of the organization and an evaluation of the results, to the extent appropriate, by the Joint Commission staff. Thereafter, Joint Commission staff shall transmit the report and recommendations to the Accreditation Committee for action, as provided in paragraph II.C of these procedures.
6. Or preliminarily accredit the organization.
7. Or deny Preliminary Accreditation to those organizations applying under Early Survey Policy Option 1.

III. Conditional Accreditation

A. Survey to Determine Implementation of the ESC. Within approximately six months from the date the organization is notified of its Conditional Accreditation decision, the Joint Commission shall conduct a survey of the organization to determine the degree to which deficiencies have been corrected or improvements implemented, although the Joint Commission may shorten that time period, as appropriate.

B. Review and Determination by Joint Commission Staff. Joint Commission staff shall review the survey findings, survey documents, and any other relevant materials or information received from any source. In accordance with decision rules approved by the Accreditation Committee, the Joint Commission staff shall do the following:

1. Determine or recommend to the Accreditation Committee that the organization be accredited, as described in paragraph VII of these procedures.
2. Or recommend to the Accreditation Committee that the organization be preliminarily denied accreditation.
3. Or defer consideration while additional information regarding the organization's compliance status is gathered and reviewed by the Joint Commission staff. At the conclusion of this review, one of the recommendations outlined in paragraph III.D of these procedures shall be made to the Accreditation Committee.

C. Action by the Accreditation Committee. Following review of the recommendations of the Joint Commission staff, the Accreditation Committee shall do the following:

1. Accredit the organization, as described in paragraph VII of these procedures.
2. Or preliminarily deny accreditation to the organization.
3. Or defer consideration while additional information regarding the organization's compliance status is gathered and reviewed by the Joint Commission staff.
4. Or order a resurvey or partial resurvey of the organization and an evaluation of the results, to the extent appropriate, by the Joint Commission staff. Thereafter, Joint Commission staff shall transmit the report and recommendation to the Accreditation Committee for action, as provided in paragraph III.C of these procedures.

D. Charges to the Organization. The full costs of the Conditional Accreditation process shall be paid by the organization that receives Conditional Accreditation.

IV. Review Hearing Panels

A. Right to a Hearing Before a Review Hearing Panel. An organization that has been preliminarily denied accreditation* or Preliminary Accreditation pursuant to paragraph II.B.3, II.B.7, II.C.3, II.C.7, or III.C.2 of these procedures is entitled to a hearing in which to make a detailed presentation before a Review Hearing Panel if the Joint Commission receives the organization's written request for the hearing within five business days after the organization receives the written notice of the Accreditation Committee's decision, including confirmation of a decision by the president, or his or her designee, to preliminarily deny accreditation, as provided in paragraph I.D of these procedures. A Review Hearing Panel shall be composed of two health care professionals who are not on the Accreditation Committee and one member of the Accreditation Committee who is familiar with the organization's decision.

B. Notice of the Time and Place of the Presentation Before a Review Hearing Panel. The presentation before the Review Hearing Panel shall be held at the Joint Commission's headquarters except when the president of the Joint Commission, or his or her designee, determines otherwise for good cause. At least 30 calendar days before the presentation, the Joint Commission shall send the organization written notice of the time and place of the hearing and copies of any supplemental materials or information received from any source that the organization does not already have and that might affect any accreditation decision. The notice shall advise the organization of the agenda to be followed and, if feasible, of the identity and professional qualifications of the panel members. At least 10 calendar days before the scheduled hearing date, the organization must submit to the Joint Commission any materials it wishes to be considered by the Review Hearing Panel.

C. Procedure for the Conduct of a Hearing. A Review Hearing Panel may proceed with only two of the three panel members present, provided one of them is the member of the Accreditation Committee. Representatives of the organization may make oral and written presentations and may be accompanied by legal counsel. Presentations or information concerning actions taken by the organization subsequent to the survey upon which the Preliminary Denial of Accreditation decision was based are not considered relevant to the validity of the decision. A Joint Commission surveyor who participated in the survey will ordinarily appear at the hearing.

---

* The Preliminary Denial of Accreditation decision, if subsequently changed to other than Denial of Accreditation following review and action by the Accreditation Committee, is no longer disclosable as part of the organization's accreditation decision history.

APP

D. Report of Review Hearing Panel. After a hearing has been completed, the Review Hearing Panel shall review the facts regarding the original Preliminary Denial of Accreditation decision. The panel will submit a written report of its findings on factual matters for consideration by the Accreditation Committee.

E. Charges to the Organization. The organization will be charged a nominal fee for the conduct of a Review Hearing Panel.

V. Second Consideration by the Accreditation Committee

A. Scope of Review. The report of the Review Hearing Panel shall be considered by the Accreditation Committee.

B. Decision. Following such consideration, the Accreditation Committee shall do the following:
1. Accredit or preliminarily accredit the organization, as described in paragraph VII of these procedures
   or
2. Conditionally accredit the organization
   or
3. Deny accreditation to the organization
   or
4. Defer consideration while additional information regarding the organization's compliance status is gathered and reviewed by Joint Commission staff
   or
5. Order a resurvey or partial resurvey of the organization and an evaluation of the results, to the extent appropriate, by the Joint Commission staff

VI. Review by the Board Appeal Review Committee

A. Review Request. An organization that has been denied accreditation or Preliminary Accreditation pursuant to paragraph V.B.3 of these procedures is entitled to request a review of the decision by the Board Appeal Review Committee if the Joint Commission receives the organization's request for review within five business days after the organization receives the written notice of the Accreditation Committee's decision. The Board Appeal Review Committee is composed of four members of the Board of Commissioners who are not members of the Accreditation Committee.

B. Notice of Time and Procedure for Review. The Joint Commission shall send the organization a copy of the report of the Review Hearing Panel at least 20 business days before the meeting of the Board Appeal Review Committee at which the organization's request for review will be considered. Two members of the Board Appeal Review Committee will constitute a quorum. This meeting will generally be held by telephone conference, except when it is held in conjunction with meetings of the Board of Commissioners or other committee(s) of the Board of Commissioners. The organization must submit any materials that it wishes the Board Appeal Review Committee to consider at least 10 calendar days before the scheduled meeting date. The Board Appeal Review Committee shall review the decision of the Accreditation Committee, which considered the report of the Review Hearing Panel, and any written materials submitted by the organization, and shall do one of the following:

1. Deny accreditation or Preliminary Accreditation to the organization, after finding that there is substantial evidence to support the Accreditation Committee's decision

   or

2. Make an independent evaluation of the Accreditation Committee's decision and then decide to conditionally accredit, preliminarily accredit, or accredit the organization, as described in paragraph VII of these procedures

The action taken by the Board Appeal Review Committee shall constitute the final accreditation decision of the Joint Commission.

C. Participation. No member of the Accreditation Committee or of the Review Hearing Panel who participated in an accreditation decision or review of findings on factual matters concerning an organization shall participate in any deliberations or votes of the Board Appeal Review Committee in its review of that accreditation decision or report of findings on factual matters. This provision shall not preclude any commissioner who participated in a review hearing as a member of the Review Hearing Panel from presenting and responding to questions about the report of that Review Hearing Panel to the Board Appeal Review Committee.

VII. Procedure Relating to Not Compliant Standards and Determination of Corrected Not Compliant Standards

A. A decision of the Joint Commission staff pursuant to paragraph I.A.1, I.B.2.c, or I.C.2.c of these procedures, of the Accreditation Committee pursuant to paragraph II.B.1, II.C.1, or III.C.1 of these procedures, or of a Board Appeal Review Committee, as provided in paragraph VI.B of these procedures, to accredit an organization may be made contingent upon satisfactory correction of not compliant standards or, when appropriate, upon compliance with interim life safety measures. The organization may be conditionally accredited or its accreditation may be withdrawn if it does not correct or document the correction of the specified not compliant standards within the time specified in the notice of the decision to the organization, or, when applicable, fails to demonstrate compliance with the interim life safety measures. Joint Commission staff (through the use of surveys, partial surveys, or through other means, such as ESC and MOS) shall determine whether the organization has corrected the not compliant standards within the time provided or, when applicable, has demonstrated compliance with interim life safety measures and shall report its findings to the organization. If the Joint Commission staff determines that the organization has not corrected the not compliant standards within the time provided or, when applicable, has not demonstrated compliance with interim life safety measures, the organization's status will change to Provisional Accreditation. The Joint Commission shall report its findings to the organization and, after reviewing any comments of the organization, as appropriate and in accordance with decision rules approved by the Accreditation Committee, do the following:

1. Provide another opportunity to the organization to correct or document the correction of not compliant standards, as provided in any applicable decision rules approved by the Accreditation Committee

   or

2. Determine or recommend that the organization be placed in Conditional Accreditation status with a conditional follow-up survey in approximately four months or at another time as appropriate

   or

3. Recommend to the Accreditation Committee that the organization be preliminarily denied accreditation, if certain not compliant standards, specified in decision rules approved by the Accreditation Committee, have not been corrected or the correction of which has not been documented after the specified number of opportunities given to the organization to do so, and, when applicable and as specified in decision rules approved by the Accreditation Committee, the organization has failed to demonstrate compliance with interim life safety measures

B. If the Joint Commission staff determines to recommend to the Accreditation Committee that the organization be preliminarily denied accreditation in accordance with paragraph VII.A.3, or be conditionally accredited in accordance with VII.A.2, the staff shall submit its recommendation and any comments of the organization to the Accreditation Committee for action, as provided in paragraph II.B.1 through II.B.7.

VIII. Final Accreditation Decision

A. The action taken by the Joint Commission staff shall constitute the final decision of the Joint Commission to do the following:

1. Accredit the organization, when taken pursuant to paragraph I.A.1, I.B.2.c, or I.C.2.c of these procedures

   or

2. Conditionally accredit the organization, when taken pursuant to paragraph I.A.3 or VII.A.2 of these procedures

   or

3. Preliminarily accredit the organization, when taken pursuant to paragraph I.A.6 of these procedures

B. The action taken by the Accreditation Committee shall constitute the final decision of the Joint Commission to do the following:

1. Accredit the organization, when taken pursuant to paragraph II.B.1, II.C.1, or III.C.1 of these procedures

   or

2. Conditionally accredit the organization, when taken pursuant to paragraph II.B.2 or II.C.2 of these procedures
   or
3. Deny accreditation to the organization, when taken pursuant to paragraph II.B.3, II.C.3, III.C.2, or VII.B of these procedures, and the organization does not request the opportunity to make a presentation before a Review Hearing Panel pursuant to paragraph IV.A of these procedures
   or
4. Preliminarily accredit the organization, when taken pursuant to paragraph II.B.6 of these procedures
   or
5. Deny Preliminary Accreditation to the organization, when taken pursuant to paragraph II.B.7 of these procedures, and the organization applying for Early Survey Policy Option 1 or 2 does not request the opportunity to make a presentation before a Review Hearing Panel pursuant to paragraph IV.A of these procedures

C. The action taken by the Board Appeal Review Committee shall constitute the final decision of the Joint Commission to accredit the organization, conditionally accredit the organization, or deny accreditation, when taken pursuant to paragraph VI.B of these procedures

IX. Status of the Organization Pending a Final Decision and Effective Date of a Final Decision

A. The accreditation status of an accredited organization shall continue in effect pending any final accreditation decision.

B. A final decision to accredit, preliminarily accredit, or conditionally accredit an organization that follows an initial Accreditation Committee decision of Preliminary Denial of Accreditation pursuant to paragraph II.B shall be considered effective as of the first day after completion of the organization's survey from which the decision results.

C. A final decision to deny accreditation or Provisional Accreditation to an organization shall become effective as follows:
   1. As of the date of the decision made by the Board Appeal Review Committee pursuant to paragraph VI.B of these procedures
      or
   2. At the expiration of the time during which an organization may, but does not, request a review by the Board Appeal Review Committee, pursuant to paragraph VI.A of these procedures
      or
   3. At the expiration of the time during which an organization may, but does not, request the opportunity to make a presentation before a Review Hearing Panel pursuant to paragraph IV.A of these procedures
      or

APP

4. On receipt by the Joint Commission, before a final decision, of notification from the organization that it withdraws its request for review of a Preliminary Denial of Accreditation decision before a Review Hearing Panel or its request for appeal of a Denial of Accreditation decision before the Board Appeal Review Committee

APP

X. Notice

Any notice required by these accreditation procedures to be given to an organization shall be addressed to the organization at its post office address as shown in Joint Commission records and shall be sent to the organization by certified letter as forwarded by a recognized package delivery service. Any notice required to be given to the Joint Commission by the organization shall be sent by the organization in the same manner and shall be addressed to the Office of the Executive Vice President for Accreditation Operations, Joint Commission on Accreditation of Healthcare Organizations, One Renaissance Boulevard, Oakbrook Terrace, IL 60181.

Sentinel Events

I. Sentinel Events

In support of its mission to continuously improve the safety and quality of health care provided to the public, the Joint Commission reviews organizations' activities in response to sentinel events in its accreditation process, including all full accreditation surveys and random unannounced surveys.

- A sentinel event is an unexpected occurrence involving death or serious physical or psychological injury, or the risk thereof. Serious injury specifically includes loss of limb or function. The phrase *or the risk thereof* includes any process variation for which a recurrence would carry a significant chance of a serious adverse outcome.
- Such events are called *sentinel* because they signal the need for immediate investigation and response.
- The terms *sentinel event* and *medical error* are not synonymous; not all sentinel events occur because of an error, and not all errors result in sentinel events.

II. Goals of the Sentinel Event Policy

The policy has four goals:
1. To have a positive impact in improving resident care, treatment, and services and preventing sentinel events
2. To focus the attention of an organization that has experienced a sentinel event on understanding the causes that underlie the event, and on changing the organization's systems and processes to reduce the probability of such an event in the future
3. To increase the general knowledge about sentinel events, their causes, and strategies for prevention
4. To maintain the confidence of the public and accredited organizations in the accreditation process

III. Standards Relating to Sentinel Events
Standards

Each Joint Commission accreditation manual contains standards in the "Improving Organization Performance" (PI) chapter that relate specifically to the management of sentinel events. These standards are PI.1.10, PI.2.20, PI.2.30, and PI.3.10.

Organization-Specific Definition of Sentinel Event

The Improving Organization Performance standard, PI.2.30, requires each accredited organization to define *sentinel event* for its own purposes in establishing mechanisms to identify, report, and manage these events. While this definition must be consistent with the general definition of sentinel event as published by the Joint Commission, accredited organizations have some latitude in setting more specific parameters to define *unexpected, serious,* and *the risk thereof.* At a minimum, an organization's definition must include those events that are subject to review under the Sentinel Event Policy as defined in Section IV of this chapter.

Expectations Under the Standards for an Organization's Response to a Sentinel Event

Accredited organizations are expected to identify and respond appropriately to all sentinel events (as defined by the organization in accordance with the preceding paragraph) occurring in the organization or associated with services that the organization provides, or provides for. Appropriate response includes conducting a timely, thorough, and credible root cause analysis; developing an action plan designed to implement improvements to reduce risk; implementing the improvements; and monitoring the effectiveness of those improvements.

Root Cause Analysis

Root cause analysis is a process for identifying the basic or causal factors that underlie variation in performance, including the occurrence or possible occurrence of a sentinel event. A root cause analysis focuses primarily on systems and processes, not on individual performance. It progresses from special causes* in clinical processes to common causes† in organizational processes and identifies potential improvements in processes or systems that tend to decrease the likelihood of such events in the future or determines, after analysis, that no such improvement opportunities exist.

Action Plan

The product of the root cause analysis is an action plan that identifies the strategies that the organization intends to implement to reduce the risk of similar events occurring in the future. The plan should address responsibility for implementation, oversight, pilot testing as appropriate, time lines, and strategies for measuring the effectiveness of the actions.

Survey Process

When conducting an accreditation survey, the Joint Commission seeks to evaluate the organization's compliance with the applicable standards and to score those standards based on performance throughout the organization over time (for example, the preceding 12 months for a full accreditation survey). Surveyors are instructed not to seek out specific sentinel events beyond those already known to the Joint Commission.

If, in the course of conducting the usual survey activities, a sentinel event is identified, the surveyor will take the following steps:

---

* **Special cause** is a factor that intermittently and unpredictably induces variation over and above what is inherent in the system. It often appears as an extreme point (such as a point beyond the control limits on a control chart) or some specific, identifiable pattern in data.

† **Common cause** is a factor that results from variation inherent in the process or system. The risk of a common cause can be reduced by redesigning the process or system.

- Inform the CEO that the event has been identified
- Inform the CEO the event will be reported to the Joint Commission for further review and follow-up under the provisions of the Sentinel Event Policy

During the on-site survey, the surveyor(s) will assess the organization's compliance with sentinel event–related standards in the following ways:
- Review the organization's process for responding to a sentinel event
- Interview the organization's leaders and staff about their expectations and responsibilities for identifying, reporting, and responding to sentinel events
- Ask for an example of a root cause analysis that has been conducted in the past year to assess the adequacy of the organization's process for responding to a sentinel event. Additional examples may be reviewed if needed to more fully assess the organization's understanding of, and ability to conduct, root cause analyses. In selecting an example, the organization may choose a "closed case" or a "near miss"* to demonstrate its process for responding to a sentinel event.

SE

IV. Reviewable Sentinel Events

Definition of Occurrences That Are Subject to Review by the Joint Commission Under the Sentinel Event Policy

The definition of a reviewable sentinel event takes into account a wide array of occurrences applicable to a wide variety of health care organizations. Any or all occurrences might apply to a particular type of health care organization. Thus, not all of the following occurrences might apply to your particular organization. The subset of sentinel events that is subject to review by the Joint Commission includes any occurrence that meets any of the following criteria:
- The event has resulted in an unanticipated death or major permanent loss of function, not related to the natural course of the resident's illness or underlying condition[†‡]

  or

---

* **Near miss** Used to describe any process variation that did not affect an outcome but for which a recurrence carries a significant chance of a serious adverse outcome. Such a near miss falls within the scope of the definition of a sentinel event but outside the scope of those sentinel events that are subject to review by the Joint Commission under its Sentinel Event Policy

[†] A distinction is made between an adverse outcome that is primarily related to the natural course of the resident's illness or underlying condition (not reviewed under the Sentinel Event Policy) and a death or major permanent loss of function that is associated with the treatment (including "recognized complications") or lack of treatment of that condition, or otherwise not clearly and primarily related to the natural course of the resident's illness or underlying condition (reviewable). In indeterminate cases, the event will be presumed reviewable and the organization's response will be reviewed under the Sentinel Event Policy according to the prescribed procedures and time frames without delay for additional information such as autopsy results.

[‡] *Major permanent loss of function* means sensory, motor, physiologic, or intellectual impairment not present on admission requiring continued treatment or life-style change. When major permanent loss of function cannot be immediately determined, applicability of the policy is not established until either the resident is discharged with continued major loss of function, or two weeks have elapsed with persistent major loss of function, whichever occurs first.

- The event is one of the following (even if the outcome was not death or major permanent loss of function unrelated to the natural course of the resident's illness or underlying condition):
  - ○ Suicide of a resident in a setting where the resident receives around-the-clock care, treatment, and services (for example, hospital, residential treatment center, crisis stabilization center)
  - ○ Unanticipated death of a full-term infant
  - ○ Infant abduction or discharge to the wrong family
  - ○ Rape*
  - ○ Hemolytic transfusion reaction involving administration of blood or blood products having major blood group incompatibilities
  - ○ Surgery on the wrong resident or wrong body part†

Examples of reviewable sentinel events and nonreviewable events are provided in Table 1 (page SE-5).

How the Joint Commission Becomes Aware of a Sentinel Event

Each organization is encouraged, but not required, to report to the Joint Commission any sentinel event meeting the preceding criteria for reviewable sentinel events. Alternatively, the Joint Commission might become aware of a sentinel event by some other means such as communication from a resident, a family member, an employee of the organization, a surveyor, or through the media.

Reasons for Reporting a Sentinel Event to the Joint Commission

Although self-reporting a sentinel event is not required and there is no difference in the expected response, time frames, or review procedures, whether the organization voluntarily reports the event or the Joint Commission becomes aware of the event by some other means, there are several advantages to the organization that self-reports a sentinel event:

- Reporting the event enables the addition of the "lessons learned" section to the Joint Commission's Sentinel Event Database, thereby contributing to the general knowledge about sentinel events and to the reduction of risk for such events in many other organizations

---

* *Rape*, as a reviewable sentinel event, is defined as unconsented sexual contact involving a resident and another resident, staff member, or other perpetrator while being treated or on the premises of the health care organization, including oral, vaginal, or anal penetration or fondling of the resident's sex organ(s) by another individual's hand, sex organ, or object. One or more of the following must be present to determine reviewability:
- Any staff-witnessed sexual contact as described above
- Sufficient clinical evidence obtained by the organization to support allegations of unconsented sexual contact
- Admission by the perpetrator that sexual contact, as described above, occurred on the premises

† All events of surgery on the wrong resident or wrong body part are reviewable under the policy, regardless of the magnitude of the procedure or the outcome.

Table 1. Examples of Reviewable and Nonreviewable Sentinel Events*

SE

Examples of Sentinel Events That are Reviewable Under the Joint Commission's Sentinel Event Policy

Any patient death, paralysis, coma, or other major permanent loss of function associated with a medication error.

Any suicide of a patient in a setting where the resident is housed around-the-clock, including suicides following elopement from such a setting.

Any elopement, that is unauthorized departure, of a patient from an around-the-clock care setting resulting in a temporally related death (suicide or homicide) or major permanent loss of function.

Any procedure on the wrong patient, wrong side of the body, or wrong organ.

Any intrapartum (related to the birth process) maternal death.

Any perinatal death unrelated to a congenital condition in an infant having a birth weight greater than 2,500 grams.

Assault, homicide, or other crime resulting in patient death or major permanent loss of function.

A resident fall that results in death or major permanent loss of function as a direct result of the injuries sustained in the fall.

Hemolytic transfusion reaction involving major blood group incompatibilities.

> **Note:** An adverse outcome that is *directly related* to the natural course of the resident's illness or underlying condition, for example, terminal illness present at the time of presentation, is **not** reportable **except** for suicide in, or following elopement from, a 24-hour care setting (*see* above).

Examples of Sentinel Events That are Nonreviewable Under the Joint Commission's Sentinel Event Policy

Any "near miss."

Full return of limb or bodily function to the same level as prior to the adverse event by discharge or within two weeks of the initial loss of said function.

Any sentinel event that has not affected a recipient of care (patient, client, resident).

Medication errors that do not result in death or major permanent loss of function.

Suicide other than in an around-the-clock care setting or following elopement from such a setting.

* **Note:** *This list may not apply to all settings.*

continued on next page

SE

Table 1. Examples of Reviewable and Nonreviewable Sentinel Events* *(continued)*

A death or loss of function following a discharge "against medical advice (AMA)."

Unsuccessful suicide attempts.

Unintentionally retained foreign body without major permanent loss of function.

Minor degrees of hemolysis with no clinical sequelae.

> **Note:** In the context of its performance improvement activities, an organization may choose to conduct intensive assessment, for example, root cause analysis, for some nonreportable events. Please refer to the "Improving Organization Performance" chapter of this Joint Commission accreditation publication.

* **Note:** *This list may not apply to all settings.*

- Early reporting provides an opportunity for consultation with Joint Commission staff during the development of the root cause analysis and action plan
- The organization's message to the public that it is doing everything possible to ensure that such an event does not happen again is strengthened by its acknowledged collaboration with the Joint Commission to understand how the event happened and what can be done to reduce the risk of such an event in the future

Required Response to a Reviewable Sentinel Event

If the Joint Commission becomes aware (either through voluntary self-reporting or otherwise) of a sentinel event that meets the preceding criteria (*see* page SE-3) and the event has occurred in an accredited organization, the organization is expected to do the following:

- Prepare a thorough and credible root cause analysis and action plan within 45 calendar days of the event or of becoming aware of the event
- Submit to the Joint Commission its root cause analysis and action plan, or otherwise provide for Joint Commission evaluation of its response to the sentinel event under an approved protocol (see Section VI), within 45 calendar days of the known occurrence of the event

The Joint Commission will then determine whether the root cause analysis and action plan are acceptable. If the determination that an event is reviewable under the Sentinel Event Policy occurs more than 45 calendar days following the known occurrence of the event, the organization will be allowed 15 calendar days for its response. If the organization fails to submit an acceptable root cause analysis within the 45 calendar days (or within 15 calendar days, if the 45 calendar days have already elapsed), it will be at risk for being placed on Accreditation Watch by the Accreditation Committee. An organization that experiences a sentinel event that does not meet the criteria for review under the Sentinel Event Policy is expected to complete a root cause analysis but does not need to submit it to the Joint Commission.

Review of Root Cause Analyses and Action Plans

A root cause analysis will be considered acceptable if it has the following characteristics:

- The analysis focuses primarily on systems and processes, not on individual performance
- The analysis progresses from special causes in clinical processes to common causes in organizational processes
- The analysis repeatedly digs deeper by asking "Why?"; then, when answered, "Why?" again, and so on
- The analysis identifies changes that could be made in systems and processes (either through redesign or development of new systems or processes), which would reduce the risk of such events occurring in the future
- The analysis is thorough and credible

To be thorough, the root cause analysis must include the following:

- A determination of the human and other factors most directly associated with the sentinel event and the process(es) and systems related to its occurrence
- An analysis of the underlying systems and processes through a series of "Why?" questions to determine where redesign might reduce risk
- An inquiry into all areas appropriate to the specific type of event as described in Table 2 (*see* page SE-9)
- An identification of risk points and their potential contributions to this type of event
- A determination of potential improvement in processes or systems that would tend to decrease the likelihood of such events in the future, or a determination, after analysis, that no such improvement opportunities exist

To be credible, the root cause analysis must do the following:

- Include participation by the leadership of the organization and by individuals most closely involved in the processes and systems under review
- Be internally consistent (that is, not contradict itself or leave obvious questions unanswered)
- Provide an explanation for all findings of "not applicable" or "no problem"
- Include consideration of any relevant literature

An action plan will be considered acceptable if it does the following:

- Identifies changes that can be implemented to reduce risk or formulates a rationale for not undertaking such changes
- Identifies, in situations where improvement actions are planned, who is responsible for implementation, when the action will be implemented (including any pilot testing), and how the effectiveness of the actions will be evaluated

All root cause analyses and action plans will be considered and treated as confidential by the Joint Commission. A detailed listing of the minimum scope of root cause analysis for specific types of sentinel events is included in Table 2.

Accreditation Watch Designation

An organization is placed on Accreditation Watch when a reviewable sentinel event has occurred and has come to the Joint Commission's attention, and a thorough and credible root cause analysis of the sentinel event and action plan has not been completed in specified time frames. Although Accreditation Watch status is not an official accreditation category, it can be publicly disclosed by the Joint Commission.

Follow-up Activities

After the Joint Commission has determined that an organization has conducted an acceptable root cause analysis and developed an acceptable action plan, the Joint Commission will notify it that the root cause analysis and action plan are acceptable and will assign an appropriate follow-up activity, typically a measure of success* (MOS) or follow-up survey within six months.

V. The Sentinel Event Database

To achieve the third goal of the Sentinel Event Policy, "to increase the general knowledge about sentinel events, their causes, and strategies for prevention," the Joint Commission collects and analyzes data from the review of sentinel events, root cause analyses, action plans, and follow-up activities. These data and information form the content of the Joint Commission's Sentinel Event Database.The Joint Commission is committed to developing and maintaining this Sentinel Event Database in a fashion that protects the confidentiality of the organization, the caregiver, and the resident. Included in this database are three major categories of data elements:
1. Sentinel event data
2. Root cause data
3. Risk reduction data

Aggregate data relating to root causes and risk-reduction strategies for sentinel events that occur with significant frequency will form the basis for future error-prevention advice to organizations through Sentinel Event Alert and other media. The Sentinel Event Database is also a major component of the evidence base for the National Patient Safety Goals.

VI. Procedures for Implementing the Sentinel Event Policy

Voluntary Reporting of Reviewable Sentinel Events to the Joint Commission

If an organization wishes to report an occurrence in the subset of sentinel events that are subject to review by the Joint Commission, the organization will be asked to complete a form to be sent to the Joint Commission's Office of Quality Monitoring by mail or by facsimile transmission (630/792-5636). Copies of the sentinel

---

* For more information about MOS, *see* "The New Joint Commission Accreditation Process" chapter in this book.

Table 2. Minimum Scope of Root Cause Analysis for Specific Types of Sentinel Events

Detailed inquiry into these areas is expected when conducting a root cause analysis for the specified type of sentinel event. Inquiry into areas not checked (or listed) should be conducted as appropriate to the specific event under review.

	Suicide (24-Hour Care)	Medication Error	Procedural Complication	Wrong-Site Surgery	Treatment Delay	Restraint Death	Elopement Death	Assault/Rape/ Homicide	Transfusion Death	Infant Abduction
Behavioral assessment process*	X					X	X	X		
Physical assessment process†	X		X	X	X	X	X			
Patient identification process		X		X					X	
Patient observation procedures	X					X	X	X	X	
Care planning process	X		X			X	X			
Continuum of care	X				X	X				
Staffing levels	X	X	X	X	X	X	X	X	X	X
Orientation and training of staff	X	X	X	X	X	X	X	X	X	X
Competency assessment/ credentialing	X	X	X		X	X	X	X	X	X
Supervision of staff‡		X	X		X	X			X	
Communication with patient/family	X			X	X	X	X			X
Communication among staff members	X	X	X	X	X	X			X	X
Availability of information	X	X	X	X	X	X			X	
Adequacy of technological support		X	X							
Equipment maintenance/ management		X	X				X			
Physical environment§	X	X	X				X	X	X	X
Security systems and processes	X						X	X		X
Control of medications: Storage/access		X							X	
Labeling of medications		X							X	

* Includes the process for assessing a patient's risk to self (and to others, in cases of assault, rape, or homicide where a patient is the assailant).

† Includes search for contraband.

‡ Includes supervision of physicians in training.

§ Includes furnishings; hardware (e.g., bars, hooks, rods); lighting; distractions.

event reporting form can be obtained by calling the Sentinel Event Hotline at 630/792-3700 or the Office of Quality Monitoring at 630/792-5642. This form can also be accessed via the Joint Commission Web site at http://www.jcaho.org.

Reviewable Sentinel Events That Are Not Reported by the Organization

If the Joint Commission becomes aware of a sentinel event subject to review under the Sentinel Event Policy that was not reported to the Joint Commission by the organization, the CEO of the organization is contacted, and a preliminary assessment of the sentinel event is made. An event that occurred more than one year before the date the Joint Commission became aware of the event will not, in most cases, be reviewed under the Sentinel Event Policy. In such a case, a written response will be requested from the organization, including a summary of processes in place to prevent similar occurrences.

Determination That a Sentinel Event Is Reviewable Under the Sentinel Event Policy

SE

Based on available factual information received about the event, Joint Commission staff will apply the preceding definition (page SE-3) to determine whether the event is reviewable under the Sentinel Event Policy. Challenges to a determination that an event is reviewable will be resolved through consultation with senior staff in the Division of Accreditation Operations.

Initial On-Site Review of a Sentinel Event

An initial on-site review of a sentinel event will usually not be conducted unless it is determined that there is a potential ongoing threat to resident health or safety or potentially significant noncompliance with Joint Commission standards. If an on-site (for-cause) review is conducted, the organization will be billed an appropriate amount based on the established fee schedule to cover the costs of conducting such a survey.

Disclosable Information

If the Joint Commission receives an inquiry about the accreditation status of an organization that has experienced a reviewable sentinel event, the organization's accreditation status will be reported in the usual manner without making reference to the sentinel event. If the inquirer specifically references the specific sentinel event, the Joint Commission will acknowledge that it is aware of the event and currently is working or has worked with the organization through the sentinel event review process.

Initiation of Accreditation Watch

If the Joint Commission becomes aware that an organization has experienced a reviewable sentinel event, but the organization fails to submit or otherwise make available an acceptable root cause analysis and action plan, or otherwise provide for Joint Commission evaluation of its response to the sentinel event under an approved protocol (within 45 calendar days of the event, or of its becoming aware of the event, or within 15 calendar days if the determination that the event is reviewable under the Sentinel Event Policy occurs more than 45 calendar days following the known occurrence of the event, unless Joint Commission staff for good reason has agreed to a short extension of time), a recommendation will be made to the Accreditation Committee to place the organization on Accreditation Watch. If the Accreditation Committee places the organization on Accreditation Watch, the organization will then be permitted an additional 15 calendar days to submit an acceptable root cause analysis and action plan, or otherwise provide for Joint Commission evaluation of its response to the sentinel event under an approved protocol.

The organization will be offered advisory assistance in performing a root cause analysis of the event.

Accreditation Watch status is considered publicly disclosable information.

In all cases of an organization refusing to permit review of information regarding a reviewable sentinel event in accordance with the Sentinel Event Policy and its approved protocols, the initial response by the Joint Commission is assignment of Accreditation Watch. Continued refusal can result in loss of accreditation.

Submission of Root Cause Analysis and Action Plan

The organization that experiences a sentinel event subject to the Sentinel Event Policy is asked to submit two documents (in addition to the sentinel event reporting form discussed on page SE-8): (1) the complete root cause analysis, including its findings; and (2) the resulting action plan that describes the organization's risk reduction strategies and a strategy for evaluating their effectiveness. The template, "A Framework for a Root Cause Analysis and Action Plan in Response to a Sentinel Event," is available to organizations as an aid in organizing the steps in a root cause analysis and developing an action plan. This three-page form can be obtained by calling the Sentinel Event Hotline at 630/792-3700 or by accessing it on the Joint Commission Web site at http://www.jcaho.org.

The root cause analysis and action plan are not to include the resident's name or the names of caregivers involved in the sentinel event.

Alternatively, if the organization has concerns about waivers of confidentiality protections as a result of sending the root cause analysis documents to the Joint Commission, the following alternative approaches to a review of the organization's response to the sentinel event are acceptable:

1. A review of the root cause analysis and action plan documents brought to Joint Commission headquarters by organization staff, then taken back to the organization on the same day.
2. An on-site visit by a specially trained surveyor to review the root cause analysis and action plan.
3. An on-site visit by a specially trained surveyor to review the root cause analysis and findings without directly viewing the root cause analysis documents through a series of interviews and a review of relevant documentation. For purposes of this review activity, *relevant documentation* includes, at a minimum, any documentation relevant to the organization's process for responding to sentinel events, the resident's medical record, and the action plan resulting from the analysis of the subject sentinel event. The latter serves as the basis for appropriate follow-up activity.
4. When the organization affirms that it meets specified criteria respecting the risk of waiving confidentiality protections for root cause analysis information shared with the Joint Commission, an on-site visit by a specially trained surveyor is conducted to do the following:
   a. Interviews and review relevant documentation, including the resident's medical record, to obtain information about the following:

- The process the organization uses in responding to sentinel events
- The relevant policies and procedures preceding and following the organization's review of the specific event, and the implementation thereof, sufficient to permit inferences about the adequacy of the organization's response to the sentinel event

b. A standards-based survey of the resident care, treatment, and services and the organization management functions relevant to the sentinel event under review

Any one of the four alternatives will result in a sufficient charge to the organization to cover the average direct costs of the visit. Inquiries about the fee should be directed to the Joint Commission's pricing unit at 630/792-5115.

The Joint Commission must receive a request for review of an organization's response to a sentinel event using any of these alternative approaches within at least five business days of the self-report of a reviewable event or of the initial communication by the Joint Commission to the organization that it has become aware of a reviewable sentinel event.

The Joint Commission's Response

Staff assesses the acceptability of the organization's response to the reviewable sentinel event, including the thoroughness and credibility of any root cause analysis information reviewed and the organization's action plan. If the root cause analysis and action plan are found to be thorough and credible, the response will be accepted and an appropriate follow-up activity will be assigned.

If the response is unacceptable, staff will provide consultation to the organization on the criteria that have not yet been met and will allow an additional 15 calendar days beyond the original submission period for the organization to resubmit its response. This additional time is provided only if the organization's initial submission of its root cause analysis and action plan was within the time frame outlined previously.

If the response continues to be unacceptable, staff will recommend to the Accreditation Committee that the organization be placed on Accreditation Watch and be required to address the inadequacies and to submit, or make available for review, a new root cause analysis and action plan within 15 calendar days of notification that the Accreditation Committee has found the response to be unacceptable and has placed the organization on Accreditation Watch, or staff will provide for further Joint Commission evaluation of the organization's response to the event.

Depending on the organization's initial response to the Accreditation Watch decision, the Joint Commission will determine whether an on-site visit should be made to help the organization conduct an appropriate root cause analysis and develop an action plan.

When the organization's response (initial or revised) is found to be acceptable, the Joint Commission issues a letter that does the following:

- Reflects the Joint Commission's determination to (1) continue or modify the organization's current accreditation status and (2) terminate the Accreditation Watch if previously assigned
- Assigns an appropriate follow-up activity, typically an MOS or a follow-up visit to be conducted within six months

If on review the organization's response is still not acceptable or the organization fails to respond, staff will recommend to the Accreditation Committee that the organization be placed in Preliminary Denial of Accreditation. If approved by the Accreditation Committee, this accreditation decision would be considered publicly disclosable information, and the process for resolution of Preliminary Denial of Accreditation would be initiated.

Action Plan Follow-up Activity

The follow-up activity will assess (based on applicable standards) the following:

- The organization's response to additional relevant information obtained since completion of the root cause analysis
- The implementation of system and process improvements identified in the action plan
- The means by which the organization will continue to assess the effectiveness of those efforts
- The organization's response to data collected to measure the effectiveness of the actions
- The resolution of any outstanding requirements for improvement

A decision to maintain or change the organization's accreditation status as a result of the follow-up activity or to assign additional follow-up requirements will be based on existing decision rules unless otherwise determined by the Accreditation Committee.

Handling Sentinel Event–Related Documents

The handling of any submitted root cause analyses and action plans is restricted to specially trained staff in accordance with procedures designed to protect the confidentiality of the documents.

Upon completion of the Joint Commission review of any submitted root cause analyses and action plans, and the abstraction of the required data elements for the Joint Commission's Sentinel Event Database, the original root cause analysis documents and any copies will be destroyed. Upon request, the original documents will be returned to the organization.

The action plan resulting from the analysis of the sentinel event will initially be retained to serve as the basis for the follow-up activity. After the action plan has been implemented to the satisfaction of the Joint Commission as determined through follow-up activities, the Joint Commission will destroy the action plan.

Oversight of the Sentinel Event Policy

The Accreditation Committee of the Joint Commission's Board of Commissioners is responsible for overseeing the implementation of this policy and procedure. In addition to reviewing and deciding individual cases involving Accreditation Watch, the Accreditation Committee periodically audits root cause analyses and action plans reviewed by staff. For the purposes of these audits, the Joint Commission temporarily retains random samples of these documents. Upon completion of the audit, these documents are also destroyed.

SE

For more information about the Joint Commission's Sentinel Event Policy and procedures, visit the Joint Commission's Web site at http://www.jcaho.org or call the Sentinel Event Hotline at 630/792-3700.

National Patient Safety Goals

This chapter addresses the National Patient Safety Goals and requirements. Organizations providing care relevant to each of the goals will be responsible for implementing the applicable requirements or, with Joint Commission approval, effective alternatives.

As with Joint Commission standards, accredited organizations are evaluated for continuous compliance with the specific requirements associated with the National Patient Safety Goals. Compliance with these requirements is assessed by the Joint Commission through on-site surveys and Evidence of Standards Compliance (ESC). In mid-cycle, the organization also assesses its own compliance in the Periodic Performance Review (PPR).* Organizations are judged to be either compliant or not compliant with each goal. If an organization does not fully comply with all the requirements associated with a goal, the organization will be assigned a requirement for improvement for the goal in the same way that noncompliance with an element of performance (EP) for a standard generates a requirement for improvement for that standard. Failure to resolve a requirement for improvement for a goal can ultimately lead to loss of accreditation.†

---

* For those programs required to complete a PPR.

† **Note:** *You might notice that some goals appear to be misnumbered or "missing" from the numerical sequence. This is not a typographical error. Some goals do not apply to long term care and therefore have not been included in this chapter.*

The purpose of the Joint Commission's National Patient Safety Goals is to promote specific improvements in resident safety. The goals highlight problematic areas in health care and describe evidence and expert-based solutions to these problems. Recognizing that sound system design is intrinsic to the delivery of safe, high-quality health care, the goals focus on systemwide solutions, wherever possible.

Although the requirements associated with the National Patient Safety Goals are generally more prescriptive than Joint Commission standards requirements, organizations may request Joint Commission approval of specific alternative approaches to meeting National Patient Safety Goal requirements. The Joint Commission also provides guidance on how to achieve effective compliance with each goal's requirements. This guidance includes detailed answers to Frequently Asked Questions (FAQs).

NP SG

The National Patient Safety Goals are derived primarily from informal recommendations made in the Joint Commission's safety newsletter, *Sentinel Event Alert.* The Sentinel Event database, which contains de-identified aggregate information on sentinel events reported to the Joint Commission, is the primary, but not the sole, source of information from which the alerts, as well as the National Patient Safety Goals, are derived. A broadly representative Sentinel Event Advisory Group works with Joint Commission staff on a continuing basis to determine priorities for, and develop, goals and associated requirements. As part of this development process, candidate goals and requirements are sent to the field for review and comment. Selected existing and new goals and requirements are annually recommended by the Advisory Group to the Joint Commission's Board of Commissioners for final review and approval. The Advisory Group also assists the Joint Commission in evaluating potential alternatives to goal requirements that have been suggested by individual organizations.

Goal 1

Improve the accuracy of resident identification.

Requirement 1A

Use at least two resident identifiers (neither to be the resident's room number) whenever administering medications or blood products; taking blood samples and other specimens for clinical testing, or providing any other treatments or procedures.

Note: *The preceding requirement is not scored here. It is scored at standard PC.5.10, EP 4. See page PC-24.*

Requirement 1B

A Prior to the start of any invasive procedure, conduct a final verification process, such as a "time out," to confirm the correct resident, procedure, and site, using active—not passive—communication techniques.

Goal 2

Improve the effectiveness of communication among caregivers.

Requirement 2A

For verbal or telephone orders or for telephonic reporting of critical test results, verify the complete order or test result by having the person receiving the order or test result "read-back" the complete order or test result.

Note: *The preceding requirement is not scored here. It is scored at standard IM.6.50, EP 4. See page IM-22.*

Requirement 2B

Standardize a list of abbreviations, acronyms and symbols that are *not* to be used throughout the organization.

Note: *The preceding requirement is not scored here. It is scored at standard IM.3.10, EP 2. See page IM-16.*

NP SG

Goal 3

Improve the safety of using medications.

Requirement 3A

Remove concentrated electrolytes (including, but not limited to, potassium chloride, potassium phosphate, sodium chloride > 0.9%) from resident care units.

Note: *The preceding requirement is not scored here. It is scored at standard MM.2.20, EP 9. See page MM-12.*

Requirement 3B

Standardize and limit the number of drug concentrations available in the organization.

Note: *The preceding requirement is not scored here. It is scored at standard MM.2.20, EP 8. See page MM-12.*

Requirement 3C

A Identify and, at a minimum, annually review a list of look-alike/sound-alike drugs used in the organization, and take action to prevent errors involving the interchange of these drugs.

Goal 5

Improve the safety of using infusion pumps.

Requirement 5A

A Ensure free-flow protection on all general-use and PCA (resident controlled analgesia) intravenous infusion pumps used in the organization.

Goal 7

Reduce the risk of health care–associated infections.

Requirement 7A

Comply with current Centers for Disease Control and Prevention (CDC) hand hygiene guidelines.*

Note: *The preceding requirement is not scored here. It is scored at standard IC.4.10, EP 2. See page IC-11.*

Requirement 7B

A Manage as sentinel events all identified cases of unanticipated death or major permanent loss of function associated with a health care–associated infection.

Goal 8

Accurately and completely reconcile medications across the continuum of care.

Requirement 8A

A During 2005, for full implementation by January 2006, develop a process for obtaining and documenting a complete list of the resident's current medications upon the resident's admission to the organization and with the involvement of the resident. This process includes a comparison of the medications the organization provides to those on the list.

Requirement 8B

A A complete list of the resident's medications is communicated to the next provider of service when it refers or transfers a resident to another setting, service, practitioner, or level of care within or outside the organization.

Goal 9

Reduce the risk of resident harm resulting from falls.

Requirement 9A

A Assess and periodically reassess each resident's risk for falling, including the potential risk associated with the resident's medication regimen, and take action to address any identified risks.

Requirement 9B

A Implement a fall-reduction program, including a transfer protocol, and evaluate the effectiveness of the program.

Goal 10

Reduce the risk of influenza and pneumococcal disease in institutionalized older adults.

Requirement 10A

A Develop and implement a protocol for administration and documentation of the flu vaccine.

Requirement 10B

A Develop and implement a protocol for administration and documentation of the pneumococcus vaccine.

Requirement 10C

A Develop and implement a protocol to identify new cases of influenza and to manage an outbreak.

---

* Organizations are required to comply with all 1A, 1B, and 1C CDC recommendations or requirements.

**NP
SG**

Accreditation Participation Requirements

This chapter includes specific requirements for participation in the accreditation process and for maintaining an accreditation award. These differ from survey eligibility criteria in that the accreditation process may be initiated even when all Accreditation Participation Requirements (APRs) have not yet been met.

For an organization seeking accreditation for the first time, compliance with the APRs is assessed during the initial survey. For the accredited organization, compliance with these requirements is assessed throughout the accreditation cycle through on-site surveys, the Periodic Performance Review (PPR), Evidence of Standards Compliance (ESC), and periodic updates of organization-specific data and information. Organizations are either compliant or not compliant with APRs. When an organization does not comply with an APR, the organization will be assigned a requirement for improvement in the same context that noncompliance with a standard or element of performance (EP) generates a requirement for improvement. However, refusal to permit performance of an unscheduled or unannounced for-cause survey (APR 3) or falsification of information (APR 10), will immediately lead to Preliminary Denial of Accreditation. All requirements for improvement can impact the accreditation decision and follow-up requirements, as determined by established accreditation decision rules. Failure to resolve a requirement for improvement can ultimately lead to loss of accreditation.

APR

Application for Accreditation

APR 1

When requested, the organization provides the Joint Commission with all official records and reports of public or publicly recognized licensing (for example, a state license), examining, reviewing, or planning bodies.*

Element of Performance for APR 1

A 1. The organization provides the Joint Commission with all official records and reports of licensing, examining, reviewing, or planning bodies.

APR

APR 2

The organization immediately reports any changes in the information provided in the application for accreditation and any changes made between surveys.†

Rationale for APR 2

An organization that experiences a significant change in ownership or control, location, capacity, or the categories of services offered must notify the Joint Commission in writing not more than 30 days after such changes. The Joint Commission may decide that the organization must be resurveyed when a significant merger or consolidation has taken place. The Joint Commission continues the organization's accreditation until it determines whether a resurvey is necessary. Failure to provide timely notification to the Joint Commission of ownership, merger or consolidation, and service changes may result in interruption or loss of accreditation.

Element of Performance for APR 2

A 1. The organization notifies the Joint Commission not more than 30 days before or after a significant change in ownership or control, location, capacity, or the categories of services offered.

Acceptance of Survey

APR 3

An organization permits the performance of an unscheduled or unannounced for-cause survey‡ at the discretion of the Joint Commission.

---

* *See also* page APP-19 in the "Accreditation Policies and Procedures" chapter.

† *See also* page APP-37.

‡ *See also* page APP-39 for an explanation of the difference between an unscheduled and unannounced for-cause survey. In addition, *see* the last paragraph of "Continuous Compliance" on page APP-36.

Rationale for APR 3

The Joint Commission may perform either an unscheduled or unannounced for-cause survey when it becomes aware of potentially serious patient care or safety issues in an organization. Either type of survey can take place at any point in an organization's three-year accreditation cycle. An unscheduled or unannounced survey can either include all of the organization's services or address only those areas where a serious concern may exist. In addition, the Joint Commission conducts unannounced surveys on a random sample of accredited organizations at 9 to 30 months following the accreditation date. An organization's failure to permit an unscheduled or unannounced survey is grounds for withdrawal of accreditation.

Elements of Performance for APR 3

A 1. The organization permits the performance of an unscheduled for-cause survey.

A 2. The organization permits the performance of an unannounced for-cause survey.

APR

Performance Measurement*

APR 4 ▬▬▬▬▬▬▬▬▬▬▬▬▬▬▬▬▬▬▬▬▬▬▬▬

The organization selects and uses performance measures relevant to the services provided and populations served.

Rationale for APR 4

Each Medicare/Medicaid–certified Skilled Nursing Facility/Nursing Facility (SNF/NF) required to collect and submit Minimum Data Set (MDS) data to a state agency per Centers for Medicare & Medicaid Services (CMS) regulation must share monthly Facility Quality Indicator (QI) Profiles, Quality Measure (QM) reports, CMS Form 2567 reports, Plans of Correction, and/or publicly reported Quality Measure reports, as appropriate, with Joint Commission surveyors at the time of survey and discuss how the data were used to identify and prioritize performance improvement activities.

A long term care organization not required to collect MDS data must participate in a performance measurement accepted for use in the accreditation process and use accepted performance measures from the performance measurement system.

---

* Organizations are encouraged to keep up-to-date on any changes in ORYX requirements by reviewing recent issues of *Joint Commission Perspectives*® or going to the Performance Measurement area on the Joint Commission's Web site at http://www.jcaho.org/pms/index.htm.

Elements of Performance for APR 4

A 1. **For Medicare/Medicaid-certified Skilled Nursing Facility/Nursing Facility only:** If the organization is required to collect and submit Minimum Data Set (MDS) data to a state agency per Centers for Medicare & Medicaid Services (CMS) regulation, it shares monthly Facility Quality Indicator (QI) Profiles, Quality Measure (QM) reports, CMS Form 2567 reports, "Plans of Correction," and/or publicly reported Quality Measure reports as appropriate, at the time of survey and discusses how the data were used to identify and prioritize performance improvement activities.

2. Not applicable.

A 3. **For long term care organizations not required to collect MDS data:** The organization participates in a performance measurement accepted for use in the accreditation process and uses accepted performance measures from the performance measurement system.

APR

APR 5

A non-Medicare/Medicaid certified long term care organization selects and uses accepted performance measures from at least one listed performance measurement system.

Rationale for APR 5

The organization identifies the appropriate number of clinical measures that meet Joint Commission requirements. The organization submits data for its measures to the performance measurement system(s) at least quarterly, and such submissions identify monthly data points. An organization applying for initial survey must notify the Joint Commission of its measure selection(s) no later than the time of survey. Each organization must also notify the Joint Commission of any subsequent additions or changes to its measure selections. An individual measure must be used for at least four consecutive quarters before it can be replaced. For purposes of reporting to the Joint Commission, an organization will be expected to do the following:

- Continue to use a measure if the data suggest an unstable pattern of performance or otherwise identify an opportunity for improvement
  or
- Change to a new measure if the data reflect continuing stable and satisfactory performance

Elements of Performance for APR 5

A 1. The organization has selected a sufficient number of performance measures to meet current ORYX requirements.

A 2. The organization notifies the Joint Commission of its performance measures selections by the date requested.

A 3. The organization notifies the Joint Commission of any changes in its performance measures selections.

A 4. Each individual performance measure is used for at least four consecutive quarters.

APR 6

A non-Medicare/Medicaid certified long term care organization ensures that aggregate data for the selected measures are submitted to the Joint Commission at least quarterly.

Rationale for APR 6

Organization-specific aggregate data, reported as monthly data points, must be submitted four times per year by established deadlines from the performance measurement system to the Joint Commission for use in the accreditation process, as required by the Joint Commission. The Joint Commission has defined the type and format of performance measurement data to be submitted in a fashion consistent with nationally recognized standards.

The submission of organization-specific data will be performed by the selected performance measurement system(s) and will include comparative data for other organizations in the same performance measurement system that have selected the same performance measures.

Element of Performance for APR 6

A 1. The organization ensures that aggregate data for the selected performance measures are submitted four times a year in accordance with established timelines to the Joint Commission.

APR 7

Not applicable.

Public Information Interviews

APR 8

The organization provides notice of an upcoming full accreditation survey and of the opportunity for a Public Information Interview (PII).*

Rationale for APR 8

An organization must provide an opportunity for the public to participate in a public information interview during a full survey. The public includes the following:
- Residents and their families

---

* *See also* pages APP-22 and APP-25.

- Resident advocates and advocacy groups
- Members of the community for whom services are provided
- Organization personnel and staff

The organization is responsible for making the public information interview process widely known and effective as a source of compliance information in the accreditation process. The Joint Commission requires an organization scheduled for a full survey to post announcements of the survey date, the opportunity for a PII, and how to request an interview. To maximize participation, postings must be made throughout the organization in the form provided by the Joint Commission (*see* the Public Notice Form on page APP-23). Organizations should post notices in public eating areas, on bulletin boards near major entrances, and in treatment or residential areas. In addition, if all staff members are not likely to see such postings, the organization must provide each staff member with a written announcement of the survey.

APR

The organization must also provide potential PII participants with sufficient advance notice. The Joint Commission requires that organizations post public notices at least 30 days before the scheduled survey date. Notices must remain posted until the survey is completed.

The organization should also promptly initiate community advertising or other communications as soon as it receives notice of the survey date. Appropriate steps to take in notifying the community of the opportunity for PIIs include the following:

- Informing all advocacy groups (such as organized patient groups and unions) that have substantively communicated with the organization in the previous 12 months
- Reaching other members of the community, for example, through a public service announcement on radio or television, a classified advertisement in a local newspaper, or a notice in a community newsletter or other publication
- Informing individuals who inquire about the survey of the survey date(s) and opportunity to participate

Element of Performance for APR 8
A 1. The organization provides notice of an upcoming full survey and of the opportunity of a PII.

APR 9
The organization notifies the Joint Commission of any requests for a PII.*

Rationale for APR 9
The organization must promptly forward to the Joint Commission all written requests to participate in a PII. Organizations receiving an oral request should instruct the individual(s) to make the request in writing and mail it to the Joint

---

* *See also* pages APP-22–APP-25.

Commission. The organization should provide the individual(s) needing assistance in doing this with the necessary support. The organization is responsible for notifying the interviewee(s) of the exact date, time, and place of the PII.

Elements of Performance for APR 9

A 1. The organization notifies the Joint Commission of any requests for a PII.

A 2. The organization notifies any interviewee(s) of the exact date, time, and place of the PII.

Misrepresentation of Information

APR 10 ▄▄▄▄▄▄▄▄
The organization does not misrepresent information in the accreditation process.*

Rationale for APR 10
Information provided by the organization and used by the Joint Commission for the accreditation process must be accurate and truthful. Such information can be provided in the following ways:
- Provided orally
- Obtained through direct observation by Joint Commission surveyors
- Derived from documents supplied by the organization to the Joint Commission
- Involve data submitted electronically by the organization through the performance measurement system to the Joint Commission

The Joint Commission requires each organization seeking accreditation to engage in the accreditation process in good faith. Any organization that fails to participate in good faith by falsifying information presented in the accreditation process might have its accreditation denied or removed by the Joint Commission.

For the purpose of this requirement, falsification is defined as the fabrication, in whole or in part, and through commission or omission, of any information provided by an applicant or accredited organization to the Joint Commission. This includes any redrafting, reformatting, or content deletion of documents. However, the organization may submit additional material that summarizes or otherwise explains the original information submitted to the Joint Commission. These additional materials must be properly identified, dated, and accompanied by the original documents.

Element of Performance for APR 10
A 1. The organization provides accurate and truthful information throughout the accreditation process.

---

* *See also* page APP-10.

APR 11 ━━━━━━━━━━━━━━━━━━━━━━━━━━━━━━━━

The organization does not publicly misrepresent its accreditation status or the scope of facilities and services to which the accreditation applies.*

Rationale for APR 11

Organizations accredited by the Joint Commission must be accurate when describing to the public the nature and meaning of their accreditation. On request, the Joint Commission's Department of Communications will provide accredited organizations with appropriate guidelines for characterizing the accreditation award. An organization may not engage in any false or misleading advertising with respect to the accreditation award. Any such advertising may be grounds for denying or revoking accreditation.

Elements of Performance for APR 11

A 1. The organization accurately represents its accreditation status as to the scope of facilities and services to which the accreditation applies.

A 2. The organization does not engage in any false or misleading advertising with respect to the accreditation award.

APR 12 ━━━━━━━━━━━━━━━━━━━━━━━━━━━━━━━━

Accredited organizations or organizations seeking accreditation are not permitted to use Joint Commission full-time, part-time, or intermittent surveyors to provide any accreditation-related consulting services.

Rationale for APR 12

Consulting services include, but are not limited to, the following:
- Helping an organization to meet Joint Commission standards
- Helping an organization to complete its PPR
- Assisting an organization to remedy areas identified in its PPR as needing improvement
- Conducting mock surveys for an organization
- Providing consultation to an organization to address Priority Focus Process (PFP) information

Element of Performance for APR 12

A 1. The organization does not use Joint Commission full-time, part-time, or intermittent surveyors to provide any accreditation-related consulting services.

---

* *See also* pages APP-11–APP-12.

Survey Observers

APR 13 ▬▬▬▬▬▬▬▬▬

An organization that applies for survey is obligated to accept Joint Commission surveyor management staff and/or a member of the Board of Commissioners to observe a survey under two specific circumstances:

- Observation and mentoring of surveyors as part of surveyor management and development
- Preceptorship of new surveyors

The observer will not participate in the on-site survey process in any fashion, including the scoring of standards compliance. The presence of an observer will not result in any additional charge to the organization nor will it be accepted as de facto grounds for score revisions or decision appeal.

APR

Element of Performance for APR 13

A 1. The organization accepts Joint Commission surveyor management staff and/or a member of the Board of Commissioners to observe a survey under either of the two specific circumstances.

Periodic Performance Review

APR 14 ▬▬▬▬▬▬▬▬▬

The organization fulfills the Periodic Performance Review requirement at the midpoint of its accreditation cycle.

Rationale for APR 14

Full Periodic Performance Review

The organization must complete and transmit to the Joint Commission a PPR and plan of action and identify appropriate measures of success (MOS) at the 18-month point in the accreditation cycle. The organization also participates in a conference call with Joint Commission staff to reach final agreement on the elements of the plan of action and measures of success.

The plan of action addresses all standards areas identified as being not in compliance. At the time of the organization's triennial survey, the surveyors will validate whether the MOS data indicate that performance has been sustained.

The results of the PPR do not affect an organization's accreditation decision at the 18-month point of the accreditation cycle. In the unlikely event that the Joint Commission or the organization identifies a continuing situation that represents a potential threat to health or safety through the PPR, a special announced survey will be initiated to facilitate resolution of the situation.

Option 1

If the organization selects option 1 as an alternative to the full PPR, the organization must attest that, after careful consideration with legal counsel, the organization has decided not to participate in the full PPR and instead will complete a PPR and plan of action and identify appropriate measures of success at the 18-month point in the accreditation cycle. The organization may elect to participate in a conference call related to standards issues with Joint Commission staff at the 18-month in the accreditation cycle. The plan of action addresses all standards areas identified as being not in compliance. At the time of the organization's triennial survey, the surveyors will validate whether the MOS data indicate that performance has been sustained.

Option 2

If the organization selects option 2 as an alternative to the full PPR it must attest that, after careful consideration with legal counsel, the organization has decided not to participate in the full PPR and instead intends to undergo a limited survey at the midpoint in its accreditation cycle. Following the survey, the organization must submit a plan of action with appropriate MOS for any recommendation cited at the survey. The organization also participates in a conference call with Joint Commission staff to reach final agreement on the elements of the plan of action and MOS. At the time of the organization's triennial survey, the surveyors will validate whether the MOS data indicate that performance has been sustained.

Option 3

If the organization selects option 3 as an alternative to the full PPR, it must attest that, after careful consideration with legal counsel, it has decided not to participate in the full PPR and instead intends to undergo a limited survey at the midpoint in its accreditation cycle. Following the survey, the organization may elect to participate in a conference call to discuss standards-related issues with Joint Commission staff. At the time of the organization's triennial survey, the surveyors will receive no information relating to the organization's option 3 survey findings.

Elements of Performance for APR 14

A 1. The organization completes the full PPR and plan of action at the 18-month point in the accreditation cycle.

OR

The organization attests that, after careful consideration with legal counsel, it has decided not to participate in the full PPR and completes option 1.

OR

The organization attests that, after careful consideration with legal counsel, it has decided not to participate in the full PPR and completes option 2 at the midpoint in the accreditation cycle.

OR

The organization attests that, after careful consideration with legal counsel, it has decided not to participate in the full PPR and completes option 3 at the midpoint in the accreditation cycle.

A 2. For the full PPR and Option 2, the organization participates in a conference call with the Joint Commission staff to reach final agreement on the elements of the plan of action.

Long Term Care–Medicare/Medicaid Certified Only

APR 15

The organization notifies the Joint Commission within 24 hours when, at any time during the accreditation cycle, any state agency Skilled Nursing Facility/Nursing Facility survey has resulted in termination from the Medicare/Medicaid program.

Element of Performance for APR 15

A 1. The Joint Commission has been notified that the SNF/NF has been terminated from the Medicare/Medicaid program.

APR

APR

Ethics, Rights, and Responsibilities

Overview

The **goal** of the ethics, rights, and responsibilities function is to improve care, treatment, services, and outcomes by recognizing and respecting the rights of each resident and by conducting business in an ethical manner. Care, treatment, and services are provided in a way that respects and fosters dignity, autonomy, positive self regard, civil rights, and involvement of residents. Care, treatment, and services consider the resident's abilities and resources, the relevant demands of his or her environment, and the requirements and expectations of the providers and those they serve. The family is involved in care, treatment, and services decisions with the resident's approval.

An organization's adherence to ethical care and business practices significantly affects the resident's experience of and response to care, treatment, and services. The standards in this chapter address the following processes and activities related to ethical care and business practices:

- Managing the organization's relationships with residents and the public in an ethical manner
- Considering the values and preferences of residents, including the decision to discontinue care, treatment, and services
- Helping residents understand and exercise their rights
- Informing residents of their responsibilities in care, treatment, and services
- Recognizing the organization's responsibilities under law

Residents deserve care, treatment, and services that safeguard their personal dignity and respect their cultural, psychosocial, and spiritual values. These values often influence the resident's perceptions and needs. By understanding and respecting these values, providers can meet care, treatment, and services needs and preferences.

Standards

The following is a list of all standards for this function. They are presented here for your convenience without footnotes or other explanatory text. If you have a question about a term used here, please check the Glossary.

Note: *A revised standard numbering system is being used with the reformatted standards. This revised numbering system will allow for more flexibility to add standards while maintaining the current label for each standard.*

RI

Organization Ethics

RI.1.10   The organization follows ethical behavior in its care, treatment, and services and business practices.

RI.1.20   The organization addresses conflicts of interest.

RI.1.30   The integrity of decisions is based on identified care, treatment, and service needs of the residents.

RI.1.40   When care, treatment, and services are subject to internal or external review that results in the denial of care, treatment, services, or payment, the organization makes decisions regarding the provision of ongoing care, treatment, and services, or discharge based on the assessed needs of the residents.

Individual Rights

RI.2.10   The organization respects the rights of residents.

RI.2.20   Residents receive information about their rights.

RI.2.30   Residents are involved in decisions about care, treatment, and services provided.

RI.2.40   Informed consent is obtained.

RI.2.50   Consent is obtained for recording or filming made for purposes other than the identification, diagnosis, or treatment of the residents.

RI.2.60   Not applicable

RI.2.70   Residents have the right to refuse care, treatment, and services in accordance with law and regulation.

RI.2.80   The organization addresses the wishes of the resident relating to end of life decisions.

RI.2.90   Residents and, when appropriate, their families are informed about the outcomes of care, treatment and services that have been provided, including unanticipated outcomes.

RI.2.100   The organization respects the resident's right to and need for effective communication.

RI.2.110   Residents have a right to unlimited contact with visitors and others.

RI.2.120   The organization addresses the resolution of complaints from residents and their families.

RI.2.130   The organization respects the needs of residents for confidentiality, privacy, and security.

RI.2.140   Residents have a right to an environment that preserves dignity and contributes to a positive self image.

RI.2.150   Residents have the right to be free from mental, physical, sexual, and verbal abuse, neglect, and exploitation.

RI.2.160   Residents have the right to pain management.

RI.2.170   Residents have a right to access protective and advocacy services.

RI.2.180   The organization protects research subjects and respects their rights during research, investigation, and clinical trials involving human subjects.

RI.2.190   In organizations that provide opportunities for work, a defined policy addresses situations in which residents work.

RI.2.200   Residents have a right to exercise citizenship privileges.

RI.2.210   Residents have a right to a quality of life that supports independent expression, choice, and decision making, consistent with applicable law and regulation.

RI.2.220   Residents receive care that respects their personal values, beliefs, cultural and spiritual preferences, and life-long patterns of living.

RI.2.230   Residents have a right to freedom from chemical or physical restraint.

RI.2.240   Residents can participate or refuse to participate in social, spiritual, or community activities and groups.

RI

RI.2.250   As appropriate to their care or service plan, residents can access transportation services.

RI.2.260   Residents have a right to a resident council.

RI.2.270   Residents can select their medical, dental, and other licensed independent practitioner care providers.

RI.2.280   Residents have a right to communicate with their medical, dental, and other licensed independent practitioner care providers.

RI.2.290   Residents have a right to manage or delegate management of personal financial affairs.

RI.2.300   Not applicable

RI.2.310   Not applicable

RI.2.320   Not applicable

Individual Responsibilities

RI.3.10   Residents are given information about their responsibilities while receiving care, treatment, and services.

Understanding the Parts of This Chapter

To help you navigate this reformatted standards chapter, it may be helpful to think of its parts this way:

- The **standard** is the "goal"
- The **rationale** explains why it's important to achieve this goal
- The **elements of performance** identify the step(s) needed to achieve this goal

These parts are defined as follows.

Standard A statement that defines the performance expectations and/or structures or processes that must be in place for an organization to provide safe, high-quality care, treatment, and services. An organization is either "compliant" or "not compliant" with a standard.

Accreditation decisions are based on simple counts of the standards that are determined to be "not compliant."

Rationale A statement that provides background, justification, or additional information about a standard. A standard's rationale is not scored. In some instances, the rationale for a standard is self-evident. Therefore, not every standard has a written rationale.

Elements of performance (EPs) The specific performance expectations and/or structures or processes that must be in place for an organization to provide safe, high-quality care, treatment, and services. The scoring of EP compliance determines an organization's overall compliance with a standard. EPs are evaluated on the following scale:

> 0   Insufficient compliance
> 1   Partial compliance
> 2   Satisfactory compliance
> NA Not applicable

You will find a **measure of success** icon—**⑩**—next to some EPs. Measures of success (MOS) need to be developed for certain EPs when a standard is judged to be out of compliance through either the Periodic Performance Review (PPR) or the onsite survey. An MOS is defined as a quantifiable measure, usually related to an audit, that can be used to determine whether an action has been effective and is being sustained.*

Assessing Your Compliance

Once you are familiar with the parts of this chapter, you can begin to assess your compliance with its requirements. The scoring category designations are provided next to each EP for your convenience. If you would like to assess your organization's performance, mark your scores for the EPs and standards by following the simple steps described below.

---

* For more information about MOS, *see* "The New Joint Commission Accreditation Process" chapter in this book.

Two components are scored for each EP: (1) compliance with the requirement itself **and** (2) compliance with the track record* for that requirement. Scoring has been simplified and track record achievements (which have always been part of the scoring) have been appropriately modified.

Note: *Some standards and EPs do not apply to a particular type of organization; these standards and EPs are marked "not applicable" and the related text is not included. Your organization is not expected to comply with standards and EPs marked "not applicable."*

In addition, some standards and EPs that do apply to organizations may not apply to the specific care, treatment, and services that your individual organization provides. Although these standards and EPs are included in the book, you are not expected to comply with them. If you are unsure about the standards or EPs that apply to your organization, please contact the Joint Commission's Standards Interpretation Group at 630/792-5900.

RI

Step 1: Score Your Compliance with Each Element of Performance

Before you can determine your compliance with the standards, you must score your compliance with each EP. There are three scoring criterion categories: A, B, and C (described below). Please note that for each EP scoring criterion category, your organization must meet the performance requirement itself and the track record achievements (*see* "Track Record Achievements").

Category A

These EPs relate to the presence or absence of the requirement(s) and are scored either yes (2) or no (0); however, score 1 for partial compliance is also possible based on track record achievements.

If an A EP has multiple components designated by bullets, your organization must be compliant with all the bullets to receive a score of 2. If your organization does not meet one or more requirements in the bullets, you will receive a score of 0.

Category B

Category B EPs are scored in two steps:
1. As with category A EPs, category B EPs relate to the presence or absence of the requirement(s). If your organization *does not meet* the requirement(s), the EP is scored 0; there is no need to assess your compliance with the principles of good process design.
2. If your organization *does meet* the requirement(s), but there is concern about the quality or comprehensiveness of the effort, then and only then should you assess the qualitative aspect of the EP. That is, review the applicable principles of good process design and ask how the principles were applied in the situation under discussion. Good process design has the following characteristics:

---

* **Track record** The amount of time that an organization has been in compliance with a standard, EP, or other requirement.

- Is consistent with your organization's mission, values, and goals
- Meets the needs of patients
- Reflects the use of currently accepted practices (doing the right thing, using resources responsibly, using practice guidelines)
- Incorporates current safety information and knowledge such as sentinel event data and National Patient Safety Goals
- Incorporates relevant performance improvement results

This two-part evaluation applies to both simple and bulleted B EPs. First, the EPs are assessed to determine whether the requirements are present. If the EP has multiple components designated by bullets, as with the category A EPs, your organization must meet the requirements in *all* the bulleted items to get a score of 2. If your organization meets *none* of the requirements in the bullets, it receives a score of 0. If your organization meets *at least one, but not all,* of the bulleted requirements, it receives a score of 1 for the EPs.

Use the following rules to determine your EP score:
- Your EP score is 0 if your organization does not meet the requirement(s); you *do not* need to assess your compliance with the preceding applicable principles of good process design
- Your EP score is 1 if your organization does meet the requirement(s) but considered only *some* of the preceding applicable principles of good process design
- Your EP score is 2 if your organization does meet the requirement(s) *and* considered *all* the preceding principles of good process design

Category C

C EPs are scored 0, 1, or 2 based on the number of times your organization does not meet the EP. These EPs are frequency based and require totaling the number of occurrences (that is, results of performance or nonperformance) related to a particular EP. Each situation discovered by a surveyor(s) will be counted as a separate occurrence.

Note: *Multiple events of the same type related to a single resident and single practitioner/staff member are counted as* one occurrence only.

Use the following rules to determine your EP score:
- Your EP score is 2 if you find one or fewer occurrences of noncompliance with the EP
- Your EP score is 1 if you find two occurrences of noncompliance with the EP
- Your EP score is 0 if you find three or more occurrences of noncompliance with the EP

If an EP in the C category has multiple requirements designated by bullets, the following scoring guidelines apply:
- If there are fewer than two findings in all bullets, the EP is scored 2
- If there are three or more findings in all bullets, the EP is scored 0
- In all other combinations of findings, the EP is scored 1

Track Record Achievements

In addition to meeting the requirement(s) in each EP, regardless of category, your organization must also meet the following track record achievements:

Score	Initial Survey	Full Survey
2	4 months or more	12 months or more
1	2 to 3 months	6 to 11 months
0	Fewer than 2 months	Fewer than 6 months

Sample Sizes

If during an onsite survey, your organization has been found to be not compliant with one or more standards, you must demonstrate Evidence of Standards Compliance (ESC) for each standard that is not compliant. The ESC must address compliance at the EP level; when an EP within a noncompliant standard requires an MOS, your organization must demonstrate achievement with the MOS when completing the ESC.

RI

Note: *Not every EP requires an MOS. EPs that do require an MOS are clearly marked in this chapter. Organizations are required to demonstrate achievement with an MOS only for EPs within a noncompliant standard that require an MOS. Organizations do not need to demonstrate achievement with an MOS for any EP within a compliant standard.*

When demonstrating achievement with an MOS during the ESC process, your organization is **required** to use the following sample sizes, which were established because of their statistical significance, their relative simplicity in application, and their sensitivity to an organization's population size:

- For a population size of fewer than 30 cases,* sample 100% of available cases
- For a population size of 30 to 100 cases, sample 30 cases
- For a population size of 101 to 500 cases, sample 50 cases
- For a population size greater than 500 cases, sample 70 cases

Note: *Organizations are* encouraged, but not required, *to follow this sample size when demonstrating achievement with an MOS for an EP within a noncompliant standard after conducting a full, Option 1, or Option 2 PPR.*

When conducting PPR (optional use) or demonstrating an ESC (mandatory use), use the following percentages to determine your EP score: 90% through 100% of your sample size is in compliance = score 2; 80% through 89% of your sample size is in compliance = score 1; less than 80% of your sample size is in compliance = score 0.

In addition, the following information should govern your organization's selection of samples:

- The appropriate sample size should be determined by the specific population related to the survey findings

---

* *Case* refers to a single instance in which a situation related to a survey finding occurs. For example, if a survey finding was related to **pain assessment**, then a case would be any resident record. If a survey finding was related to **pain management**, a case would be any resident record for residents receiving pain management.

- The sampling approach should involve either systematic random sampling (for example, your organization selects every second or third case for review) or simple random sampling (for example, your organization uses a series of random numbers generated by a computer to identify the cases to be reviewed)
- If your organization chooses not to use these sample sizes while conducting PPR options 1 or 2, you should make sure that your sample size is sufficiently large enough to ensure statistical significance
- When submitting a clarifying ESC, if your organization selects records as part of its sample, the records should be from a period of no more than three months before the last date of the survey
- Assessment of MOS compliance is conducted for a four-month period following the date of ESC approval. Your organization should select records as a part of your sample following the date of ESC approval and use the required sample sizes. MOS percentage compliance rates are derived from the average of all four months.

Step 2: Use Your EP Scores to Gauge Your Compliance with the Standards

Now that you have evaluated and scored each EP for a particular standard, use these simple rules to determine your compliance with the standard itself:

- Your organization is not in compliance (that is, "not compliant") with the standard if any EP is scored 0
- Otherwise, your organization is in compliance with a standard if 65% or more of its EPs are scored 2

Standards, Rationales, Elements of Performance, and Scoring

Organization Ethics

Introduction
An organization has an ethical responsibility to the residents and community it serves. To fulfill this responsibility, ethical care, treatment, and services practices and ethical business practices must go hand in hand. Furthermore, the organization provides care, treatment, and services within its scope, stated mission and philosophy, and applicable law and regulation.

The organization's system of ethics supports honest and appropriate interactions with residents. The system of ethics also includes residents whenever possible in decisions about their care, treatment, and services, including ethical issues.

RI

Standard RI.1.10
The organization follows ethical behavior in its care, treatment, and services and business practices.

Elements of Performance for RI.1.10
B   1.   The organization identifies ethical issues and issues prone to conflict.

B   2.   The organization develops and implements a process to handle these issues when they arise.

B Ⓜ 3.   The organization's policies and procedures reflect ethical practices for marketing, admission, transfer, discharge, and billing.

B   4.   Marketing materials accurately represent the organization and address the care, treatment, and services that the organization can provide, directly or by contractual arrangement.

C Ⓜ 5.   Residents receive information about charges for which they will be responsible.

B   6.   The effectiveness and safety of care, treatment, and services does not depend on the resident's ability to pay.

C Ⓜ 7.   The leaders ensure that care, treatment, and services are not negatively affected when the organization grants a staff member's request to be excused from participating in an aspect of the care, treatment, and services.

C Ⓜ 8.   Residents are informed whenever services, charges, or coverage change.

Standard RI.1.20

The organization addresses conflicts of interest.

Rationale for RI.1.20

Potential conflicts of interest can arise in subtle and obvious circumstances. The organization needs to be aware of potential conflicts of interest and review relationships with other entities carefully to ensure that its mission and responsibility to the residents and community it serves is not harmed by any professional, ownership, contractual, or other relationships.

Elements of Performance for RI.1.20

A　　1.　The organization defines what constitutes a *conflict of interest.*

C Ⓜ 2.　The organization discloses existing or potential conflicts of interest for those who provide care, treatment, and services as well as governance.

B　　3.　The organization reviews its relationship and its staff's relationships with other care providers, educational institutions, and payers to ensure that those relationships are within law and regulation and determine if conflicts of interest exist.

B　　4.　The organization addresses conflicts of interest when they arise.

RI

Standard RI.1.30

The integrity of decisions is based on identified care, treatment, and service needs of the residents.

Rationale for RI.1.30

Decisions are based on the residents' care, treatment, and services needs, regardless of how the organization compensates or shares financial risk with its leaders, managers, staff, and licensed independent practitioners.

Elements of Performance for RI.1.30

B　　1.　The organization has policies and procedures that address the integrity of clinical decision making.

C Ⓜ 2.　To avoid compromising the quality of care, decisions are based on the resident's identified care, treatment, and services needs and in accordance with organization policy.

B　　3.　Policies and procedures and information about the relationship between the use of care, treatment, and services and financial incentives are available to all residents, staff, licensed independent practitioners, and contracted providers, when requested.

Standard RI.1.40

When care, treatment, and services are subject to internal or external review that results in the denial of care, treatment, services, or payment, the organization makes decisions regarding the provision of ongoing care, treatment, and services, or discharge based on the assessed needs of the residents.

Rationale for RI.1.40

When an individual requests or presents for care, treatment, and services, the organization is professionally and ethically responsible for providing care, treatment, and services within its capability, mission, and applicable law and regulation. At times, indications for such care, treatment, and services can contradict the recommendations of an external entity performing a utilization review (for example, insurance companies, managed care reviewers, and federal or state payers). If such a conflict arises, care, treatment, services, and discharge decisions are made based on the residents' identified needs, regardless of the recommendations of the external agency.

Elements of Performance for RI.1.40

RI

C Ⓜ 1. The organization makes decisions regarding the provision of ongoing care, treatment, services, or discharge based on the care, treatment, and services required by the resident.

C Ⓜ 2. The resident and/or the family is involved in these decisions.

Individual Rights

Introduction

A mere list of rights cannot guarantee those rights. Rather, an organization shows its support of rights by how its staff interacts with residents and involves them in decisions about their care, treatment, and services. These standards focus on how the organization respects the culture and rights of residents during those interactions. This begins with respecting their right to treatment, care, and services.

Standard RI.2.10

The organization respects the rights of residents.

Elements of Performance for RI.2.10

B 1. The organization's policies and practices address the rights of residents to care, treatment, and services within its capability and mission and in compliance with law and regulation.

C Ⓜ 2. Each resident has a right to have his or her cultural, psychosocial, spiritual, and personal values, beliefs, and preferences respected.

C Ⓜ 3. The organization supports the right of each resident to personal dignity.

C Ⓜ 4. The organization accommodates the right to pastoral and other spiritual services for residents.

Standard RI.2.20

Residents receive information about their rights.

Elements of Performance for RI.2.20

1. Not applicable

2. Not applicable

C Ⓜ 3. Information on rights is given and explained to each resident upon admission and when any rights are changed.

C Ⓜ 4. The resident acknowledges in writing receipt of rights information and any changes to it as appropriate to the populations served or residents.

C Ⓜ 5. Information on the extent to which the organization is able, unable, or unwilling to honor advance directives is given upon admission if the resident has an advance directive.

C Ⓜ 6. The resident has the right to access, request amendment to, and receive an accounting of disclosures regarding his or her own health information as permitted under applicable law.

B 7. Regardless of payment method, residents have access to at least appropriate and timely care; their attending physician; all staff, including administrative staff; care-planning and discharge-planning processes; uniform policies and practices for providing care throughout the organization; and comparable provision of care, treatment, and services to all residents under applicable state plan or other payer source.

B 8. The organization has policies and practices about transfers, including room-to-room transfers; discharges; and providing services consistent with the applicable state plan or other payer source.

C Ⓜ 9. Upon admission, residents are informed about the organization's policies and procedures regarding the handling of life-threatening emergencies. (*See* standard PC.9.20 regarding policies and procedures for life-threatening emergencies.)

Standard RI.2.30

Residents are involved in decisions about care, treatment, and services provided.

Rationale for RI.2.30

Making decisions about care, treatment, and services sometimes presents questions, conflicts, or other dilemmas for the organization and the residents, family, or other decision makers. These dilemmas may involve issues about admission;

care, treatment, and services; or discharge. The organization works with residents and, when appropriate, their families to resolve such dilemmas.

Elements of Performance for RI.2.30

C Ⓜ 1. Residents are involved in decisions about their care, treatment, and services.

C Ⓜ 2. Residents are involved in resolving dilemmas about care, treatment, and services.

C Ⓜ 3. A surrogate decision maker, as allowed by law, is identified when a resident cannot make decisions about his or her care, treatment, and services.

C Ⓜ 4. The legally responsible representative approves care, treatment, and services decisions.*

C Ⓜ 5. The family, as appropriate and as allowed by law, with permission of the resident or surrogate decision maker, is involved in care, treatment, and services decisions.

6. Through 9. Not applicable

B 10. Family or surrogate decision makers, as allowed by law, are actively involved under the following circumstances:
   - When the resident has been legally judged incompetent
   - When the resident's physician determines he or she is medically incapable of understanding or making decisions

C Ⓜ 11. The organization helps in the process of assigning a legal guardian to a resident for health decision making, when necessary.

C Ⓜ 12. The organization identifies those authorized for resolving conflicts related to transfer and discharge.

C Ⓜ 13. The organization identifies those authorized for resolving conflicts related to room and roommate assignments.

Standard RI.2.40 ▬▬▬▬▬▬▬▬▬▬▬▬▬▬▬▬

Informed consent is obtained.

Rationale for RI.2.40

The goal of the informed consent process is to establish a mutual understanding between the resident and the physician or other provider or practitioner who provides the care, treatment, and services about the care, treatment, and services that the resident receives. This process allows each resident to fully participate in decisions about his or her care, treatment, and services.

---

* In some states, law dictates that urgent care, family planning, and/or behavioral health services can be provided to a minor without the approval or consent of a parent or guardian.

Elements of Performance for RI.2.40

B 1. The organization's policies describe the following:
- Which procedures or care, treatment, and services require informed consent
- The process used to obtain informed consent
- How informed consent is to be documented in the record
- When a surrogate decision maker, rather than the resident, may give informed consent
- When procedures or care, treatment, and services normally requiring informed consent may be given without informed consent

C Ⓜ 2. Informed consent is obtained and documented in accordance with the organization's policy.

B 3. A complete informed consent process includes a discussion of the following elements:*
- The nature of the proposed care, treatment, services, medications, interventions, or procedures
- Potential benefits, risks, or side effects, including potential problems related to recuperation
- The likelihood of achieving care, treatment, and services goals
- Reasonable alternatives to the proposed care, treatment, and services
- The relevant risks, benefits, and side effects related to alternatives, including the possible results of not receiving care, treatment, and services
- When indicated, any limitations on the confidentiality of information learned from or about the resident

Standard RI.2.50

Consent is obtained for recording or filming† made for purposes other than the identification, diagnosis, or treatment of the residents.

Rationale for RI.2.50

Recording or filming of care, treatment, and services provided to residents can be useful for many purposes, but such recording or filming is likely to compromise the resident's privacy and confidentiality. Therefore, the organization should obtain consent from the resident for recording or filming.

---

* Documentation of the items listed in EP 3 may be in a form, progress notes, or elsewhere in the record.

† Recording or filming refers to photographic, video, electronic, or audio media.

Elements of Performance for RI.2.50

C Ⓜ 1. When recording or filming are to be used only for internal organizational purposes (for example, performance improvement and education), there is documentation of consent, which may be obtained as part of general consent to treatment or another form, if a statement is included in the form regarding the use of recordings or filming for such internal purposes.

C Ⓜ 2. When recording or films are made for external purposes that will be heard or seen by the public (for example, commercial filming, television programs, marketing), there is documentation of a specific, separate consent that includes the circumstances of the use of the recording or film.

C Ⓜ 3. Except for the circumstances set forth in EP 4 (below), there is documentation of consent before recording or filming.

C Ⓜ 4. The following occurs in situations in which the resident is unable to give informed consent before recording or filming:
- The recording or filming may occur before consent, provided it is within the established policy of the organization and the policy is established through an appropriate ethical mechanism (for example, an ethics committee) that includes community input
- The recording or film remains in the organization's possession and is not used for any purpose until and unless consent is obtained
- If consent for use cannot subsequently be obtained, the recording or film is either destroyed or the nonconsenting resident must be removed from the recording or film

A 5. Residents have the right to request cessation of recording or filming.

A 6. Residents have the right to rescind consent for use up until a reasonable time before the recording or film is used.

C Ⓜ 7. Anyone who engages in recording or filming (who is not already bound by the organization's confidentiality policy) signs a confidentiality statement to protect the resident's identity and confidential information.

Standard RI.2.60

Not applicable

Standard RI.2.70

Residents have the right to refuse care, treatment, and services in accordance with law and regulation.

Elements of Performance for RI.2.70

A 1. Residents have the right to refuse care, treatment, and services in accordance with law and regulation.

A 2. When the resident is not legally responsible, the surrogate decision maker, as allowed by law, has the right to refuse care, treatment, and services on the resident's behalf.

3. Not applicable

C Ⓜ 4. The resident's right to refuse care, treatment, and services is consistent with the most current advance directive information obtained from the resident or family upon admission.

Standard RI.2.80

The organization addresses the wishes of the resident relating to end of life decisions.

Elements of Performance for RI.2.80

B 1. Policies, in accordance with law and regulation, address advance directives and the framework for forgoing or withdrawing life-sustaining treatment and withholding resuscitative services.

C Ⓜ 2. Adults are given written information about their rights to accept or refuse medical or surgical treatment, including forgoing or withdrawing life-sustaining treatment or withholding resuscitative services.

A 3. The existence or lack of an advance directive does not determine an individual's access to care, treatment, and services.

C Ⓜ 4. Documentation indicates whether or not the resident has signed an advance directive.

A 5. The resident has the option to review and revise advance directives.

C Ⓜ 6. Appropriate staff are aware of the advance directive if one exists.

C Ⓜ 7. The organization helps or refers the residents for assistance in formulating advance directives upon request.

B 8. The organization has a mechanism for health care professionals and designated representatives to honor advance directives within the limits of the law and the organization's capabilities.

C Ⓜ 9. The organization documents and honors the resident's wishes concerning organ donation within the limits of the law or organization capacity.

10. Through 18. Not applicable

B 19. Organization policy requires residents to be informed about the laws governing advance directives, including "do not hospitalize" orders; "do-not-resuscitate" orders; and organ-donation request procedures.

C Ⓜ 20. The organization determines residents' wishes about organ donation when they are admitted.

C Ⓜ 21. The policies are consistently implemented.

Standard RI.2.90

Residents and, when appropriate, their families are informed about the outcomes of care, treatment, and services that have been provided, including unanticipated outcomes.

Elements of Performance for RI.2.90

At a minimum, the resident and, when appropriate, his or her family are informed about the following (EPs 1–2):

C Ⓜ 1. Outcomes of care, treatment, and services that have been provided that the resident (or family) must be knowledgeable about to participate in current and future decisions affecting the resident's care, treatment, and services

C Ⓜ 2. Unanticipated outcomes of care, treatment, and services that relate to sentinel events considered reviewable* by the Joint Commission

C Ⓜ 3. The responsible licensed independent practitioner or his or her designee informs the resident (and when appropriate, his or her family) about those unanticipated outcomes of care, treatment, and services (see EP 2).[†]

Standard RI.2.100

The organization respects the resident's right to and need for effective communication.

Rationale for RI.2.100

The resident has the right to receive information in a manner that he or she understands. This includes communication between the organization and the resident, as well as communication between the resident and others outside the organization.

Elements of Performance for RI.2.100

B 1. The organization respects the right and need of residents for effective communication.

B 2. Written information provided is appropriate to the age; understanding; and, as appropriate to the population served, the language of the resident.

C Ⓜ 3. The organization facilitates provision of interpretation (including translation services) as necessary.

C Ⓜ 4. The organization addresses the needs of those with vision, speech, hearing, language, and cognitive impairments.

---

* See the "Sentinel Events" chapter of this manual for a definition of reviewable sentinel events.

[†] In settings where there is no licensed independent practitioner, the staff member responsible for the care of the resident is responsible for sharing information about such outcomes.

B   5.   The organization offers telephone and mail service as appropriate to the setting and population.

Standard RI.2.110

Residents have a right to unlimited contact with visitors and others.

Rationale for RI.2.110

Residents have the right to privately communicate with persons of their choice in the organization or the community.

Elements of Performance for RI.2.110

B   1.   The organization establishes liberal visiting hours that are limited only by the residents' personal preferences.

C Ⓜ   2.   The organization clearly communicates rules and regulations about visitors and visiting hours.

A   3.   The organization provides space for residents to receive visitors in comfort and privacy.

C Ⓜ   4.   The organization supports the right of residents to choose with whom they want to talk.

C Ⓜ   5.   The organization complies with law and regulation for visitors allowed immediate access to residents and exempted from normal visiting hours.

C Ⓜ   6.   Residents can refuse to talk to persons not associated with the organization or not directly involved in his or her care. Such persons include visitors, vendors, accreditation surveyors, and representatives of community organizations.

C Ⓜ   7.   The organization ensures that residents' privacy and security are considered in all interactions.

Standard RI.2.120

The organization addresses the resolution of complaints from residents and their families.

Elements of Performance for RI.2.120

C Ⓜ   1.   The organization informs residents, families, and staff about the internal complaint/grievance resolution process upon admission.

C Ⓜ   2.   The organization receives; reviews; and, when possible, resolves complaints from residents and their families.

C Ⓜ   3.   The organization responds to individuals making a significant (as defined by the organization) or recurring complaint.

C Ⓜ 4. The organization informs residents about their right to file a complaint with the state authority.

C Ⓜ 5. Residents can freely voice complaints and recommend changes without being subject to coercion; discrimination; reprisal; or unreasonable interruption of care, treatment, and services.

B 6. The organization prominently posts a description of the complaint/grievance process in the facility.

C Ⓜ 7. If the organization does not resolve the complaint/grievance to the resident's or family's satisfaction, it refers them to other sources of assistance, such as ombudsman, legal services, or adult protective services programs.

B 8. The organization's written admission guidelines list other sources of assistance, including ombudsman, legal services, or adult protective services programs, for complaint resolution.

RI

C Ⓜ 9. The organization provides these guidelines to residents and families on admission.

Standard RI.2.130

The organization respects the needs of residents for confidentiality, privacy, and security.

Rationale for RI.2.130

This standard and its EPs allow flexibility in how an organization can accomplish this requirement. Privacy, safety, and security can be demonstrated in various ways, for example, via policies and procedures, practices, or the design of the environment.

Elements of Performance for RI.2.130

C Ⓜ 1. The organization protects confidentiality of information about residents.

C Ⓜ 2. The organization respects the privacy of residents.

C Ⓜ 3. Residents who desire private telephone conversations have access to space and telephones appropriate to their needs and the care, treatment, and services provided.

C Ⓜ 4. The organization provides for the safety and security of residents and their property.

C Ⓜ 5. Residents who are married or have significant others are given a reasonable degree of privacy.

C Ⓜ 6. The organization obtains documented resident/family consent when confidential information needs to be posted in the organization.

Standard RI.2.140 ━━━━━━━━━━━━━━━━━━━━━━━━━━━━

Residents have a right to an environment that preserves dignity and contributes to a positive self image.

Rationale for RI.2.140

The organization creates a supportive environment for all residents. Additionally, residents can have items such as pictures, clothing, photos, radios, furniture, afghans, and the like to help them personalize their living space. Staff recognizes that the need for such items may change over time and supports the unique needs of each resident.

Elements of Performance for RI.2.140

B   1.   The environment of care supports the positive self-image of residents and preserves their human dignity.

B   2.   The organization provides sufficient storage space to meet the personal needs of the residents.

B   3.   The organization allows residents to keep and use personal clothing and possessions, unless this infringes on others' rights or is medically or therapeutically contraindicated (as appropriate to the setting or service).

B   4.   The environment's essential components include the following:
- A homelike atmosphere
- Sufficient space with access to personal living space
- Appropriate communication about room and roommate assignments or changes
- Environmental adaptations to help those with dementia, cognitive impairment, or temporary confusion
- Appropriate accommodations for married couples and clients with significant others regardless of sexual orientation, unless any limitations consistent with the organization's mission and philosophy have been disclosed to the resident at the time of or before admission

Standard RI.2.150 ━━━━━━━━━━━━━━━━━━━━━━━━━━━━

Residents have the right to be free from mental, physical, sexual, and verbal abuse, neglect, and exploitation.*

Note: *See standard PC.3.10, which addresses assessing and reporting of abuse, neglect, and exploitation.*

Elements of Performance for RI.2.150

B   1.   The organization addresses how it will, to the best of its ability, protect residents from real or perceived abuse; neglect, including involuntary seclusion; or exploitation from anyone, including staff, students, volunteers, other residents, visitors, or family members.

---

* **Exploitation** Taking advantage of another for one's own advantage or benefit.

C Ⓜ 2. All allegations, observations, or suspected cases of abuse, neglect, or exploitation that occur in the organization are investigated by the organization.

Standard RI.2.160

Residents have the right to pain management.

Rationale for RI.2.160

Residents may experience pain. Unrelieved pain has adverse physical and psychological effects. The organization respects and supports the right of residents to pain management. In accordance with the organization's mission, this may occur through referral.

Element of Performance for RI.2.160

B 1. The organization plans, supports, and coordinates activities and resources to ensure that pain is recognized and addressed appropriately and in accordance with the care, treatment, and services provided, including the following:
- Assessing for pain
- Educating all relevant providers about assessing and managing pain
- Educating residents and families, when appropriate, about their roles in managing pain and the potential limitations and side effects of pain treatments

Standard RI.2.170

Residents have a right to access protective and advocacy services.

Elements of Performance for RI.2.170

C Ⓜ 1. When the organization serves a population of residents who often need protective services (that is, guardianship and advocacy services, conservatorship, and child or adult protective services), it provides resources to help the family and the courts determine the resident's needs for such services.

B 2. When appropriate, the organization maintains a list of names, addresses, and telephone numbers of pertinent state client advocacy groups such as the state authority and the protection and advocacy network.

C Ⓜ 3. The list is given to residents when requested.

B 4. The organization develops and implements policies and procedures for the above requirements.

Applicable to Long Term Care Programs Participating in Research
Standard RI.2.180 ▬▬▬▬▬▬▬▬▬▬▬▬▬▬▬▬▬

The organization protects research subjects and respects their rights during research, investigation, and clinical trials involving human subjects.

Rationale for RI.2.180

An organization that conducts research, investigations, or clinical trials involving human subjects knows that its first responsibility is to the health and well-being of the research subjects. To protect and respect the research subjects' rights, the organization reviews all research protocols. If another institution's Institutional Review Board (IRB) reviews the research protocols, the organization does not need to perform this activity.

Elements of Performance for RI.2.180

C Ⓜ 1. The organization reviews all research protocols in relation to its mission, values, and other guidelines and weighs the relative risks and benefits to the research subjects.

C Ⓜ 2. The organization provides residents who are potential subjects in research, investigation, and clinical trials with adequate information* to participate or refuse to participate in research.

C Ⓜ 3. Residents are informed that refusing to participate or discontinuing participation at any time will not compromise their access to care, treatment, and services not related to the research.

C Ⓜ 4. Consent forms address the above elements of performance; indicate the name of the person who provided the information and the date the form was signed; and address the participant's right to privacy, confidentiality, and safety.

C Ⓜ 5. Subjects are told the extent to which their personally identifiable private information will be held in confidence.

C Ⓜ 6. All information given to subjects is in the medical record or research file along with the consent forms.

C Ⓜ 7. If a research-related injury (that is, physical, psychological, social, financial, or otherwise) occurs, the principal investigator attempts to address any harmful consequences the subject may have experienced as a result of research procedures.

C Ⓜ 8. The organization obtains and maintains a copy of the consent form.

RI

---

* **Adequate information** includes an explanation of the purpose of the research and expected duration of the subject's participation; a description of expected benefits, potential discomforts, and risks; alternative services that might prove advantageous to the resident; and a full explanation of the procedures to be followed.

Standard RI.2.190 ▬▬▬▬▬▬▬▬▬▬▬▬▬▬▬▬▬▬▬▬▬▬▬

In organizations that provide opportunities for work, a defined policy addresses situations in which residents work.

Rationale for RI.2.190

Residents may be offered the opportunity to perform work for the organization (for example, work therapy programs in grounds keeping or the library) that does not endanger them, other residents, or staff. If the organization asks residents to perform such tasks (work), they have the right to refuse.

Elements of Performance for RI.2.190

B　　1.　Policies and procedures address situations in which residents work.

C Ⓜ 2.　Policies and procedures are implemented.

C Ⓜ 3.　Wages paid to residents are in accordance with applicable law and regulation.

C Ⓜ 4.　Work is addressed in the care, treatment, and services plan.

C Ⓜ 5.　Work is performed voluntarily.

Standard RI.2.200 ▬▬▬▬▬▬▬▬▬▬▬▬▬▬▬▬▬▬▬▬▬

Residents have a right to exercise citizenship privileges.

Element of Performance for RI.2.200

C Ⓜ 1.　The organization helps residents with citizenship privileges to exercise their citizenship privileges, including arranging for them to vote.

Standard RI.2.210 ▬▬▬▬▬▬▬▬▬▬▬▬▬▬▬▬▬▬▬▬▬

Residents have a right to a quality of life that supports independent expression, choice, and decision making, consistent with applicable law and regulation.

Elements of Performance for RI.2.210

B　　1.　Residents receive care that respects their independence, expression of choice, and decision making.

C Ⓜ 2.　The organization supports residents in making choices about the planned course of care, treatment, and services.

C Ⓜ 3.　The organization honors the resident's health beliefs and expectations.

Standard RI.2.220 ▬▬▬▬▬▬▬▬▬▬▬▬▬▬▬▬▬▬▬▬▬

Residents receive care that respects their personal values, beliefs, cultural and spiritual preferences, and life-long patterns of living.

Elements of Performance for RI.2.220

C Ⓜ 1. The organization respects residents' personal values, beliefs, and cultural and spiritual preferences.

C Ⓜ 2. The organization respects residents' life-long patterns of living, including lifestyle choices related to sexual orientation.

Standard RI.2.230

Residents have a right to freedom from chemical or physical restraint.

Rationale for RI.2.230

The organization avoids the use of restraints if at all possible.

Note: *The use of restraints is consistent with requirements in the "Provision of Care, Treatment, and Services" chapter.*

Element of Performance for RI.2.230

B 1. Organization policies and procedures support the resident's right to be free from restraints.

Standard RI.2.240

Residents can participate or refuse to participate in social, spiritual, or community activities and groups.

Element of Performance for RI.2.240

C Ⓜ 1. The organization supports each resident's right to participate or refuse to participate in social, spiritual, or community activities and groups.

Standard RI.2.250

As appropriate to their care or service plan, residents can access transportation services.

Elements of Performance for RI.2.250

C Ⓜ 1. The organization arranges transportation for residents to and from physician or dentist appointments and other activities identified in their care or services plan.

C Ⓜ 2. The organization arranges for an appropriate attendant, as necessary, when transporting residents.

Standard RI.2.260

Residents have a right to a resident council.

Elements of Performance for RI.2.260

A   1.   The organization establishes a resident council.

B   2.   Residents are involved in planning and running the resident council.

C Ⓜ   3.   Residents are informed of council meetings and invited to attend.

C Ⓜ   4.   When a resident cannot attend or chooses not to attend the resident council, the organization has a way to send that resident's concerns to the council and provide feedback to the residents.

C Ⓜ   5.   When a resident council is not a suitable forum for resolving particular complaints or addressing certain cases, the organization provides a resident representative or advocate.

Standard RI.2.270 ━━━━━━━━━━━━━━━━━━━━━━━━━━━

Residents can select their medical, dental, and other licensed independent practitioner care providers.

RI

Elements of Performance for RI.2.270

C Ⓜ   1.   The organization supports each resident's right to choose an attending physician, dentist, and other licensed independent practitioner.

C Ⓜ   2.   The organization supports resident requests for a different licensed independent practitioner both on admission and throughout the course of care.

C Ⓜ   3.   The organization makes reasonable attempts to respond to these requests.

Note: *In facilities with a closed medical staff (such as Veterans Affairs or chronic disease hospitals), the choice may be limited to the licensed independent practitioners in the system.*

Standard RI.2.280 ━━━━━━━━━━━━━━━━━━━━━━━━━━━

Residents have a right to communicate with their medical, dental, and other licensed independent practitioner care providers.

Elements of Performance for RI.2.280

C Ⓜ   1.   The organization supports the residents' right to know their medical, dental, and other licensed independent practitioner care providers.

C Ⓜ   2.   The organization provides residents and families with names and telephone numbers of the physician or other practitioner primarily responsible for their care.

C Ⓜ   3.   The organization provides residents and families with names and professional status of individuals responsible for authorizing and performing procedures and treatments, when appropriate.

C Ⓜ 4. The organization helps residents make and keep appointments.

C Ⓜ 5. The organization considers residents' possible impairments when providing information.

Standard RI.2.290
Residents have a right to manage or delegate management of personal financial affairs.

Elements of Performance for RI.2.290
C Ⓜ 1. Residents can access and use available funds.

C Ⓜ 2. Residents who authorize the organization to manage their funds do so in writing.

C Ⓜ 3. When the organization manages a resident's personal funds, the resident has ready and reasonable access to those funds.

C Ⓜ 4. When the organization manages a resident's personal funds, it gives the resident at least quarterly an accurate accounting of all financial transactions on the resident's behalf.

C Ⓜ 5. The organization involves the legal guardian, durable power of attorney, or family, as appropriate.

Standard RI.2.300
Not applicable

Standard RI.2.310
Not applicable

Standard RI.2.320
Not applicable

Individual Responsibilities

Introduction
The safety of health care delivery is enhanced when residents, as appropriate to their condition, are partners in the health care process. Additionally, organizations are entitled to reasonable and responsible behavior on the part of the residents, within their capabilities, and their families. The organization identifies the responsibilities of the residents and their families and educates them about these responsibilities, particularly in regard to facilitating the safe delivery of care, treatment, and services.

The statement of responsibilities includes at least the following:

- **Providing information.** Residents and families, as appropriate, must provide, to the best of their knowledge, accurate and complete information about present complaints, past illnesses, hospitalization, medications, and other matters relating to their health. Residents and their families must report perceived risks in their care and unexpected changes in their condition. They can help the organization understand their environment by providing feedback about service needs and expectations.

- **Asking questions.** Residents and families, as appropriate, must ask questions when they do not understand their care, treatment, and services or what they are expected to do.

- **Following instructions.** Residents and their families must follow the care, treatment, and services plan developed. They should express any concerns about their ability to follow the proposed care plan or course of care, treatment, and services. The organization makes every effort to adapt the plan to the specific needs and limitations of the residents. When such adaptations to the care, treatment, and services plan are not recommended, residents and their families are informed of the consequences of the care, treatment, and services alternatives and not following the proposed course.

- **Accepting consequences.** Residents and their families are responsible for the outcomes if they do not follow the care, treatment, and services plan.

- **Following rules and regulations.** Residents and their families must follow the organization's rules and regulations.

- **Showing respect and consideration.** Residents and their families must be considerate of the organization's staff and property, as well as other residents and their property.

- **Meeting financial commitments.** Residents and their families should promptly meet any financial obligation agreed to with the organization.

Standard RI.3.10

Residents are given information about their responsibilities while receiving care, treatment, and services.

Elements of Performance for RI.3.10

B 1. The organization has a policy that defines the mechanism for communicating responsibilities of residents.

B 2. The policy includes the responsibilities for providing information, asking questions, following instructions, accepting consequences, following rules and regulations, showing respect and consideration, and meeting financial commitments.

C Ⓜ 3. Residents are informed about their responsibilities verbally, in writing, or both, based on organization policy.

C Ⓜ 4. Residents are informed about their responsibilities initially and as needed thereafter.

Provision of Care, Treatment, and Services*

Overview

Care, treatment, and services are provided through the successful coordination and completion of a series of processes that include appropriate initial assessment of needs; development of a plan for care, treatment, and services; the provision of care, treatment, and services; ongoing assessment of whether the care, treatment, and services provided are meeting the resident's needs; and either the successful discharge of the resident or referral or transfer of the resident for continuing care, treatment, and services.

The provision of care, treatment, and services to residents consists of four core processes or elements:
1. Assessing resident needs
2. Planning care, treatment, and services
3. Providing the care, treatment, and services the resident needs
4. Coordinating care, treatment, and services

These core elements may also include the following activities:
- Providing access to the appropriate levels of care and/or disciplines for residents
- Providing interventions based on the plan for care, treatment, and services
- Teaching residents what they need to know about their care, treatment, and services
- Coordinating care, treatment, and services, if needed, when the resident is referred, transferred, or discharged

The elements that make up the provision of care, treatment, and services are related to each other through an integrated and cyclical process that may occur over minutes, hours, days, weeks, months, or years, depending on the setting and the needs of the resident. This cyclical process may occur among multiple organizations or within a single organization. The standards in this chapter address the processes in this cycle, including those provided for resident populations with unique needs or residents who are receiving interventions or services that are problem prone.

The core processes or elements of the provision of care, treatment, and services should not be seen as separate steps, rather as interrelated activities in an integrated and ongoing care process. The activities related to the provision of care, treatment, and services should be capable of moving easily between elements as required to meet residents' needs and maintain the continuity of care, treatment, and services.

PC

---

* This chapter is a compilation of the former "Assessment," "Care," "Education," and "Continuum of Care" chapters.

Standards

The following is a list of all standards for this function. They are presented here for your convenience without footnotes or other explanatory text. If you have a question about a term used here, please check the Glossary.

Note: *A revised standard numbering system is being used with the reformatted standards. The revised numbering system will allow for more flexibility to add standards while maintaining the current label for each standard.*

Entry to Care, Treatment, and Services

PC.1.10   The organization accepts for care, treatment, and services only those residents whose identified, care, treatment, and service needs it can meet.

Assessment

PC.2.10   Not applicable

PC.2.20   The organization defines in writing the data and information gathered during assessment and reassessment.

PC.2.30 Through PC.2.110   Not applicable

PC.2.120   The organization defines in writing the time frame(s) for conducting the initial assessment(s).

PC.2.130   Initial assessments are performed as defined by the organization.

PC.2.140   Not applicable

PC.2.150   Residents are reassessed as needed.

Additional Standard for Victims of Abuse

PC.3.10   Residents who may be victims of abuse, neglect, or exploitation are assessed. (*See* standard RI.2.150.)

PC.3.20 Through PC.3.220   Not applicable

Diagnostic Services

PC.3.230   Diagnostic testing necessary for determining the resident's health care needs is performed.

PC

Planning Care, Treatment, and Services

PC.4.10   Development of a plan for care, treatment, and services is individualized and appropriate to the resident's needs, strengths, limitations, and goals.

Providing Care, Treatment, and Services

PC.5.10   The organization provides care, treatment, and services for each resident according to the plan for care, treatment, and services.

PC.5.20   Not applicable

PC.5.30   The attending physician prescribes the medical requirements of care for the residents he or she admits.

PC.5.40   The attending physician visits the resident in accordance with the resident's needs and at least once during the 30 days after admission.

PC.5.50   Care, treatment, and services are provided in an interdisciplinary, collaborative manner.

PC.5.60   The organization coordinates the care, treatment, and services provided to a resident as part of the plan for care, treatment, and services and consistent with the organization's scope of care, treatment, and services.

PC.5.70   Not applicable

Education

PC.6.10   The resident receives education and training specific to the resident's needs and as appropriate to the care, treatment, and services provided.

PC.6.20   Not applicable

PC.6.30   The resident receives education and training specific to the resident's abilities as appropriate to the care, treatment, and services provided by the organization.

PC.6.40   Not applicable

PC.6.50   The organization provides academic education to children and youth as needed.

PC.6.60   Not applicable

Nutritional Care
PC.7.10   The organization has a process for preparing and/or distributing food and nutrition products.

Pain
PC.8.10   Pain is assessed in all residents.

Restorative Services
PC.8.20   When necessary, residents receive appropriate restorative services, including assistance with activities of daily living, such as eating, dressing, grooming, bathing, oral hygiene, ambulation, and toilet activities.

Preventive Care
PC.8.30   Residents at risk for health-related complications receive appropriate preventive care.

Social and Diversional Activities
PC.8.40   Residents are helped so they can participate in social and diversional activities according to their functional levels.

Access to the Outdoors
PC.8.50   Not applicable

PC.8.60   Not applicable

End-of-Life Care
PC.8.70   Comfort and dignity are optimized during end-of-life care.

Specific Procedures

Administering Blood and Blood Components
PC.9.10   Blood and blood components are administered safely, as appropriate to the settings.

Responding to Life-Threatening Emergencies
PC.9.20   The organization responds to life-threatening emergencies according to organization policy and procedure.

PC.9.30 Through PC.11.70   Not applicable

Restraint and Seclusion
PC.11.80   The organization designs a system to achieve a restraint-free environment.

PC.11.90   When alternatives to restraint are ineffective, restraint is safely and appropriately used.

PC.11.100 Through PC.12.190   Not applicable

Standards for Additional Special Procedures

Sedation and Anesthesia Care for Subacute Services
PC.13.10   Licensed independent practitioners define the scope of assessment for operative or other procedures and/or the administration of moderate or deep sedation or anesthesia.

PC.13.20   Operative or other procedures and/or the administration of moderate or deep sedation or anesthesia are planned.

PC.13.30   Residents are monitored during the procedure and/or administration of moderate or deep sedation or anesthesia.

PC.13.40   Residents are monitored immediately after the procedure and/or administration of moderate or deep sedation or anesthesia.

PC

Additional Special Procedures
PC.13.50 Through PC.14.30   Not applicable

Discharge or Transfer from the Organization
PC.15.10   A process addresses the needs for continuing care, treatment, and services after discharge or transfer.

PC.15.20   The transfer or discharge of a resident to another level of care, treatment, and services, different professionals, or different settings is based on the resident's assessed needs and the organization's capabilities.

PC.15.30   When residents are transferred or discharged, appropriate information related to the care, treatment, and services provided is exchanged with other service providers.

PC.15.40   Residents are not transferred or discharged unless they meet specific criteria in accordance with law and regulation.

PC.15.50   The organization tells residents and their families of its bed-hold policy.

Waived Testing
PC.16.10   The organization establishes policies and procedures that define the context in which waived test results are used in resident care, treatment, and services.

PC.16.20   The organization identifies the staff responsible for performing and supervising waived testing.

PC.16.30   Staff performing tests have adequate, specific training and orientation to perform the tests and demonstrate satisfactory levels of competence.

PC.16.40   Approved policies and procedures governing specific testing-related processes are current and readily available.

PC.16.50   Quality control checks, as defined by the organization, are conducted on each procedure.

PC.16.60   Appropriate quality control and test records are maintained.

PC

Understanding the Parts of This Chapter

To help you navigate this reformatted standards chapter, it may be helpful to think of its parts this way:

- The **standard** is the "goal"
- The **rationale** explains why it's important to achieve this goal
- The **elements of performance** identify the step(s) needed to achieve this goal

These parts are defined as follows.

Standard A statement that defines the performance expectations and/or structures or processes that must be in place for an organization to provide safe, high-quality care, treatment, and services. An organization is either "compliant" or "not compliant" with a standard.

Accreditation decisions are based on simple counts of the standards that are determined to be "not compliant."

Rationale A statement that provides background, justification, or additional information about a standard. A standard's rationale is not scored. In some instances, the rationale for a standard is self-evident. Therefore, not every standard has a written rationale.

Elements of performance (EPs) The specific performance expectations and/or structures or processes that must be in place for an organization to provide safe, high-quality care, treatment, and services. The scoring of EP compliance determines an organization's overall compliance with a standard. EPs are evaluated on the following scale:

0	Insufficient compliance
1	Partial compliance
2	Satisfactory compliance
NA	Not applicable

You will find a **measure of success** icon—Ⓜ—next to some EPs. Measures of success (MOS) need to be developed for certain EPs when a standard is judged to be out of compliance through either the Periodic Performance Review (PPR) or the onsite survey. An MOS is defined as a quantifiable measure, usually related to an audit, that can be used to determine whether an action has been effective and is being sustained.*

Assessing Your Compliance

Once you are familiar with the parts of this chapter, you can begin to assess your compliance with its requirements. The scoring category designations are provided next to each EP for your convenience. If you would like to assess your organization's performance, mark your scores for the EPs and standards by following the simple steps described below.

---

* For more information about MOS, *see* "The New Joint Commission Accreditation Process" chapter in this book.

Two components are scored for each EP: (1) compliance with the requirement itself **and** (2) compliance with the track record* for that requirement. Scoring has been simplified and track record achievements (which have always been part of the scoring) have been appropriately modified.

Note: *Some standards and EPs do not apply to a particular type of organization; these standards and EPs are marked "not applicable" and the related text is not included. Your organization is not expected to comply with standards and EPs marked "not applicable."*

In addition, some standards and EPs that do apply to organizations may not apply to the specific care, treatment, and services that your individual organization provides. Although these standards and EPs are included in the book, you are not expected to comply with them. If you are unsure about the standards or EPs that apply to your organization, please contact the Joint Commission's Standards Interpretation Group at 630/792-5900.

Step 1: Score Your Compliance with Each Element of Performance

PC

Before you can determine your compliance with the standards, you must score your compliance with each EP. There are three scoring criterion categories: A, B, and C (described below). Please note that for each EP scoring criterion category, your organization must meet the performance requirement itself and the track record achievements (*see* "Track Record Achievements").

Category A

These EPs relate to the presence or absence of the requirement(s) and are scored either yes (2) or no (0); however, score 1 for partial compliance is also possible based on track record achievements.

If an A EP has multiple components designated by bullets, your organization must be compliant with all the bullets to receive a score of 2. If your organization does not meet one or more requirements in the bullets, you will receive a score of 0.

Category B

Category B EPs are scored in two steps:
1. As with category A EPs, category B EPs relate to the presence or absence of the requirement(s). If your organization *does not meet* the requirement(s), the EP is scored 0; there is no need to assess your compliance with the principles of good process design.
2. If your organization *does meet* the requirement(s), but there is concern about the quality or comprehensiveness of the effort, then and only then should you assess the qualitative aspect of the EP. That is, review the applicable principles of good process design and ask how the principles were applied in the situation under discussion. Good process design has the following characteristics:

---

* **Track record** The amount of time that an organization has been in compliance with a standard, EP, or other requirement.

- Is consistent with your organization's mission, values, and goals
- Meets the needs of patients
- Reflects the use of currently accepted practices (doing the right thing, using resources responsibly, using practice guidelines)
- Incorporates current safety information and knowledge such as sentinel event data and National Patient Safety Goals
- Incorporates relevant performance improvement results

This two-part evaluation applies to both simple and bulleted B EPs. First, the EPs are assessed to determine whether the requirements are present. If the EP has multiple components designated by bullets, as with the category A EPs, your organization must meet the requirements in *all* the bulleted items to get a score of 2. If your organization meets *none* of the requirements in the bullets, it receives a score of 0. If your organization meets *at least one, but not all,* of the bulleted requirements, it receives a score of 1 for the EPs.

Use the following rules to determine your EP score:
- Your EP score is 0 if your organization does not meet the requirement(s); you *do not* need to assess your compliance with the preceding applicable principles of good process design
- Your EP score is 1 if your organization does meet the requirement(s) but considered only *some* of the preceding applicable principles of good process design
- Your EP score is 2 if your organization does meet the requirement(s) *and* considered *all* the preceding principles of good process design

Category C

C EPs are scored 0, 1, or 2 based on the number of times your organization does not meet the EP. These EPs are frequency based and require totaling the number of occurrences (that is, results of performance or nonperformance) related to a particular EP. Each situation discovered by a surveyor(s) will be counted as a separate occurrence.

Note: *Multiple events of the same type related to a single resident and single practitioner/staff member are counted as* one occurrence only.

Use the following rules to determine your EP score:
- Your EP score is 2 if you find one or fewer occurrences of noncompliance with the EP
- Your EP score is 1 if you find two occurrences of noncompliance with the EP
- Your EP score is 0 if you find three or more occurrences of noncompliance with the EP

If an EP in the C category has multiple requirements designated by bullets, the following scoring guidelines apply:
- If there are fewer than two findings in all bullets, the EP is scored 2
- If there are three or more findings in all bullets, the EP is scored 0
- In all other combinations of findings, the EP is scored 1

Track Record Achievements

In addition to meeting the requirement(s) in each EP, regardless of category, your organization must also meet the following track record achievements:

Score	Initial Survey	Full Survey
2	4 months or more	12 months or more
1	2 to 3 months	6 to 11 months
0	Fewer than 2 months	Fewer than 6 months

Sample Sizes

If during an onsite survey, your organization has been found to be not compliant with one or more standards, you must demonstrate Evidence of Standards Compliance (ESC) for each standard that is not compliant. The ESC must address compliance at the EP level; when an EP within a noncompliant standard requires an MOS, your organization must demonstrate achievement with the MOS when completing the ESC.

Note: *Not every EP requires an MOS. EPs that do require an MOS are clearly marked in this chapter. Organizations are required to demonstrate achievement with an MOS only for EPs within a noncompliant standard that require an MOS. Organizations do not need to demonstrate achievement with an MOS for any EP within a compliant standard.*

When demonstrating achievement with an MOS during the ESC process, your organization is **required** to use the following sample sizes, which were established because of their statistical significance, their relative simplicity in application, and their sensitivity to an organization's population size:

- For a population size of fewer than 30 cases,* sample 100% of available cases
- For a population size of 30 to 100 cases, sample 30 cases
- For a population size of 101 to 500 cases, sample 50 cases
- For a population size greater than 500 cases, sample 70 cases

Note: *Organizations are encouraged, but not required, to follow this sample size when demonstrating achievement with an MOS for an EP within a noncompliant standard after conducting a full, Option 1, or Option 2 PPR.*

When conducting PPR (optional use) or demonstrating an ESC (mandatory use), use the following percentages to determine your EP score: 90% through 100% of your sample size is in compliance = score 2; 80% through 89% of your sample size is in compliance = score 1; less than 80% of your sample size is in compliance = score 0.

In addition, the following information should govern your organization's selection of samples:

- The appropriate sample size should be determined by the specific population related to the survey findings

---

* *Case* refers to a single instance in which a situation related to a survey finding occurs. For example, if a survey finding was related to **pain assessment**, then a case would be any resident record. If a survey finding was related to **pain management**, a case would be any resident record for residents receiving pain management.

- The sampling approach should involve either systematic random sampling (for example, your organization selects every second or third case for review) or simple random sampling (for example, your organization uses a series of random numbers generated by a computer to identify the cases to be reviewed)
- If your organization chooses not to use these sample sizes while conducting PPR options 1 or 2, you should make sure that your sample size is sufficiently large enough to ensure statistical significance
- When submitting a clarifying ESC, if your organization selects records as part of its sample, the records should be from a period of no more than three months before the last date of the survey
- Assessment of MOS compliance is conducted for a four-month period following the date of ESC approval. Your organization should select records as a part of your sample following the date of ESC approval and use the required sample sizes. MOS percentage compliance rates are derived from the average of all four months.

Step 2: Use Your EP Scores to Gauge Your Compliance with the Standards

Now that you have evaluated and scored each EP for a particular standard, use these simple rules to determine your compliance with the standard itself:

PC

- Your organization is not in compliance (that is, "not compliant") with the standard if any EP is scored 0
- Otherwise, your organization is in compliance with a standard if 65% or more of its EPs are scored 2

Standards, Rationales, Elements of Performance, and Scoring

Entry to Care, Treatment, and Services

Agreeing to provide care, treatment, and services for a resident should be based both on the resident's needs and the scope of the services provided by the organization. To do this, the organization does the following:

- Establishes criteria to determine entry eligibility
- Defines the minimum information necessary to determine the resident's eligibility for entry to a program or service
- Defines the appropriate professionals and settings needed to provide the services offered consistent with the organization's mission
- Makes entry decisions for appropriate care, treatment, and services offered by the organization based on these criteria

When subacute services are offered, the organization identifies the philosophy and scope of services that it provides to meet the needs of this medically complex population.

PC

Standard PC.1.10

The organization accepts for care, treatment, and services only those residents whose identified care, treatment, and service needs it can meet.

Elements of Performance for PC.1.10

B   1. The organization has a defined written process that includes the following:
- The information to be gathered to determine eligibility for entrance into the organization
- The populations of residents accepted or not accepted by the organization, for example, programs designed to treat adults that do not treat young children
- The criteria to determine eligibility for entry into the system
- The procedures for accepting referrals

C Ⓜ   2. Residents are screened for appropriateness at the point of first contact (including contact by phone) with the organization.

B   3. The interdisciplinary team is consulted when necessary to determine whether a prospective resident meets admission criteria.

C Ⓜ   4. If a resident is not accepted after referral and preadmission screening, the reasons for denying admission are stated.

B   5. The staff refers the resident to another appropriate organization, making reasonable referral efforts.

B   6.   The staff explains to the referring organization its reasons for not accepting the resident and, when possible, suggests a more appropriate organization.

B   7.   When warranted by need, separate specialized screening, assessment, and reassessment processes are identified for the various populations served.

     8.   Not applicable

C ⓜ   9.   The organization accepts residents for care, treatment, and services according to established processes.

Assessment

The goal of assessment is to determine the appropriate care, treatment, and services to meet a resident's initial needs as well as his or her changing needs while in the setting.

Identifying and delivering appropriate care, treatment, and services depends on three processes:

PC

1. *Collecting data* about each resident's health history; physical, functional, and psychosocial status; and needs as appropriate to the setting and circumstances
2. *Analyzing data* to produce information about residents' needs for care, treatment, and services and to identify the need for additional data
3. *Making care, treatment, and services decisions* based on information developed about each resident's needs and his or her response to care, treatment, and services

Qualified staff assesses each resident's care needs throughout the resident's contact with the organization through assessments or screenings. These activities may also identify the need for additional assessments or planning. These assessments are as follows:
- Defined by the organization
- Individualized to meet each resident's needs
- Address the needs of special populations

The process defined by the organization identifies the resident's physical, cognitive, behavioral, emotional, and psychosocial status. This assessment identifies facilitating factors and possible barriers to the resident reaching his or her goals, including the presenting problems and needs, such as the following:
- Symptoms that might be associated with a disease, condition, or treatment (such as pain, nausea, or dyspnea)
- Social barriers, including cultural and language barriers
- Social and environmental factors
- Physical disabilities
- Vision and hearing impairments and disabilities
- Developmental disabilities

- Communicative disorders
- Cognitive disorders
- Emotional, behavioral, and mental disorders
- Substance abuse, dependence, and other addictive behaviors

The depth and frequency of the assessment or screening depend on a number of factors, including the resident's needs; program goals; and the care, treatment, and services provided. Assessment or screening activities may vary between settings, as defined by the clinical and other leaders of the organization. Resident screenings, assessments, and reassessments need to be done and documented within a reasonable time frame to identify the resident's needs and determine whether these needs are being met.

Information gathered at the first contact can indicate the need for more data or a more intensive assessment of the resident's physical, psychological, cognitive, and communicative skills or development or social functioning. At a minimum, the need for further assessment is determined by the care, treatment, and services sought; the client's presenting condition(s); and whether the client agrees to care, treatment, and services.

PC

Standard PC.2.10
Not applicable

Standard PC.2.20
The organization defines in writing the data and information gathered during assessment and reassessment.

Elements of Performance for PC.2.20

B   1.   The organization's written definition of the data and information gathered during assessment and reassessment includes the following:
- The scope of assessment and reassessment activities by each discipline
- The content of the assessment and reassessment
- The criteria for when an additional or more in-depth assessment is done*

B   2.   The screening, assessment, and reassessment activities described are within the scope of practice, state licensure laws, applicable regulations, or certification of the discipline doing the assessment.

A   3.   If applicable, separate specialized assessment and reassessment information is identified for the various populations served.

   4. Through 11. Not applicable

---

* For example, nutritional or functional risk assessments may be defined for at-risk residents. In such cases, nutritional risk criteria should be developed by dieticians or other qualified individuals, and functional risk criteria should be developed by rehabilitation specialists or other qualified individuals.

B   12. The information defined by the organization to be gathered during the initial assessment(s) includes the following, as relevant to the care, treatment, and services:
- Current diagnosis(es)
- Pertinent history
- Medication history, including drug allergies and sensitivities
- Current medications, including prescribed and over-the-counter medications
- Current treatments

The information defined by the organization to be gathered during the initial assessment(s) also includes the following (EPs 13–20):

B   13. The resident's physical and neuropsychiatric status, including the following:
- Musculoskeletal status
- Cardiorespiratory status
- Gastrointestinal status
- Integumentary status
- Foot care needs
- Mental, affective, and cognitive status and needs

PC

B   14. The resident's communication status, including the following:
- Ability to hear
- Ability to speak
- Predominant language(s)
- Modes of expression

B   15. The resident's functional status, including the following:
- Ability to perform activities of daily living
- Mobility, balance, and strength
- Ability to swallow
- Physical limitations and precautions
- Rehabilitation status, needs, and potential
- Orientation

B   16. The resident's activity status, needs, and potential, including the following:
- Personal preferences regarding schedules and grooming
- The resident's activity and recreational skills, based on his or her cognitive abilities and the limitations of his or her illness or treatment
- Hobbies, recreational interests, associated needs, and potential
- Ability to participate in structured and group activities

B   17. The resident's nutritional* and hydration status and needs, including the following:
- Potential nutritional risk, deficiencies, and needs
- Cultural, religious, or ethnic food preferences
- Nutrient-intake patterns and special dietary requirements
- Dietary/food allergies
- Food and fluid consumption
- Bowel and urinary output
- Skin integrity
- Swallowing problems
- Appropriate laboratory tests
- Weight (at least monthly)
- Criteria used to evaluate weight gain and loss to determine the need for further assessment

B   18. The resident's dental status and oral health, including the following:
- Dental status and oral health, including the condition of the oral cavity, teeth, and tooth-supporting structures
- The presence or absence of natural teeth or dentures and the ability to function with or without natural teeth or dentures

PC

B   19. The resident's pain, including the following:
- Pain status, including its origin, location, severity, and alleviating and exacerbating factors
- Current treatment for pain and response to treatment

B   20. The resident's psychosocial and spiritual status, including the following:
- Cultural and ethnic factors that influence care, treatment, and services
- Current emotional status
- Social skills
- Current living situation
- Family relationships and circumstances
- Relevant past history of roles
- Response to stress caused by the illness and required treatment
- Spiritual orientation, status, and needs
- The dying resident's concerns related to hope, despair, guilt, or forgiveness

B   21. In addition, when the bereavement process is a significant factor, the psychosocial assessment includes the social, spiritual, and cultural variables that influence the perceptions and expressions of grief by the resident or family.

---

* The content of the nutritional screening criteria that the organization develops (which may include the minimum data set [MDS]), is at the discretion of the organization but should be contained in an approved policy. The standards also reflect that, based on the results of the nutrition screen, further nutrition assessment is completed when indicated and the resident is reassessed at determined intervals.

Standards PC.2.30 Through PC.2.110 ▬▬▬▬▬▬▬▬▬▬

Not applicable

Standard PC.2.120 ▬▬▬▬▬▬▬▬▬▬▬▬▬▬▬▬▬▬▬▬

The organization defines in writing the time frame(s) for conducting the initial assessment(s).

Elements of Performance for PC.2.120

A   1.   The organization defines the time frame(s) for conducting the initial assessment(s).

2. Through 7. Not applicable

At a minimum, the organization specifies the following time frames for assessments:

A Ⓜ 8.   Each resident's initial Minimum Data Set/interdisciplinary assessment is to be completed within 14 days of admission or as required by law and regulation.

A   9.   For subacute services, the organization initiates assessments within 24 hours of admission and completes them within 48 hours after admission for all disciplines pertinent to the reason for admission.

A   10. The attending physician or licensed independent practitioner performs a *medical assessment*. These time frames apply for all admissions and re-admissions. Any previous medical history does not have to be completely redone. It can be updated with information about the most recent illness and hospitalization since the date the last history was taken within a time frame appropriate to the resident's condition. This time frame must not exceed 24 hours before admission or within 72 hours after admission.

Durable, legible originals or reproductions of a medical history and physical examination, obtained from the attending physician or licensed independent practitioner and completed within 30 days before admission or readmission, are acceptable, provided that there is a summary of the resident's condition and course of care during the interim period, and the summary also includes the resident's current physical/psychosocial status.

A   11. If the attending physician or licensed independent practitioner other than the attending physician performed the medical assessment that is being transferred, and that assessment was performed within 30 days before admission, then within 24 hours before admission or within 72 hours after admission (48 hours for subacute services), the attending physician or attending licensed independent practitioner must do the following:
• Review the physical examination
• Conduct a second medical assessment to confirm the information and findings

PC

- Update any information and findings as necessary, including a summary of the resident's condition and course of care during the interim period and the current physical/psychosocial status
- Sign and date the additional information to attest to its currency

A 12. The assessment findings are recorded in the medical record on admission within time frames noted in EP 11.

A 13. Each resident's oral health assessment is to be performed and documented within 90 days before admission or within 14 days after admission.

Standard PC.2.130

Initial assessments are performed as defined by the organization.

Elements of Performance for PC.2.130

C Ⓜ 1. Each resident is assessed per organization policy.

C Ⓜ 2. Each resident's initial assessment is conducted within the time frame specified by the needs of the resident, organization policy, and law and regulation.

A 3. A registered nurse assesses the resident's need for nursing care in all settings, as required by law, regulation, or organization policy.

C Ⓜ 4. Residents who exhibit symptoms of dementia are evaluated, and a differential diagnosis is established.

C Ⓜ 5. The evaluation* of residents who exhibit symptoms of dementia is performed by a neurologist, a psychiatrist, or a geriatrician, if available, or another qualified physician.

Standard PC.2.140

Not applicable

Standard PC.2.150

Residents are reassessed† as needed.

---

* Guidelines for conducting such an evaluation are available from the "Guidelines for Dignity" from the Alzheimer's Association. The guidelines include a history and physical examination; a mental status evaluation; a neurologic examination; a blood workup; a psychiatric evaluation; a neuropsychiatric assessment; a psychological assessment; CT/MRI, as indicated; and any reversible causes for the presenting symptoms.

† The scope and intensity of any further assessments are based on the resident's diagnosis; the setting; the resident's desire for care, treatment, and services; and the resident's response to any previous care, treatment, and services.

Rationale for PC.2.150

Each resident may be reassessed for many reasons, including the following:
- To evaluate his or her response to care, treatment, and services
- To respond to a significant change in status and/or diagnosis or condition
- To satisfy legal or regulatory requirements
- To meet time intervals specified by the organization
- To meet time intervals determined by the course of the care, treatment, and services for the resident

Elements of Performance for PC.2.150

C Ⓜ 1. Each resident is reassessed as needed.

C Ⓜ 2. When the organization provides subacute services, reassessment occurs in conjunction with the interdisciplinary care plan schedule (every two weeks for the first quarter, every month for the second quarter, and quarterly thereafter) or in response to change(s) in the resident's condition.

Additional Standard for Victims of Abuse

Standard PC.3.10

Residents who may be victims of abuse, neglect, or exploitation are assessed. (*See* standard RI.2.150.)

PC

Rationale for PC.3.10

Victims of abuse, neglect, or exploitation may come to an organization in a variety of ways. The resident may be unable or may be reluctant to speak of the abuse, and it may not be obvious to the casual observer. Staff needs to be able to identify abuse, neglect, and exploitation as well as the extent and circumstances of the abuse, neglect, or exploitation, to give the resident appropriate care.

Criteria for identifying and assessing victims of abuse, neglect, or exploitation should be used throughout the organization. The assessment of the resident must be conducted within the context of the requirements of the law to preserve evidentiary materials and support future legal actions.

Elements of Performance for PC.3.10

A 1. The organization develops or adopts criteria* for identifying victims in each of the following situations:
- Physical assault
- Rape
- Sexual molestation
- Domestic abuse
- Elder neglect or abuse
- Child neglect or abuse
- Exploitation

---

* The Family Violence Prevention Fund is one resource that can be contacted for further information at http://www.fvpf.org.

B   2.   Appropriate staff* is educated about abuse, neglect, or exploitation and how to refer as appropriate.

A   3.   A list of private and public community agencies that provide or arrange for assessment and care of abuse victims is maintained to facilitate appropriate referrals.

B   4.   Victims of abuse, neglect, or exploitation are identified using the criteria developed or adopted by the organization at entry into the system and on an ongoing basis.

B   5.   The organization's staff refers appropriately or conducts the assessment of victims of abuse, neglect, or exploitation.

A   6.   All cases of possible abuse, neglect, or exploitation are reported to appropriate agencies according to organization policy and law and regulation.

A   7.   All cases of possible abuse, neglect, or exploitation are immediately reported in the organization.

PC

Standards PC.3.20 Through PC.3.220 ━━━━━━━━━

Not applicable

Diagnostic Services

Standard PC.3.230 ━━━━━━━━━━━━━━━━━

Diagnostic testing† necessary for determining the resident's health care needs is performed.

Elements of Performance for PC.3.230

C Ⓜ   1.   Diagnostic testing and procedures are performed as ordered.

C Ⓜ   2.   Diagnostic testing and procedures are performed in a timely manner as defined by the organization.

C Ⓜ   3.   When a test report requires clinical interpretation, relevant information is provided with the request.

         4.   Not applicable

---

* Staff should be able to screen for abuse and neglect as indicated by the resident's needs or conditions. The organization may define who conducts the full assessment for alleged or suspected abuse or neglect or refer to another organization.

† Diagnostic testing includes laboratory, radiologic, electrodiagnostic, and other functional tests and imaging technologies.

A   5.   Radiologic and other diagnostic services, including pathology and clinical laboratory services, are available 24 hours a day, seven days a week.

Planning Care, Treatment, and Services

Planning includes creating an initial plan for care, treatment, and services appropriate to the resident's specific assessed needs and then revising or maintaining the plan based on the resident's response. Planning for care, treatment, and services is individualized to meet the resident's unique needs and circumstances. Performed by qualified individuals, planning for care, treatment, and services involves using an interdisciplinary approach and involving the resident to the extent possible.

The plan may be modified or terminated based on reassessment; the resident's need for further care, treatment, and services; or the achievement of plan of care goals. This modification may result in planning for the resident's transfer to another setting or service or discharge from the organization.

An interdisciplinary approach is used to plan and manage care, treatment, and services and ultimately guide the outcomes of care, treatment, and services. This approach may draw from internal staff and external consultants from the areas of activities, dietetic, medical, nursing, pharmacy, rehabilitation, social services, and other disciplines whose roles and responsibilities are determined by the following:

- Professional skills, competence, and credentials
- The component of care, treatment, and services being provided
- Licensure, certification, regulation, scope of practice, and job description

PC

Standard PC.4.10

Development of a plan for care, treatment, and services is individualized and appropriate to the resident's needs, strengths, limitations, and goals.

Rationale for PC.4.10

Planning care, treatment, and services is not limited to developing a written plan. Rather, planning is a dynamic process that addresses the execution of care, treatment, and services. The plan for care, treatment, and services must be consistently re-evaluated to ensure that the resident's needs are met. Planning for care, treatment, and services includes the following:

- Integrating assessment findings in the care-planning process
- Developing a plan for care, treatment, and services that includes resident care goals that are reasonable and measurable
- Regularly reviewing and revising the plan for care, treatment, and services
- Determining how the planned care, treatment, and services will be provided
- Documenting the plan for care, treatment, and services
- Monitoring the effectiveness of care planning and the provision of care, treatment, and services
- Involving residents and/or families in care planning

Elements of Performance for PC.4.10

B   1.   Care, treatment, and services are planned to ensure that they are appropriate to the resident's needs.

B   2.   Development of a plan for care, treatment, and services is based on the data from assessments.

B   3.   The interdisciplinary team identifies and prioritizes each resident's care needs based on the analysis of assessment data.

C Ⓜ 4.   An individualized, interdisciplinary plan for care, treatment, and services is developed by an interdisciplinary team representing all appropriate health care professionals as soon as possible after admission, but no later than 7 calendar days after comprehensive assessments are completed.

C Ⓜ 5.   When subacute care is provided, the interdisciplinary care plan is completed no later than 72 hours after comprehensive assessments are completed (which occurs within 72 hours of admission).

       6.   Not applicable

B   7.   The plan identifies the following:
- The care, treatment, and settings
- The frequency at which care, treatment, and services and interventions will occur
- The team members responsible for providing care, treatment, and services
- The financial implications of care, treatment, and services
- Interventions to facilitate the resident's return to the community or discharge to an appropriate level of care

C Ⓜ 8.   An interim plan for care, treatment, and services is developed for each resident immediately after the resident is admitted.

B   9.   A process is in place for gathering input, collaborating on care plan development, and reporting the final plan to team members not available to participate in care planning.

A   10.   Policies and procedures define how care plans can be modified between team meetings.

B   11.   The organization implements a process for evaluating the plan for care, treatment, and services and its effectiveness, which includes the following:
- 90-day evaluation intervals or more frequent intervals in response to a significant change in the resident's physical, communicative, psychosocial, functional, or emotional status
- Care plan revisions that reflect the resident's current needs, problems, goals, care, treatment, and services
- Review and revision by the interdisciplinary team of all components of care, treatment, and services needed by the resident

C Ⓜ 12. Evaluation of the resident is based on the resident care goals and the resident's plan for care, treatment, and services.

C Ⓜ 13. The goals of care, treatment, and services are revised when necessary.

B 14. Plans for care, treatment, and services are regularly reviewed and revised when necessary.

B 15. When subacute care is provided, the interdisciplinary team revises care plans in collaboration with residents, family, and the individual responsible for financial resource monitoring.

C Ⓜ 16. When subacute care is provided, the care plan review occurs every two weeks for the first quarter, every month for the second quarter, and quarterly thereafter or more frequently when indicated by change in the resident's condition.

Providing Care, Treatment, and Services

Caring for residents involves providing individualized, planned, and appropriate interventions in settings responsive to specific individual needs. "Care" includes care, treatment, services, rehabilitation, habilitation, or another intervention provided to the resident by the organization.

The goal of providing effective care, treatment, and services is met when the following are performed well:
- Intervening in a collaborative manner (in light of assessed resident needs)
- Educating the resident
- Promoting health and providing appropriate preventive care
- Providing supportive care, treating a disease or condition, and/or treating symptoms (such as pain, nausea, or dyspnea) using accepted professional standards of practice
- Meeting the resident's nourishment needs, if appropriate to the setting
- Helping residents with appropriate restorative services, including assistance with activities of daily living, such as eating, dressing, grooming, bathing, oral hygiene, ambulation, and toilet activities
- Rehabilitating physical, communicative, or psychosocial impairment or maintaining the resident's level of functioning
- Coordinating the care, treatment, and services provided to a resident
- Optimizing comfort and dignity during end-of-life care
- Involving families as indicated and acceptable to the resident

All interventions should respect and encourage the resident's ability to make choices, to develop and maintain a sense of achievement about attaining their personal health goals, and to choose to continue or modify participation in the care process.

The activities comprising care, treatment, and services may be performed by a variety of staff whose roles and responsibilities are determined by the component of

PC

care, treatment, and services being provided; relevant licensure; law and regulation; registration; certification; scope of practice; job description; or privileges. The actions or interventions may also be carried out by the resident, family, volunteers, or other caregivers.

Standard PC.5.10

The organization provides care, treatment, and services for each resident according to the plan for care, treatment, and services.

Elements of Performance for PC.5.10

C Ⓜ 1.   The organization provides care, treatment, and services for each resident according to the plan for care, treatment, and services.

2.   Not applicable

3.   Not applicable

A   4.   The organization uses at least two resident identifiers, neither to be the resident's room number, whenever taking blood samples or administering medications, blood, or blood products.

Standard PC.5.20

Not applicable

Standard PC.5.30

The attending physician prescribes the medical requirements of care for the residents he or she admits.

Elements of Performance for PC.5.30

C Ⓜ 1.   Orders* are obtained from the physician or other authorized individuals according to law and regulation and professional practice acts before providing care, treatment, and services.

C Ⓜ 2.   The order is tailored to each resident's needs and includes all elements required by law and regulation.

C Ⓜ 3.   All orders are renewed or updated to reflect the following:
  - Changes in the care, treatment, and services being provided
  - Changes in the resident's physical or psychosocial condition
  - The resident's response to care, treatment, and services
  - The resident's outcome related to care, treatment, and services
  - Changes in diagnosis, treatment (including procedures and medications), and equipment

---

* These orders may be verbal or written and include prescriptions.

- The minimum review time frame defined by the organization
- Applicable law and regulation

C Ⓜ 4. The organization provides care, treatment, and services according to the most recent order.

C Ⓜ 5. Each attending physician designates an alternate physician whom the organization can contact to obtain regular or emergency care when the attending physician is not available.

Standard PC.5.40

The attending physician visits the resident in accordance with the resident's needs and at least once during the 30 days after admission.

Elements of Performance for PC.5.40

B 1. The attending physician visits the resident in accordance with the resident's needs.

C Ⓜ 2. The attending physician visits the resident at least once during the 30 days after admission.

C Ⓜ 3. For planned stays of less than 30 days, the resident's attending physician visits the resident at least once before discharge.

C Ⓜ 4. The resident is seen within 72 hours of admission when the long term care physician is different from the resident's primary physician.

C 5. Physicians' visiting schedules comply with law, regulation, and organization policy regarding the following:
- Frequency and timing of visits
- Visits by physician assistants or advanced practice registered nurses instead of attending physicians

Standard PC.5.50

Care, treatment, and services are provided in an interdisciplinary, collaborative manner.

Rationale for PC.5.50

A collaborative, interdisciplinary approach to meeting the resident's needs and goals helps coordinate care, treatment, and services and achieve optimal outcomes. The mix of disciplines involved and the intensity of the collaboration will vary as appropriate to each resident and the scope of services provided by the organization. An interdisciplinary approach should not be interpreted as a requirement for the signing of other individual's notes.

PC

Elements of Performance for PC.5.50

B   1.   Care, treatment, and services are provided in an interdisciplinary, collaborative manner* as appropriate to the needs of the resident and the organization's scope of services.

       2.   Not applicable

B   3.   Changes in the resident's condition are communicated to the physician or other authorized health care professionals, the resident, and his or her family.

C Ⓜ   4.   Information from consultation and evaluation reports is communicated to the physician.

C Ⓜ   5.   The organization provides this information on a timely basis as defined by the organization and required by law and regulation.

Standard PC.5.60

The organization coordinates the care, treatment, and services provided to a resident as part of the plan for care, treatment, and services and consistent with the organization's scope of care, treatment, and services.

Rationale for PC.5.60

Throughout the provision of care, treatment, and services, residents should be matched with appropriate internal and external resources to meet their ongoing needs in a timely manner. Care, treatment, and services should be coordinated between providers and between settings, independent of whether they are provided directly or through written agreement.

Elements of Performance for PC.5.60

B   1.   The organization coordinates the care, treatment, and services provided through internal resources to a resident.

B   2.   When external resources are needed, the organization participates in coordinating care, treatment, and services with these resources.

B   3.   The organization has a process to receive or share relevant resident information to facilitate appropriate coordination and continuity when residents are referred to other care, treatment, and service providers.

B   4.   There is a process to resolve duplication or conflict with either internal or external resources.

---

* The process is designed to ensure coordinated participation of all appropriate health care professionals from the appropriate settings and includes identifying interdisciplinary team members' responsibilities, holding interdisciplinary team meetings, providing for resolution of differences among interdisciplinary team members, documenting interdisciplinary team members' participation in the medical record, and discussing and modifying the resident's interdisciplinary care plan.

B   5.   The plan of care, treatment, and services is designed to occur in a time frame that meets the resident's health needs.

     6.   Not applicable

B   7.   Services are made available directly or through arrangement to meet the following resident needs:
- 24-hour emergency dental services
- Spiritual services
- Behavioral health services,* including counseling on a continuing basis in individual, family, and group services, as appropriate
- Activity services for ambulatory and nonambulatory residents at various functional levels as well as those who are unable to attend group activities
- Assistance with guardianship and conservatorship, when indicated
- Services to facilitate family support, social work, nursing care, dental care, rehabilitation, primary physician care, or discharge

Standard PC.5.70
Not applicable

PC

Education

Standard PC.6.10
The resident receives education and training specific to the resident's needs and as appropriate to the care, treatment, and services provided.

Rationale for PC.6.10
Residents must be given sufficient information to make decisions and to take responsibility for self-management activities related to their needs. Residents and, as appropriate, their families are educated to improve individual outcomes by promoting healthy behavior and appropriately involving residents in their care, treatment, and services decisions.

Elements of Performance for PC.6.10
B   1.   Education provided is appropriate to the resident's needs.

C Ⓜ   2.   The assessment of learning needs addresses cultural and religious beliefs, emotional barriers, desire and motivation to learn, physical or cognitive limitations, and barriers to communication as appropriate.

---

* These services may be provided by various disciplines (for instance, social workers, psychologists, clinical nurse specialists, or other appropriately educated consultants).

B   3.   As appropriate to the resident's condition and assessed needs and the organization's scope of services, the resident is educated about the following:

- The plan for care, treatment, and services
- His or her condition or illness and preventive interventions
- Basic health practices and safety
- The safe and effective use of medications
- Nutrition interventions, modified diets, or oral health
- Safe and effective use of medical equipment or supplies when provided by the organization
- Understanding pain, the risk for pain, the importance of effective pain management, the pain assessment process, and methods for pain management
- Habilitation or rehabilitation techniques to help them reach the maximum independence possible
- Environmental and physical plant safety issues, such as fire safety, evacuation, storage of chemical agents, and so on
- Use of nonmedical equipment, including, but not limited to, operating call lights, beds, and personal appliances
- How to carry out self-care
- Transfer techniques
- Personal safety and mobility
- Bathroom safety
- Available resources to meet identified needs and how to access such resources
- When to seek and how to obtain follow-up or continuing care, treatment, and services

PC

Standard PC.6.20

Not applicable

Standard PC.6.30

The resident receives education and training specific to the resident's abilities as appropriate to the care, treatment, and services provided by the organization.

Rationale for PC.6.30

Learning styles vary, and the ability to learn can be affected by many factors, including individual learning preferences and readiness to learn. Educational activities must be tailored to meet the resident's needs and abilities.

Elements of Performance for PC.6.30

B   1.   Education provided is appropriate to the resident's abilities.

B   2.   Education is coordinated among the disciplines providing care, treatment, and services.

B   3.   The content is presented in an understandable manner.

B   4.   Teaching methods accommodate various learning styles.

C (M) 5.   Comprehension is evaluated.

Standard PC.6.40

Not applicable

Standard PC.6.50

The organization provides academic education to children and youth as needed.

Rationale for PC.6.50

Providing academic education helps maintain the educational and intellectual development of children and youth and helps keep them from falling behind. When school-age children or youth are in the organization for long periods, state or local laws may specify the requirements for meeting their schooling needs.

Elements of Performance for PC.6.50

A   1.   The organization defines the length of stay and absence from school that would require providing educational services in accordance with applicable law and regulation.

2.   Not applicable

B   3.   Educational resources are selected based on the resident's identified needs.

Standard PC.6.60

Not applicable

Nutritional Care

This standard focuses on providing appropriate nutritional care, including food and nutrition therapy, in a timely and efficient manner using appropriate resources. Elements of nutritional care, such as screening or assessment and education, are addressed in other standards in this book.

Standard PC.7.10

The organization has a process for preparing and/or distributing food and nutrition products.

PC

Elements of Performance for PC.7.10

B   1. Food and nutrition products are provided for the resident.

C Ⓜ 2. Food and nutrition products are stored and prepared under proper conditions of sanitation, temperature, light, moisture, ventilation, and security.

C Ⓜ 3. Residents' cultural, religious, and ethnic food preferences are honored, when possible, unless contraindicated.

C Ⓜ 4. Substitutes of equal nutritional value are offered when residents refuse the food served.

C Ⓜ 5. Staff helps residents when necessary.

      6. Not applicable

      7. Not applicable

B   8. Resident communal dining areas are adequately supervised.

A   9. A food service supervisor oversees general kitchen management.

B   10. Menus are planned in advance, dated, easy to read, and posted in conspicuous areas accessible to residents.

C Ⓜ 11. Special diets and altered diet schedules are accommodated.

A   12. Cycled menus are rotated over a period of at least three weeks.

Pain

Standard PC.8.10 ▬▬▬▬▬▬▬▬▬▬▬▬▬▬▬▬▬▬

Pain is assessed in all residents.

Rationale for PC.8.10

The identification and treatment of pain is an important component of the plan of care. Individuals are assessed based upon their clinical presentation services sought and in accordance with the care, treatment, and services provided.

Elements of Performance for PC.8.10

C Ⓜ 1. A comprehensive pain assessment is conducted as appropriate to the resident's condition and the scope of care, treatment, and services provided.

      2. Not applicable

C Ⓜ 3. Regular reassessment and follow-up occur according to criteria developed by the organization.

      4. Not applicable

5. Not applicable

C Ⓜ 6. The assessment methods are appropriate to the resident's age and/or abilities.

C Ⓜ 7. When pain is identified, the resident is treated by the organization or referred for treatment.

Restorative Services

Standard PC.8.20

When necessary, residents receive appropriate restorative services, including assistance with activities of daily living, such as eating, dressing, grooming, bathing, oral hygiene, ambulation, and toilet activities.

Elements of Performance for PC.8.20

C Ⓜ 1. Appropriate supplies and equipment are available to support self-care.

C Ⓜ 2. Adaptive self-help devices are provided when needed.

C Ⓜ 3. Residents are helped with self-care activities when needed.

C Ⓜ 4. Residents are clean and well groomed.

C Ⓜ 5. Oral prostheses are clean.

C Ⓜ 6. Residents are free from discernible body odor.

C Ⓜ 7. Skin is clean and dry.

C Ⓜ 8. Residents are appropriately helped with toileting activities.

C Ⓜ 9. Residents are appropriately helped with activities of daily living, including the following:
- Bathing
- Dressing
- Eating
- Oral hygiene
- Ambulation

B 10. All reasonable steps are taken to keep residents safe from accident and injury.

PC

Preventive Care

Standard PC.8.30 ▬▬▬▬▬▬▬▬▬▬▬▬▬▬▬▬▬▬▬▬▬

Residents at risk for health-related complications receive appropriate preventive care.

Rationale for PC.8.30

Preventive measures help limit or avoid complications associated with compromised health status.

Element of Performance for PC.8.30

C Ⓜ 1. Preventive interventions are performed according to the plan for care, treatment, and services to do the following:
- Encourage and help residents to be out of bed, except when prohibited by a physician's order
- Encourage and help chair-fast residents to leave their rooms for a change of environment
- Maintain proper body position and alignment
- Implement a skin integrity program
- Implement a bowel management program
- Implement a bladder management program
- Help with ambulation, including maintenance-of-gait training
- Provide active and passive range-of-motion exercises
- Provide assistance to help prevent aspiration, dehydration, and malnutrition
- Help with coping with the effects of illness, disability, treatment, or stay in the facility

Social and Diversional Activities

Standard PC.8.40 ▬▬▬▬▬▬▬▬▬▬▬▬▬▬▬▬▬▬▬▬▬

Residents are helped so they can participate in social and diversional activities according to their functional levels.

Elements of Performance for PC.8.40

C Ⓜ 1. Residents are helped to participate in social and leisure activities according to their interests and needs.

A 2. An activity schedule is made available to all residents, staff, and visitors.

C Ⓜ 3. The schedule of activities is communicated to residents who have difficulty reading.

B   4.   The organization offers a variety of activities to meet the needs of the population served.

Access to the Outdoors

Standard PC.8.50 ▬▬▬▬▬▬▬▬▬▬▬▬▬▬▬▬▬▬▬▬▬▬
Not applicable

Standard PC.8.60 ▬▬▬▬▬▬▬▬▬▬▬▬▬▬▬▬▬▬▬▬▬▬
Not applicable

End-of-Life Care

PC

Standard PC.8.70 ▬▬▬▬▬▬▬▬▬▬▬▬▬▬▬▬▬▬▬▬▬▬
Comfort and dignity are optimized during end-of-life care.*

Rationale for PC.8.70
The resident at or near the end of his or her life has the right to physical and psychological comfort. The organization provides care that optimizes the dying resident's comfort and dignity and addresses the resident's and his or her family's psychosocial and spiritual needs.

Elements of Performance for PC.8.70
B   1.   To the extent possible, as appropriate to the resident's and family's needs and the organization's services, interventions address resident and family comfort; dignity; and psychosocial, emotional, and spiritual needs, as appropriate, about death and grief.

C Ⓜ 2.   Staff is educated about the unique needs of dying residents and their families and caregivers.

---

* Applies to all dying residents, not just hospice residents, for whom an organization may provide care, treatment, and services.

Specific Procedures

Administering Blood and Blood Components

Standard PC.9.10
Blood and blood components are administered safely, as appropriate to the setting.

Elements of Performance for PC.9.10
    1. Through 9. Not applicable

A   10. If the organization provides for the maintenance and transfusion of blood or blood components, it meets all applicable law and regulation.

Responding to Life-Threatening Emergencies

PC

Standard PC.9.20
The organization responds to life-threatening emergencies according to organization policy and procedure.

Elements of Performance for PC.9.20
B   1. The organization develops policy and procedures for responding to life-threatening emergencies such as respiratory arrest and cardiac arrest.

B   2. Policies and procedures that address life-threatening emergencies include the following:
- Availability of first aid and Basic Life Support (CPR) services
- Emergency transfer to another organization
- Placement of a phone call to 911

A   3. The organization responds to life-threatening emergencies according to organization policy and procedure.

Standards PC.9.30 Through PC.11.70
Not applicable

Restraint and Seclusion

Standard PC.11.80
The organization designs a system to achieve a restraint-free environment.

Elements of Performance for PC.11.80

A   1.   Achieving a restraint-free environment is a stated goal of the organization.

B   2.   Processes are implemented to actively pursue this goal.

A   3.   The use of physical or chemical restraints is prohibited for discipline or staff convenience or to prevent wandering.

A   4.   The use of restraints is prohibited except to facilitate or support treatment of a resident's medical symptoms.

A   5.   Residents are allowed to refuse restraints.

A   6.   The decision to use restraints is based on an assessment of the resident's needs and is never based solely on a request from a resident's representative.

B   7.   The processes emphasize alternatives to restraint, including the following:
- Restorative programs
- Management of the resident's personal environment
- Well-trained staff to support each resident
- Support of resident rights
- Recognition and respect for the resident's past interests
- Supportive devices and special equipment
- Involvement of other people in each resident's care, such as nursing assistants, housekeeping staff, secretaries, and other administrative staff, who have been trained in resident-orientation techniques

PC

Standard PC.11.90 ▬▬▬▬▬▬▬▬▬▬▬▬▬▬▬▬▬▬▬▬▬▬▬

When alternatives to restraint are ineffective, restraint is safely and appropriately used.

Elements of Performance for PC.11.90

When alternatives to restraint are ineffective and restraint is used, the organization uses a process that addresses the following elements in accordance with law and regulation:

C **Ⓜ**   1.   The use of restraint is based on the resident's assessed needs, including precipitating factors, and is documented.

C **Ⓜ**   2.   The trial of alternatives before the use of restraint is documented.

A   3.   There is a licensed independent practitioner's written order for the use of restraint.

A   4.   Time limitations for use of restraint are determined.

A   5.   The frequency of observing and assessing the resident is determined.

A   6.   Restraint devices are correctly applied.

A   7. Restraints are periodically removed or released in accordance with law and regulation and the resident's needs.

A   8. The competence of staff involved in applying such interventions is determined.

A   9. Attention is paid to the resident's needs while in restraint.

A   10. Informed consent is obtained as appropriate.

A   11. The use of the restraint is reviewed if frequent or prolonged.

A   12. The orders for restraint are reviewed within time frames defined by the organization, not to exceed 30 days.

A   13. The interdisciplinary team monitors the resident on an ongoing basis while in restraint and can request a new physician order at any time within the 30 days due to changes in the resident's condition that require removing or modifying restraint.

C Ⓜ 14. The resident and family are educated about restraints and their alternatives.

B   15. The use of restraint is measured, assessed, and reduced as part of the organization's quality improvement program, with the goal of becoming restraint free.

A   16. Restraint is used only as follows:
- When alternatives to restraint are not effective, as determined by the interdisciplinary team, with resident and family involvement as appropriate
- When absolutely necessary to ensure the safety of the resident, other residents, and staff

C Ⓜ 17. When restraint is used, the following occurs:
- Staff interaction with the resident is positive and supportive in both verbal and nonverbal ways
- Staff interacts regularly and appropriately with the resident so that the resident is not neglected

B   18. Medication to control behavior is used as part of a therapeutic plan only after appropriate assessment by professionals.

Note: *Leaving residents in bed can be considered a form of restraint and is not to be used for the staff's convenience.*

Standards PC.11.100 Through PC.12.190 ▬▬▬▬▬▬▬▬▬

Not applicable

Standards for Additional Special Procedures

Sedation and Anesthesia Care for Subacute Services

Operative or other procedures and the administration of sedation or anesthesia often occur simultaneously. However, procedures do occur without sedation, and sedation or anesthesia is administered for noninvasive procedures (hyperbaric treatment, CT scan, MRI). Therefore, the following standards address both operative or other procedures and/or the administration of moderate or deep sedation or anesthesia.

Whenever an operative or other procedure is conducted, whether or not sedation or anesthesia is administered, appropriate staff must be involved in planning for and providing care to the resident. All procedures carry risk, but that risk is increased when sedation or anesthesia is administered.

The standards for sedation and anesthesia care apply when residents in any setting receive, for any purpose, by any route, the following:
- General, spinal, or other major regional anesthesia
  or
- Moderate or deep sedation (with or without analgesia) that, in the manner used, may be reasonably expected to result in the loss of protective reflexes

PC

Because sedation is a continuum, it is not always possible to predict how an individual resident receiving sedation will respond. Therefore, each organization develops specific, appropriate protocols for the care of residents receiving sedation. These protocols are consistent with professional standards and address at least the following:
- Sufficient qualified individuals present to perform the procedure and to monitor the resident throughout administration and recovery. The individuals providing moderate or deep sedation and anesthesia have at a minimum had competency-based education, training, and experience in the following:
  1. Evaluating residents before performing moderate or deep sedation and anesthesia
  2. Performing the moderate or deep sedation and anesthesia, including rescuing residents who slip into a deeper-than-desired level of sedation or analgesia. These include the following:
     a. Moderate sedation—are qualified to rescue residents from deep sedation and are competent to manage a compromised airway and to provide adequate oxygenation and ventilation
     b. Deep sedation—are qualified to rescue residents from general anesthesia and are competent to manage an unstable cardiovascular system as well as a compromised airway and inadequate oxygenation and ventilation
- Appropriate equipment for care and resuscitation
- Appropriate monitoring of vital signs, including, but not limited to, heart rates and oxygenation using pulse oximetry equipment, respiratory frequency and adequacy of pulmonary ventilation, the monitoring of blood pressure at regular intervals, and cardiac monitoring (by EKG or use of continuous cardiac monitoring device) in residents with significant cardiovascular disease or when dysrhythmias are anticipated or detected

- Documentation of care
- Monitoring of outcomes

Definitions of four levels of sedation and anesthesia include the following:

- **Minimal sedation (anxiolysis)**
  A drug-induced state during which residents respond normally to verbal commands. Although cognitive function and coordination may be impaired, ventilatory and cardiovascular functions are unaffected.
- **Moderate sedation/analgesia ("conscious sedation")**
  A drug-induced depression of consciousness during which residents respond purposefully to verbal commands (note, reflex withdrawal from a painful stimulus is not considered a purposeful response)—either alone or accompanied by light tactile stimulation. No interventions are required to maintain a patent airway, and spontaneous ventilation is adequate. Cardiovascular function is usually maintained.
- **Deep sedation/analgesia**
  A drug-induced depression of consciousness during which residents cannot be easily aroused but respond purposefully after repeated or painful stimulation. The ability to independently maintain ventilatory function may be impaired. Residents may require assistance in maintaining a patent airway and spontaneous ventilation may be inadequate. Cardiovascular function is usually maintained.
- **Anesthesia**
  Consists of general anesthesia and spinal or major regional anesthesia. It does not include local anesthesia. General anesthesia is a drug-induced loss of consciousness during which residents are not arousable, even by painful stimulation. The ability to independently maintain ventilatory function is often impaired. Residents often require assistance in maintaining a patent airway, and positive pressure ventilation may be required because of depressed spontaneous ventilation or drug-induced depression of neuromuscular function. Cardiovascular function may be impaired.

Standard PC.13.10

Licensed independent practitioners define the scope of assessment for operative or other procedures and/or the administration of moderate or deep sedation or anesthesia.

Rationale for PC.13.10

The scope of assessment is defined to enhance the safety of the procedures' performance.

Element of Performance for PC.13.10

B   1.   The assessment includes the following:
- The resident's history
- The resident's physical status
- Diagnostic data

- The risks and benefits of procedures
- The possible need to administer blood or blood components

Standard PC.13.20 ■■■■■■■■■■■■■■■■■■■■■■■■■■■■■■■■■■■■

Operative or other procedures and/or the administration of moderate or deep sedation or anesthesia are planned.

Rationale for PC.13.20

Because the response to procedures is not always predictable and sedation-to-anes-
thesia is a continuum, it is not always possible to predict how an individual resident
will respond. Therefore, qualified individuals are trained in professional standards
and techniques to manage residents in the case of a potentially harmful event.

Elements of Performance for PC.13.20

B   1.   Sufficient numbers of qualified staff (in addition to the licensed independent practitioner performing the procedure) are present to evaluate
the resident, help with the procedure, provide the sedation and/or anesthesia, monitor, and recover the resident.

A   2.   Individuals administering moderate or deep sedation and anesthesia
are qualified and have the appropriate credentials to manage residents
at whatever level of sedation or anesthesia is achieved, either intentionally or unintentionally.

　 3.   Not applicable

B   4.   Appropriate equipment to monitor the resident's physiologic status is
available.

B   5.   Appropriate equipment to administer intravenous fluids and drugs,
including blood and blood components, is available as needed.

B   6.   Resuscitation capabilities are available.

The following must occur before the operative and other procedures or the administration of moderate or deep sedation or anesthesia (EPs 7–10):

C Ⓜ   7.   The anticipated needs of the resident are assessed to plan for the appropriate level of postprocedure care.

C Ⓜ   8.   Preprocedural education, treatments, and services are provided
according to the plan for care, treatment, and services.

A   9.   The site, procedure, and resident are accurately identified and clearly
communicated, using active communication techniques, during a final
verification process such as a time out before the start of any surgical or
invasive procedure.

A   10.   A presedation or preanesthesia assessment is conducted.

A   11. Before sedating or anesthetizing a resident, a licensed independent practitioner with appropriate clinical privileges plans or concurs with the planned anesthesia.

A   12. The resident is reevaluated immediately before moderate or deep sedation and before anesthesia induction.

Standard PC.13.30

Residents are monitored during the procedure and/or administration of moderate or deep sedation or anesthesia.

Elements of Performance for PC.13.30

A   1. Appropriate methods are used to continuously monitor oxygenation, ventilation, and circulation during procedures that may affect the resident's physiological status.

C ⓜ 2. The procedure and/or the administration of moderate or deep sedation or anesthesia for each resident is documented in the medical record.

Standard PC.13.40

Residents are monitored immediately after the procedure and/or administration of moderate or deep sedation or anesthesia.

Elements of Performance for PC.13.40

A   1. The resident's status is assessed immediately after the procedure and/or administration of moderate or deep sedation or anesthesia.

C ⓜ 2. Each resident's physiological status, mental status, and pain level are monitored.

B   3. Monitoring is at a level consistent with the potential effect of the procedure and/or sedation or anesthesia.

B   4. Residents are discharged from the recovery area and the organization by a qualified licensed independent practitioner or according to rigorously applied criteria approved by the clinical leaders.

C ⓜ 5. Residents who have received sedation or anesthesia are discharged in the company of a responsible, designated adult.

Additional Special Procedures

Standards PC.13.50 Through PC.14.30

Not applicable

Discharge or Transfer from the Organization

Residents may be discharged from the organization entirely or discharged or transferred to another level of care, treatment, and services; to different health professionals; or to settings for continued services. The organization's processes for transfer or discharge are based on the residents' assessed needs. To facilitate discharge or transfer, the organization assesses the resident's needs; plans for discharge or transfer; facilitates the discharge or transfer process; and helps ensure that continuity of care, treatment, and services is maintained.

Standard PC.15.10

A process addresses the needs for continuing care, treatment, and services after discharge or transfer.

Elements of Performance for PC.15.10

B 1. The process addresses the following:
- The reason(s) for transfer or discharge
- The conditions under which transfer or discharge can occur
- Interdisciplinary team planning
- The residents' and caregivers' knowledge of and demonstration of all necessary activities
- Assessment of the environment (home, hospital, other facility) to which the resident is being discharged
- Identification of and indication of the involvement of supportive services*
- Plan for providing necessary care, treatment, services, assistance, and instruction
- Shifting responsibility for a resident's care from one clinician, organization, organizational program, or service to another (which could include transferring complete responsibility for the resident and his or her care, treatment, and services to others or referring the resident to others, such as one or more agencies or professionals, to provide one or more specific services)
- Mechanisms for internal and external transfer
- The accountability and responsibility for the resident's safety during transfer of both the organization initiating the transfer and the organization receiving the resident

2. Not applicable

3. Not applicable

C Ⓜ 4. Residents are transferred or discharged by order of their attending physician.

PC

---

* Supportive services include community referral information and telephone numbers, needs for medical and adaptive equipment, specific instructions on medication administration and adverse effects, and follow-up appointments.

B 5. The organization follows an established process for emergency discharge resulting from medical necessity.

Standard PC.15.20

The transfer or discharge of a resident to another level of care, treatment, and services, different professionals, or different settings is based on the resident's assessed
needs and the organization's capabilities.

Rationale for PC.15.20

For some residents, effective planning addresses how needs will be met as they
move to the next level of care, treatment, and services. For other residents, planning will consist of a clear understanding of how to access services in the future
should the need arise.

Elements of Performance for PC.15.20

C Ⓜ 1. The resident's needs for continuing care to meet physical and psychosocial needs are identified.

C Ⓜ 2. Residents are told in a timely manner of the need to plan for discharge
or transfer to another organization or level of care.

C Ⓜ 3. Planning for transfer or discharge involves the resident and all appropriate licensed independent practitioners, staff, and family members
involved in the resident's care, treatment, and services.

C Ⓜ 4. When the resident is transferred, information provided to the resident
includes the following:
- The reason they are being transferred
- Information on the facility or program to which the resident is being
transferred
- Alternatives to transfer, if any

5. Not applicable

C Ⓜ 6. When the resident is discharged, information provided to residents
includes the following:
- The reason they are being discharged
- The anticipated need for continued care, treatment, and services*
after discharge

C Ⓜ 7. When indicated, the resident is educated about how to obtain further
care, treatment, and services to meet his or her identified needs.

---

* Available services include, as appropriate, special education, adult day care, case management, home health
services, hospice, long term care facilities, ambulatory care, support groups, rehabilitation services, and community mental health services.

C Ⓜ 8. When indicated and before discharge, the organization arranges for or helps the family arrange for services needed to meet the resident's needs after discharge.

C Ⓜ 9. Written discharge instructions in a form the resident can understand are given to the resident and/or those responsible for providing continuing care.

C Ⓜ 10. The organization notifies the resident's family and encourages a family member to participate in the transfer, whenever possible.

Standard PC.15.30

When residents are transferred or discharged, appropriate information related to the care, treatment, and services provided is exchanged with other service providers.

Rationale for PC.15.30

A resident may receive care, treatment, and services in many settings and may move from one organization or provider to another. To facilitate the continuity of care, treatment, and services, information is provided to any organization or provider to which the resident is accepted, transferred, or discharged.

PC

Elements of Performance for PC.15.30

C Ⓜ 1. The organization communicates appropriate information to any organization or provider to which the resident is transferred or discharged.

C Ⓜ 2. The information shared includes the following, as appropriate to the care, treatment, and services provided:
- The reason for transfer or discharge
- A summary of care, treatment, and services provided and progress toward goals
- Community resources or referrals provided to the resident

Standard PC.15.40

Residents are not transferred or discharged unless they meet specific criteria in accordance with law and regulation.

Element of Performance for PC.15.40

C Ⓜ 1. The organization permits each resident to remain in the facility and does not transfer or discharge a resident unless as follows:
- The transfer or discharge is necessary for the resident's welfare, or the organization cannot meet his or her needs
- The transfer or discharge is appropriate because the resident's health has sufficiently improved; therefore, he or she no longer needs the organization's services

- The health or safety of residents in the facility is endangered
- After reasonable and appropriate notice as defined by the organization and in accordance with applicable law and regulation, the resident has not paid for a stay at the facility
- For a resident who becomes eligible for Medicaid after admission, the organization may charge only the Medicaid-allowable charge
- The organization ceases operation
- The resident leaves against medical advice. Such a resident signs a form stating that he or she is aware of leaving against medical advice.

Standard PC.15.50

The organization tells residents and their families of its bed-hold policy.

Element of Performance for PC.15.50

B   1.   At admission or when a resident transfers to a hospital, the organization explains in writing the conditions of its bed-hold policy to the resident and a family member or legal guardian.

PC

Waived Testing

The federal regulation governing laboratory testing, known as the Clinical Laboratory Improvement Amendments of 1988 (CLIA '88), classifies testing into four complexity levels: high complexity, moderate complexity, PPM (Provider Performed Microscopy, a subset of moderate complexity), and waived testing. The high, moderate, and PPM levels, otherwise called nonwaived testing, have specific and detailed requirements regarding personnel qualifications, quality assurance, quality control, and other systems. Joint Commission requirements for the tests and laboratories or sites that perform them are located in the *Comprehensive Accreditation Manual for Laboratory and Point-of-Care Testing (CAMLAB)*.

Waived testing is the most common complexity level performed by caregivers at the resident's bedside or point of care. The same laboratory test may be available by more than one method within an organization, and those methods may be of different complexity levels. The list of methods that are approved as waived is under constant revision, so it is advisable to check the Food and Drug Administration (FDA), Centers for Disease Control and Prevention (CDC), or Centers for Medicare & Medicaid Services (CMS) Web sites for the most up-to-date information regarding test categorization and complete CLIA requirements:

- http://www.fda.gov/cdrh/clia/index.html
- http://www.phppo.cdc.gov/clia
- http://www.cms.hhs.gov/clia

CLIA '88 identifies laboratory testing as an activity that occurs, not defined as "occurring" at a specific location. Any activity that evaluates any substance removed from a human body and translates that evaluation to a result becomes a laboratory test. The results may be stated as a number, presence or absence of a cell or reaction, or an interpretation, such as what occurs when recording a urine color. Test results that are used to assess a resident's condition or make a clinical decision about a resident are governed by CLIA '88.

Tests that produce a result measured as a number are called "quantitative" and are usually performed with the assistance of some type of instrument. Tests that produce a negative or positive result, such as occult bloods and urine pregnancy screens, are termed "qualitative" and are usually known as manual tests. Any test with analysis steps that rely on the use of an instrument to produce a result is an instrument-based test.

When a resident performs a test on himself or herself (for example, whole blood glucose testing by a resident on his or her own meter cleared by the FDA for home use), the action is not regulated. Testing performed by one individual on another individual while carrying out professional responsibilities is an activity regulated by CLIA '88. This distinction is important when caring for residents who monitor their own glucose or prothrombin times with home devices.

Standard PC.16.10

The organization establishes policies and procedures that define the context in which waived test results are used in resident care, treatment, and services.

Elements of Performance for PC.16.10

B   1.   Quantitative test result reports in the clinical record are accompanied by reference intervals specific to the test method used and are appropriate to the population served.

B   2.   Criteria for confirmatory testing for each test, qualitative or quantitative, is specified in the written procedure as dictated by clinical usage and methodology limitations.

B   3.   Actual usage is consistent with the organization's policies and the manufacturer's recommendations for each waived test.

Standard PC.16.20

The organization identifies the staff responsible for performing and supervising waived testing.

Elements of Performance for PC.16.20

B   1.   Staff members who perform testing are identified.

B   2.   Staff members who direct or supervise testing are identified.

> **Note:** *These individuals may be employees of the organization, contracted staff, or employees of a contracted service.*

Standard PC.16.30 ▬▬▬▬▬▬▬▬▬▬▬

Staff performing tests have adequate, specific training and orientation to perform the tests and demonstrate satisfactory levels of competence.

Rationale for PC.16.30

For waived tests to be performed properly, the staff performing them must be qualified to do so. Staff members who perform waived testing have specific training in each test performed. This training may be acquired through organization or other training programs, such as those provided by other health care organizations or manufacturers.

Elements of Performance for PC.16.30

C Ⓜ 1. Current competence of testing staff is demonstrated.

C Ⓜ 2. Each staff member who performs testing has been trained specifically to each test he or she is authorized to perform.

C Ⓜ 3. Each staff member who performs testing has been oriented according to the organization's specific needs.

B 4. Testing that requires the use of an instrument is performed by staff with adequate and specific training on the use and care of that instrument.

C Ⓜ 5. Competence is assessed according to organization policy at defined intervals, but at least at the time of orientation and annually thereafter.

B 6. These assessments have considered the following:
- The frequency by which staff members perform tests
- The technical backgrounds of the staff
- The complexity of the test methodology and the consequences of an inaccurate result

B 7. Methods to assess current competency include at least two of the following:
- Performing a test on an unknown specimen
- Having the supervisor or qualified delegate periodically observe routine work
- Monitoring each user's quality control performance
- Having written testing that is specific to the method assessed

B 8. The organization evaluates and documents the information listed above.

Note: *All staff who perform instrument-based testing, including but not limited to physicians, licensed independent practitioners, contracted staff, and RNs, must participate in training and competence demonstrations.*

Standard PC.16.40

Approved policies and procedures governing specific testing-related processes are current and readily available.

Rationale for PC.16.40

Current and up-to-date policies and procedures are an important reference tool in managing laboratory testing activities, particularly when individual staff members perform them infrequently. Testing policies and procedures include requirements that are in compliance with the manufacturer's recommendations regarding all of the following, as applicable:

- Specimen type (for example, a method for whole blood is not used for spinal fluid)
- Storage considerations for test components (for example, compliance with directions such as store away from direct light, temperature requirements, open container expiration dates, and so forth)
- Instrument maintenance and function checks such as calibration
- Quality control frequency and type
- Result follow-up recommendations (for example, out-of-range results' recommendation for retesting)
- Tests approved by the FDA for home use only are not used for professional purposes (for example, glucose meters cleared for home use only are not used in a hospital setting by nursing staff except as resident education)

Elements of Performance for PC.16.40

B 1. Written policies and procedures address all the following items:
- Specimen collection, identification, and required labeling, as appropriate
- Specimen preservation, as appropriate
- Instrument calibration
- Quality control and remedial action
- Equipment performance evaluation
- Test performance

B 2. The policies and procedures for each item are applicable to the specific organization.

Note: *Reference to a manufacturer's manual is acceptable if appropriate modifications have been made to customize the manual's content for the organization.*

C Ⓜ 3. Current and complete policies and procedures are readily available to the person performing the test.

A 4. The director named on the waived testing certificate or a designee approves policies and procedures at defined intervals.

Standard PC.16.50 ▬▬▬▬▬▬▬▬▬▬▬▬▬▬▬▬▬▬▬▬

Quality control checks, as defined by the organization, are conducted on each procedure.

Elements of Performance for PC.16.50

B   1.   The organization has a written quality control plan that specifies how procedures will be controlled for quality, establishes timetables, and explains the rationale for choice of procedures and timetables.

B   2.   Quality control procedures are performed at least as frequently as recommended by the manufacturer, according to the organization's policies.

C Ⓜ 3.   For instrument-based waived testing, quality control requirements include two levels of control, if commercially available.

C Ⓜ 4.   Quality control procedures are performed at least once each day on each instrument used for resident testing.

B   5.   The documented quality control rationale is based on the following:
   - How the test is used
   - Reagent stability
   - Manufacturers' recommendations
   - The organization's experience with the test
   - Currently accepted guidelines

B   6.   At a minimum, manufacturers' instructions are followed.

Standard PC.16.60 ▬▬▬▬▬▬▬▬▬▬▬▬▬▬▬▬▬▬▬▬

Appropriate quality control and test records are maintained.

Elements of Performance for PC.16.60

C Ⓜ 1.   All quality control test results are documented, including internal, external, liquid, and electronic.

C Ⓜ 2.   Test results are documented.

   Note: *Test results may be located in the clinical record.*

B   3.   Quality control records, instrument problems, and individual results are correlated.

B   4.   A formal log is not required, but a functional audit trail is maintained that allows retrieval of results and associated quality control values for a minimum of two years.

Medication* Management

Overview

Medication management is often an important component in the palliative, symptomatic, and curative treatment of many diseases and conditions. A safe medication management system addresses an organization's medication processes, including the following (as applicable):

- Selection and procurement
- Storage
- Ordering and transcribing
- Preparing and dispensing
- Administration
- Monitoring

Effective and safe medication management involves multiple services and disciplines working closely together. These standards address activities involving various individuals within an organization's medication management system, including, as appropriate to the setting, licensed independent practitioners, health care professionals, and staff involved in medication management processes.

A well-planned and implemented medication management system supports resident safety and improves the quality of care by doing the following:

- Reducing practice variation, errors, and misuse
- Monitoring medication management processes in regard to efficiency, quality, and safety
- Standardizing equipment and processes across the organization to improve the medication management system
- Using evidence-based good practices to develop medication management processes
- Managing critical processes associated with medication management to promote safe medication management throughout the organization
- Handling all medications in the same manner, including sample medications

An effective medication management system includes mechanisms for reporting potential and actual errors and a process to improve medication management processes and resident safety based on this information. The most effective feedback and improvement systems usually operate in organizations with a nonpunitive culture.

---

* For the purpose of these standards, *medication* includes prescription medications; sample medications; herbal remedies; vitamins; nutraceuticals; over-the-counter drugs; vaccines; diagnostic and contrast agents used on or administered to persons to diagnose, treat, or prevent disease or other abnormal conditions; radioactive medications; respiratory therapy treatments; parenteral nutrition; blood derivatives; intravenous solutions (plain, with electrolytes and/or drugs); and any product designated by the Food and Drug Administration (FDA) as a drug. The definition of *medication* does not include enteral nutrition solutions (which are considered food products), oxygen, and other medical gases.

The medication management chapter (standards MM.1.10 through MM.8.10) addresses critical medication management processes, including those undertaken by the organization and those provided through contracted pharmacy services. When pharmacy services are provided through a contract, the contract should address responsibility for these standards and performance expectations. An organization receiving pharmacy services should monitor the performance of contracted services. When an onsite pharmacy exists, the pharmacy is responsible for the control and distribution of all medications used in the organization. When medications are dispensed by outside pharmacies, the long term care facility, in conjunction with the consultant pharmacist, designs, monitors, and determines whether the medication management system meets applicable law and regulation, accepted standards of practice, and organization policies and procedures.

Medication* Management

Medications are essential to resident care; however, their use and handling entail certain risks. The following standards identify significant risk points and offer a system for managing them. Medical evaluation of past and current drug treatments is conducted when medications are used. Treatment efficacy, impact on current functioning, and side effects are considered, including evaluations from the resident, family, or caregivers. These standards address the following components of medication management:

- Availability
- Prescribing or ordering[†]
- Preparation and dispensing
- Administration
- Monitoring of effect

---

* **Medication** Any prescription medications; sample medications; herbal remedies; vitamins; nutriceuticals; over-the-counter drugs; vaccines; diagnostic and contrast agents used on or administered to persons to diagnose, treat, or prevent disease or other abnormal conditions; radioactive medications; respiratory therapy treatments; parenteral nutrition; blood derivatives; intravenous solutions (plain, with electrolytes and/or drugs); and any product designated by the FDA as a drug. This definition of medication does not include enteral nutrition solutions, oxygen, and other medical gases.

[†] **Prescribing or ordering** Directing the preparation, dispensing, or administration of a specific medication(s) to a specific resident.

Standards

The following is a list of all standards for this chapter. They are presented here for your convenience without footnotes or other explanatory text. If you have a question about a term used here, please check the Glossary.

Note: *A revised standard numbering system is being used with the reformatted standards. This revised numbering system will allow for more flexibility to add standards while maintaining the current label for each standard.*

Resident-Specific Information

MM.1.10   Resident-specific information is readily accessible to those involved in the medication management system.

Selection and Procurement

MM.2.10   Medications available for dispensing or administration are selected, listed, and procured based on criteria.

Storage

MM.2.20   Medications are properly and safely stored throughout the organization.

MM.2.30   Emergency medications and/or supplies, if any, are consistently available, controlled, and secure in the organization's resident care areas.

MM.2.40   A process is established to safely manage medications brought into the organization by residents or their families.

Ordering and Transcribing

MM.3.10   Only medications needed to treat the resident's condition are ordered.

MM.3.20   Medication orders are written clearly and transcribed accurately.

Preparing and Dispensing

MM.4.10   All prescriptions or medication orders are reviewed for appropriateness.

MM.4.20   Medications are prepared safely.

MM.4.30   Medications are appropriately labeled.

MM.4.40   Medications are dispensed safely.

MM

MM.4.50   The organization has a system for safely providing medications to meet resident needs when the pharmacy is closed.

MM.4.60   If the organization does not operate a pharmacy but routinely administers medications, then the organization has a process for obtaining medications from a pharmacy.

MM.4.70   Medications dispensed by the organization are retrieved when recalled or discontinued by the manufacturer or the Food and Drug Administration for safety reasons.

MM.4.80   Medications returned to the pharmacy are appropriately managed.

Administering

MM.5.10   Medications are safely and accurately administered.

MM.5.20   Self-administered medications are safely and accurately administered.

MM.5.30   Not applicable

Monitoring

MM.6.10   The effects of medication(s) on residents are monitored.

MM.6.20   The organization responds appropriately to actual or potential adverse drug events and medication errors.

High-Risk Medications

MM.7.10   The organization develops processes for managing high-risk or high-alert medications.

MM.7.20   Psychotropic medication use is monitored.

MM.7.30   Not applicable

MM.7.40   Investigational medications are safely controlled and administered.

Evaluation

MM.8.10   The organization evaluates its medication management system.

Understanding the Parts of This Chapter

To help you navigate this reformatted standards chapter, it may be helpful to think of its parts this way:

- The **standard** is the "goal"
- The **rationale** explains why it's important to achieve this goal
- The **elements of performance** identify the step(s) needed to achieve this goal

These parts are defined as follows.

Standard A statement that defines the performance expectations and/or structures or processes that must be in place for an organization to provide safe, high-quality care, treatment, and services. An organization is either "compliant" or "not compliant" with a standard.

Accreditation decisions are based on simple counts of the standards that are determined to be "not compliant."

Rationale A statement that provides background, justification, or additional information about a standard. A standard's rationale is not scored. In some instances, the rationale for a standard is self-evident. Therefore, not every standard has a written rationale.

Elements of performance (EPs) The specific performance expectations and/or structures or processes that must be in place for an organization to provide safe, high-quality care, treatment, and services. The scoring of EP compliance determines an organization's overall compliance with a standard. EPs are evaluated on the following scale:

MM

0	Insufficient compliance
1	Partial compliance
2	Satisfactory compliance
NA	Not applicable

You will find a **measure of success** icon—**Ⓜ**—next to some EPs. Measures of success (MOS) need to be developed for certain EPs when a standard is judged to be out of compliance through either the Periodic Performance Review (PPR) or the onsite survey. An MOS is defined as a quantifiable measure, usually related to an audit, that can be used to determine whether an action has been effective and is being sustained.*

Assessing Your Compliance

Once you are familiar with the parts of this chapter, you can begin to assess your compliance with its requirements. The scoring category designations are provided next to each EP for your convenience. If you would like to assess your organization's performance, mark your scores for the EPs and standards by following the simple steps described below.

---

* For more information about MOS, *see* "The New Joint Commission Accreditation Process" chapter in this book.

Two components are scored for each EP: (1) compliance with the requirement itself **and** (2) compliance with the track record* for that requirement. Scoring has been simplified and track record achievements (which have always been part of the scoring) have been appropriately modified.

Note: *Some standards and EPs do not apply to a particular type of organization; these standards and EPs are marked "not applicable" and the related text is not included. Your organization is not expected to comply with standards and EPs marked "not applicable."*

In addition, some standards and EPs that do apply to organizations may not apply to the specific care, treatment, and services that your individual organization provides. Although these standards and EPs are included in the book, you are not expected to comply with them. If you are unsure about the standards or EPs that apply to your organization, please contact the Joint Commission's Standards Interpretation Group at 630/792-5900.

Step 1: Score Your Compliance with Each Element of Performance

Before you can determine your compliance with the standards, you must score your compliance with each EP. There are three scoring criterion categories: A, B, and C (described below). Please note that for each EP scoring criterion category, your organization must meet the performance requirement itself and the track record achievements (*see* "Track Record Achievements").

Category A

These EPs relate to the presence or absence of the requirement(s) and are scored either yes (2) or no (0); however, score 1 for partial compliance is also possible based on track record achievements.

If an A EP has multiple components designated by bullets, your organization must be compliant with all the bullets to receive a score of 2. If your organization does not meet one or more requirements in the bullets, you will receive a score of 0.

Category B

Category B EPs are scored in two steps:
1. As with category A EPs, category B EPs relate to the presence or absence of the requirement(s). If your organization *does not meet* the requirement(s), the EP is scored 0; there is no need to assess your compliance with the principles of good process design.
2. If your organization *does meet* the requirement(s), but there is concern about the quality or comprehensiveness of the effort, then and only then should you assess the qualitative aspect of the EP. That is, review the applicable principles of good process design and ask how the principles were applied in the situation under discussion. Good process design has the following characteristics:

---

* **Track record** The amount of time that an organization has been in compliance with a standard, EP, or other requirement.

MM

- Is consistent with your organization's mission, values, and goals
- Meets the needs of patients
- Reflects the use of currently accepted practices (doing the right thing, using resources responsibly, using practice guidelines)
- Incorporates current safety information and knowledge such as sentinel event data and National Patient Safety Goals
- Incorporates relevant performance improvement results

This two-part evaluation applies to both simple and bulleted B EPs. First, the EPs are assessed to determine whether the requirements are present. If the EP has multiple components designated by bullets, as with the category A EPs, your organization must meet the requirements in *all* the bulleted items to get a score of 2. If your organization meets *none* of the requirements in the bullets, it receives a score of 0. If your organization meets *at least one, but not all,* of the bulleted requirements, it receives a score of 1 for the EPs.

Use the following rules to determine your EP score:
- Your EP score is 0 if your organization does not meet the requirement(s); you *do not* need to assess your compliance with the preceding applicable principles of good process design
- Your EP score is 1 if your organization does meet the requirement(s) but considered only *some* of the preceding applicable principles of good process design
- Your EP score is 2 if your organization does meet the requirement(s) *and* considered *all* the preceding principles of good process design

MM

Category C

C EPs are scored 0, 1, or 2 based on the number of times your organization does not meet the EP. These EPs are frequency based and require totaling the number of occurrences (that is, results of performance or nonperformance) related to a particular EP. Each situation discovered by a surveyor(s) will be counted as a separate occurrence.

Note: *Multiple events of the same type related to a single resident and single practitioner/staff member are counted as* one occurrence only.

Use the following rules to determine your EP score:
- Your EP score is 2 if you find one or fewer occurrences of noncompliance with the EP
- Your EP score is 1 if you find two occurrences of noncompliance with the EP
- Your EP score is 0 if you find three or more occurrences of noncompliance with the EP

If an EP in the C category has multiple requirements designated by bullets, the following scoring guidelines apply:
- If there are fewer than two findings in all bullets, the EP is scored 2
- If there are three or more findings in all bullets, the EP is scored 0
- In all other combinations of findings, the EP is scored 1

Track Record Achievements

In addition to meeting the requirement(s) in each EP, regardless of category, your organization must also meet the following track record achievements:

Score	Initial Survey	Full Survey
2	4 months or more	12 months or more
1	2 to 3 months	6 to 11 months
0	Fewer than 2 months	Fewer than 6 months

Sample Sizes

If during an onsite survey, your organization has been found to be not compliant with one or more standards, you must demonstrate Evidence of Standards Compliance (ESC) for each standard that is not compliant. The ESC must address compliance at the EP level; when an EP within a noncompliant standard requires an MOS, your organization must demonstrate achievement with the MOS when completing the ESC.

Note: *Not every EP requires an MOS. EPs that do require an MOS are clearly marked in this chapter. Organizations are required to demonstrate achievement with an MOS only for EPs within a noncompliant standard that require an MOS. Organizations do not need to demonstrate achievement with an MOS for any EP within a compliant standard.*

MM

When demonstrating achievement with an MOS during the ESC process, your organization is **required** to use the following sample sizes, which were established because of their statistical significance, their relative simplicity in application, and their sensitivity to an organization's population size:

- For a population size of fewer than 30 cases,* sample 100% of available cases
- For a population size of 30 to 100 cases, sample 30 cases
- For a population size of 101 to 500 cases, sample 50 cases
- For a population size greater than 500 cases, sample 70 cases

Note: *Organizations are* encouraged, but not required, *to follow this sample size when demonstrating achievement with an MOS for an EP within a noncompliant standard after conducting a full, Option 1, or Option 2 PPR.*

When conducting PPR (optional use) or demonstrating an ESC (mandatory use), use the following percentages to determine your EP score: 90% through 100% of your sample size is in compliance = score 2; 80% through 89% of your sample size is in compliance = score 1; less than 80% of your sample size is in compliance = score 0.

In addition, the following information should govern your organization's selection of samples:

- The appropriate sample size should be determined by the specific population related to the survey findings

---

* *Case* refers to a single instance in which a situation related to a survey finding occurs. For example, if a survey finding was related to **pain assessment**, then a case would be any resident record. If a survey finding was related to **pain management**, a case would be any resident record for residents receiving pain management.

- The sampling approach should involve either systematic random sampling (for example, your organization selects every second or third case for review) or simple random sampling (for example, your organization uses a series of random numbers generated by a computer to identify the cases to be reviewed)
- If your organization chooses not to use these sample sizes while conducting PPR options 1 or 2, you should make sure that your sample size is sufficiently large enough to ensure statistical significance
- When submitting a clarifying ESC, if your organization selects records as part of its sample, the records should be from a period of no more than three months before the last date of the survey
- Assessment of MOS compliance is conducted for a four-month period following the date of ESC approval. Your organization should select records as a part of your sample following the date of ESC approval and use the required sample sizes. MOS percentage compliance rates are derived from the average of all four months.

Step 2: Use Your EP Scores to Gauge Your Compliance with the Standards

Now that you have evaluated and scored each EP for a particular standard, use these simple rules to determine your compliance with the standard itself:

- Your organization is not in compliance (that is, "not compliant") with the standard if any EP is scored 0
- Otherwise, your organization is in compliance with a standard if 65% or more of its EPs are scored 2

MM

Standard, Rationales, Elements of Performance, and Scoring

Resident-Specific Information

Standard MM.1.10

Resident-specific information is readily accessible to those involved in the medication management system.

Rationale for MM.1.10

A major cause of medication-related sentinel events and medication errors is a lack of information. Licensed independent practitioners, appropriate health care professionals, and staff who participate in the medication management system need access to important information about each resident in order to do the following:

- Facilitate continuity of care, treatment, and services
- Create an accurate medication history and a current list of medications (also known as a drug profile)
- Safely order, prepare, dispense, administer, and monitor medications, as appropriate

MM

Elements of Performance for MM.1.10

B   1.   A written policy describes the minimum amount of information about the resident that is to be available to those involved in medication management.

  Note: *The organization defines who has access to this information; see standard IM.2.10.*

A   2.   At a minimum, the information includes the following:
- The resident's age
- The resident's sex
- The resident's current medications
- The resident's diagnoses, comorbidities, and concurrently occurring conditions
- The resident's relevant laboratory values
- The resident's allergies and past sensitivities

  As appropriate to the resident, the organization also includes information regarding the following:
- Weight and height
- Pregnancy and lactation status
- Any other information required by the organization for safe medication management

C Ⓜ 3. The information is accessible when needed (except in emergency situations when time does not permit) to licensed independent practitioners, appropriate health care professionals, and staff.

Selection and Procurement

Standard MM.2.10 ━━━━━━━━━━━━━━━━━━━━━━━━━━━━━━━━

Medications available for dispensing or administration are selected, listed, and procured based on criteria.

Note 1: *This standard is applicable to all onsite pharmacies and pharmacies contracted by the long term care facility to provide medications to its residents.*

Note 2: *The formulary is synonymous with the list of medications available for use.*

Elements of Performance for MM.2.10

B 1. Licensed independent practitioners, appropriate health care professionals, and staff involved in ordering, dispensing, administering, and/or monitoring effects of medications, including the medical director, develop criteria for determining what medications are available for dispensing or administration.

A 2. At a minimum, the criteria include the indication for use, effectiveness, risks (including propensity for medication errors, abuse potential, and sentinel events), and costs.

A 3. A list of medications for dispensing or administration (including strength and dosage form) is maintained and readily available.

   Note: *Sample medications are not required to be on this list.*

B 4. Processes and mechanisms are established to monitor resident responses to a newly added medication before the medication is made available for dispensing or administration within the organization.

B 5. Medications designated as available for dispensing or administration are reviewed at least annually based on emerging safety and efficacy information.

B 6. The organization has processes to approve and procure medications that are not on the organization's medication list.

B 7. The organization has processes to address medication shortages and outages, including the following:
   - Communicating with appropriate prescribers and staff
   - Developing approved substitution protocols

MM

- Educating appropriate licensed independent practitioners, appropriate health care professionals, and staff about these protocols
- Obtaining medications in the event of a disaster

Storage

Standard MM.2.20

Medications are properly and safely stored throughout the organization.

Note: *The following EPs also apply to emergency medications. Additional requirements for emergency medications are addressed at standard MM.2.30.*

Elements of Performance for MM.2.20

A Ⓜ 1. Only approved medications are routinely stocked or stored.*

A Ⓜ 2. Medications are stored under necessary conditions to ensure stability.

A 3. Medications are secured in accordance with the organization's policy and law and regulation so that unauthorized persons cannot obtain access to them.

A 4. Controlled substances are stored to prevent diversion and according to state and federal laws and regulations.

A 5. All expired, damaged, and/or contaminated medications are segregated until they are removed from the organization.

B 6. Medications that are easy to confuse (for example, sound-alike and look-alike drugs or reagents and chemicals that may be mistaken for medications) are segregated.

A 7. Medications and chemicals used to prepare medications are accurately labeled with contents, expiration dates, and appropriate warnings.

A 8. Drug concentrations available in the organization are standardized and limited in number.

A Ⓜ 9. Concentrated electrolytes are removed from care units or areas, unless resident safety is at risk if the concentrated electrolyte is not immediately available on a specific care unit or area and specific precautions are taken to prevent inadvertent administration.

10. Not applicable

11. Not applicable

---

* **Note:** *See standard MM.2.40 for the exception to this standard: the organization has a process to safely manage medications brought in by the resident or the resident's family.*

12. Not applicable

C Ⓜ 13. All medication storage areas are periodically inspected according to the organization's policy to make sure medications are stored properly.

Standard MM.2.30

Emergency medications and/or supplies, if any, are consistently available, controlled, and secure in the organization's resident care areas.

Note: *The following requirements for emergency medications are in addition to the requirements at standard MM.2.20, which are also applicable to emergency medications.*

Elements of Performance for MM.2.30

B 1. Organization leadership, in conjunction with licensed independent practitioners and other health care professionals whose scope of practice includes the dispensing or administration of emergency medications, decides which emergency medications and/or supplies, if any, will be readily available in care areas.

2. Not applicable

B 3. Emergency medications are available in unit-dose, age-specific, and ready-to-administer forms whenever possible.

A Ⓜ 4. Emergency medications are sealed or stored in containers (for example, crash carts, tackle boxes, emergency drug kits, closed bags that are clearly labeled, and so forth) in such a way that staff can readily determine that the contents are complete and have not expired.

5. Not applicable

6. Not applicable

B 7. Emergency medications and supplies are replaced as soon as possible after their use in accordance with the organization's policies and procedures.

MM

Standard MM.2.40

A process is established to safely manage medications brought into the organization by residents or their families.

Rationale for MM.2.40

A number of valid reasons exist for allowing residents to use their own medications in a health care organization, including avoidance of interruption in therapy; a resident's use of a nonformulary medication; or a lack of alternatives to a resident's personal medication. The organization defines its responsibilities for the safe use of these medications.

Elements of Performance for MM.2.40

The organization develops a policy that addresses the use of medications brought into the organization by residents or their families. The policy specifies the following:

B   1.   When such medications can be used or administered

B   2.   A process for the identification of the medication and the visual evaluation of its integrity if medications brought in by the resident or family are allowed

A   3.   A process to inform the prescriber and resident if medications brought into the organization by residents or their families are not permitted

Ordering and Transcribing

Standard MM.3.10 ▬▬▬▬▬▬▬▬▬▬▬▬▬▬▬▬▬▬▬▬▬▬▬▬▬▬▬

Only medications needed to treat the resident's condition are ordered.

Element of Performance for MM.3.10

MM **C ⓜ** 1.   There is a documented diagnosis, condition, or indication-for-use for each medication ordered.

Standard MM.3.20 ▬▬▬▬▬▬▬▬▬▬▬▬▬▬▬▬▬▬▬▬▬▬▬▬▬▬▬

Medication orders are written clearly and transcribed accurately.

Rationale for MM.3.20

Many medication errors occur while communicating or transcribing medication orders. The organization should take steps to reduce the potential for error or misinterpretation when orders are written or verbally communicated.

Elements of Performance for MM.3.20

Written policy(ies) address the following (EPs 1–5):

B   1.   The required elements of a complete medication order

A   2.   When generic or brand names are acceptable or required as part of a medication order

A   3.   Whether or when indication for use is required on a medication order

B   4.   Any special precautions or procedures for ordering drugs with look-alike or sound-alike names

B   5.   Actions to take when medication orders are incomplete, illegible, or unclear

B 6. The organization specifies the required elements of any of the following types of orders that it deems acceptable for use:
- "As needed" (PRN) orders
- Standing orders
- Hold orders
- Automatic stop orders
- Resume orders
- Titrating orders—orders in which the dose is either progressively increased or decreased in response to the resident's status
- Taper orders—orders in which the dose is decreased by a particular amount with each dosing interval
- Range orders—orders in which the dose or dosing interval varies over a prescribed range, depending on the situation or resident's status
- Orders for compounded drugs or drug mixtures not commercially available
- Orders for medication-related devices (for example, nebulizers and catheters)
- Orders for investigational medications
- Orders for herbal products
- Orders for medications at discharge

In addition, the organization does the following:

7. Not applicable

B 8. Reviews and updates preprinted order sheets as needed

A 9. Specifies that blanket reinstatement of previous orders for medications are not acceptable

MM

Preparing and Dispensing

Standard MM.4.10 ▬▬▬▬▬▬▬▬▬▬▬▬▬▬▬▬▬▬▬▬▬▬▬▬

All prescriptions or medication orders are reviewed for appropriateness.

Note: *This standard is applicable to all onsite pharmacies and pharmacies contracted by the long term care facility to provide medications to its residents.*

Elements of Performance for MM.4.10

C Ⓜ 1. Before dispensing, removing from floor stock, or removing from an automated storage and distribution device, a pharmacist reviews all prescription or medication orders unless a licensed independent practitioner controls the ordering, preparation, and administration of the medication; or in urgent situations when the resulting delay would harm the resident, including situations in which the resident experiences a sudden change in clinical status (for example, new onset of nausea).

2. Not applicable

3. Not applicable

4. Not applicable

B 5. The organization has a process to review all prescriptions for the following:
- The appropriateness of the drug, dose, frequency, and route of administration
- Therapeutic duplication
- Real or potential allergies or sensitivities
- Real or potential interactions between the prescription and other medications, food, and laboratory values
- Other contraindications
- Variation from organizational criteria for use
- Other relevant medication-related issues or concerns

B 6. All concerns, issues, or questions are clarified with the individual prescriber before dispensing the medication.

MM

Standard MM.4.20
Medications are prepared safely.

Elements of Performance for MM.4.20

B 1. When an onsite, licensed pharmacy is available, only the pharmacy compounds or admixes all sterile medications, intravenous admixtures, or other drugs except in emergencies or when not feasible (for example, when the product's stability is short).

C Ⓜ 2. Wherever medications are prepared, staff uses safety materials and equipment while preparing hazardous medications.

C Ⓜ 3. Wherever medications are prepared, staff uses techniques to assure accuracy in medication preparation.

C Ⓜ 4. Wherever medications are prepared, staff uses appropriate techniques to avoid contamination during medication preparation, which include but are not limited to the following:
- Using clean or sterile technique as appropriate
- Maintaining clean, uncluttered, and functionally separate areas for product preparation to minimize the possibility of contamination
- Using a laminar airflow hood or other class 100 environment while preparing any intravenous (IV) admixture in the pharmacy, any sterile product made from nonsterile ingredients, or any sterile product that will not be used within 24 hours
- Visually inspecting the integrity of the medications

Standard MM.4.30 ▬▬▬▬▬▬▬▬▬▬▬▬▬▬▬▬▬▬▬▬▬▬▬▬

Medications are appropriately labeled.

Rationale for MM.4.30

A standardized method for labeling all medications will minimize errors.

Elements of Performance for MM.4.30

B   1.   Medications are labeled in a standardized manner according to organization policy, applicable law and regulation, and standards of practice.

B   2.   Any time one or more medications are prepared but are not administered immediately, the medication container* must be appropriately labeled.

A   3.   At a minimum, all medications are labeled with the following:
- Drug name, strength, amount (if not apparent from the container)
- Expiration date† when not used within 24 hours
- Expiration time when expiration occurs in less than 24 hours
- The date prepared and the diluent for all compounded IV admixtures and parenteral nutrition solutions

A   4.   When preparing individualized medications for multiple specific residents, or when the person preparing the individualized medications is not the person administering the medication, the label also includes the following:
- Resident name
- Resident location
- Directions for use and any applicable cautionary statements either on the label or attached as an accessory label (for example, "requires refrigeration," "for IM use only")

MM

Standard MM.4.40 ▬▬▬▬▬▬▬▬▬▬▬▬▬▬▬▬▬▬▬▬▬▬▬▬

Medications are dispensed safely.

Note: *This standard is applicable to all onsite pharmacies and pharmacies contracted by the long term care facility to provide medications to its residents.*

Elements of Performance for MM.4.40

B   1.   Quantities of medications are dispensed which minimize diversion yet are still consistent with the resident's needs.

B   2.   Dispensing adheres to law, regulation, licensure, and professional standards of practice, including record keeping.

---

* A container can be any storage device such as a plastic bag, syringe, bottle, or box which can be labeled and secured in such a way that it can be readily determined that the contents are intact and have not expired.

† Expiration date, also called the "beyond use date," refers to the last date that the product should be used by the resident.

C ⓂⒷ 3. Medications are dispensed in a timely manner to meet resident needs.

C Ⓜ 4. Medications are dispensed in the most ready-to-administer forms available from the manufacturer or, if feasible, in unit-doses that have been repackaged by the pharmacy or licensed repackager.

B 5. The organization consistently uses the same dose packaging system or, if a different system is used, provides education about the use of the dose packaging system to the appropriate residents.

Standard MM.4.50 ▬▬▬▬▬▬▬▬▬▬▬▬▬▬▬▬▬▬▬▬

The organization has a system for safely providing medications to meet resident needs when the pharmacy is closed.

Note: *This standard only applies when an organization has an onsite pharmacy and residents present in the organization.*

Rationale for MM.4.50

If an urgent or emergent resident need occurs, the organization must be able to provide medications to the residents in its facility.

Element of Performance for MM.4.50

B 1. The organization has a process for providing medications to meet resident needs when the pharmacy is closed.

Standard MM.4.60 ▬▬▬▬▬▬▬▬▬▬▬▬▬▬▬▬▬▬▬▬

If the organization does not operate a pharmacy but routinely administers medications, the organization has a process for obtaining medications from a pharmacy.

Elements of Performance for MM.4.60

A 1. If the organization does not operate a pharmacy, the organization has a process for obtaining medications from a pharmacy for its use in resident care.

A 2. If the organization obtains medications from a pharmacy that is not open 24 hours a day, 7 days a week, the organization has a process for obtaining medications from another source for urgent or emergent conditions when the pharmacy is closed.

Standard MM.4.70 ▬▬▬▬▬▬▬▬▬▬▬▬▬▬▬▬▬▬▬▬

Medications dispensed by the organization are retrieved when recalled or discontinued by the manufacturer or the Food and Drug Administration for safety reasons.

Note: *This standard is applicable to all onsite pharmacies and pharmacies contracted by the long term care facility to provide medications to its residents.*

MM

Elements of Performance for MM.4.70

A   1.   When the organization has been informed of a medication recall or discontinuation by the manufacturer or the FDA for safety reasons, medications within the organization are retrieved* and appropriately handled per organization policy and law and regulation.

A   2.   When the organization has been informed of a medication recall or discontinuation by the manufacturer or the FDA for safety reasons, all those ordering, dispensing, and/or administering recalled or discontinued medications are notified.

A   3.   When the organization has been informed of a medication recall or discontinuation by the manufacturer or the FDA for safety reasons, residents who may have received the medication are identified and informed of the recall or discontinuation.

Standard MM.4.80

Medications returned to the pharmacy are appropriately managed.

Rationale for MM.4.80

Medications may be returned when allowed under law and regulation and organization policy. Previously dispensed but unused, expired, or returned medications in the organization must be accounted for and controlled. The pharmacy is responsible for controlling and accounting for all unused medications returned to the pharmacy.

MM

Elements of Performance for MM.4.80

B   1.   The organization has a process in place that addresses if and when unused, expired, or returned medications will be managed by the pharmacy or by the organization.

B   2.   The organization has a process in place that addresses how medications can be returned to the pharmacy's or organization's control, including procedures that address preventing diversion of medications and account for all unused, expired, or returned medications.

B   3.   The organization has a process in place that addresses how outside sources, if any, are used for destruction of medications.

C Ⓜ   4.   These processes are implemented.

---

* Although recalls are generally by lot number, an organization may retrieve all lots of a recalled medication instead of recording and identifying medications by their lot number.

Administering

Standard MM.5.10

Medications are safely and accurately administered.

Elements of Performance for MM.5.10

Policies and procedures address the following:

1. Not applicable

B 2. Guidelines for prescriber notification in the event of an adverse drug reaction or medication error

Before administering a medication, the licensed independent practitioner or appropriate health care professional administering the medication does the following:

C Ⓜ 3. Verifies that the medication selected for administration is the correct one based on the medication order and product label

C Ⓜ 4. Verifies that the medication is stable based on visual examination for particulates or discoloration and that the medication has not expired

C Ⓜ 5. Verifies that there is no contraindication for administering the medication

C Ⓜ 6. Verifies that the medication is being administered at the proper time, in the prescribed dose, and by the correct route

C Ⓜ 7. Advises the resident or, if appropriate, the resident's family about any potential clinically significant adverse reaction or other concerns about administering a new medication

C Ⓜ 8. Discusses any unresolved, significant concerns about the medication with the resident's physician, prescriber (if different from the physician), and/or relevant staff involved with the resident's care, treatment, and services

Standard MM.5.20

Self-administered medications are safely and accurately administered.

Elements of Performance for MM.5.20

B 1. If self administration is allowed, procedures guide the safe and accurate self administration* of medications or administration of medications by a person who is not a staff member and address training, supervision, and administration documentation.

---

* Self administration includes those instances where a resident independently uses a medication, including medications that may be held by the organization for the independent use by the resident.

C Ⓜ 2. Persons who administer medications but are not staff members (for example, the resident if self-administering) receive training and appropriate information about the following:
- The nature of the medications to be administered
- How to administer medications, such as the appropriate frequency, route of administration, and dose
- The expected actions and side effects of the medications to be administered
- How to monitor the effects of the medications on the resident

C Ⓜ 3. Persons who administer medications but are not staff members (including the resident if self-administering) are determined to be competent at medication administration before being allowed to administer medications.

Standard MM.5.30
Not applicable

Monitoring

MM

Standard MM.6.10
The effects of medication(s) on residents are monitored.

Rationale for MM.6.10
Monitoring the effects of medications on residents helps to assure that medication therapy is appropriate and minimizes the occurrence of adverse events.

Elements of Performance for MM.6.10
C Ⓜ 1. Each resident's response to his or her medication is monitored according to the clinical needs of the resident and addresses the resident's response to the prescribed medication and actual or potential medication-related problems.

C Ⓜ 2. Monitoring a medication's effect on a resident includes the following:
- Gathering the resident's own perceptions about side effects and, when appropriate, perceived efficacy
- Referring to information from the resident's medical record, relevant laboratory results, clinical response, and medication profile

B 3. The organization has a process for monitoring the resident's response to the first dose(s) of a medication new to a resident while he or she is under the direct care of the organization.

4. Not applicable

c Ⓜ 5. The consultant pharmacist reviews each resident's medication regimen at least monthly.

c Ⓜ 6. The findings, conclusions, and recommendations of medication monitoring are documented and communicated to the physician, prescriber (if different from the physician), and those involved in the resident's care.

c Ⓜ 7. The pharmacy organization reviews the resident's continuing need for and frequency of PRN medications.

Standard MM.6.20 ▬▬▬▬▬▬▬▬▬▬▬▬▬▬▬▬▬▬▬▬▬▬▬▬▬▬

The organization responds appropriately to actual or potential adverse drug events and medication errors.

Elements of Performance for MM.6.20

B 1. The organization has a process to respond to actual or potential adverse drug events and medication errors.

c Ⓜ 2. Appropriate action is taken when an actual or potential adverse drug event is identified (this may be limited to calling for outside assistance depending upon the organization's services).

c Ⓜ 3. The organization or responsible individual complies with internal and external reporting requirements for actual or potential adverse drug events (for example, to the United States Pharmacopoeia [USP], the FDA, and the Institute for Safe Medication Practices [ISMP]).

MM

High-Risk Medications

High-risk or high-alert drugs are those drugs involved in a high percentage of medication errors and/or sentinel events and medications that carry a higher risk for abuse, errors, or other adverse outcomes. Lists of high-risk or high-alert drugs are available from such organizations as the ISMP, the USP, and so forth, based on national data about medication use. However, the organization needs to develop its own list of high-risk or high-alert drugs based on its unique utilization patterns or drugs and its own internal data about medication errors and sentinel events. Examples of high-risk drugs may include investigational drugs, controlled medications, medications not on the approved FDA list, medications with a narrow therapeutic range, psychotherapeutic medications, and look-alike/sound-alike medications. Medications that are new to the market or new to the organization should also be considered.

Standard MM.7.10 ▬▬▬▬▬▬▬▬▬▬▬▬▬▬▬▬▬▬▬▬▬▬▬▬▬▬

The organization develops processes for managing high-risk or high-alert medications.

Elements of Performance for MM.7.10

A   1.   The organization identifies the high-risk or high-alert medications used within the organization, if any.

B   2.   As appropriate to the services provided, the organization develops processes for procuring, storing, ordering, transcribing, preparing, dispensing, administering, and/or monitoring high-risk or high-alert medications.

Standard MM.7.20

Psychotropic medication* use is monitored.

Rationale for MM.7.20

The ongoing monitoring of the use of psychotropic medication helps to do the following:

- Determine the resident's continued need for the current psychotropic dosing regimen
- Identify, as early as possible, when the resident has achieved the optimal benefit from the drug dose
- Identify when the drug dose can be lowered or the drug discontinued or replaced with another, less potent prescription
- Identify adverse side effects
- Evaluate the effectiveness of PRN orders in managing behavior

MM

Elements of Performance for MM.7.20

B   1.   The organization uses an interdisciplinary process that includes the physician, pharmacist, nurse, and other members of the health care team involved in the resident's care to monitor psychotropic medications.

B   2.   The organization specifies that psychotropic medications are used only during the following circumstances:
- When indicated by assessment and medical necessity
- After other nonpharmacological interventions or alternatives have been considered or used
- At the lowest effective therapeutic dose

B   3.   The use of PRN orders for psychotropic medications is periodically reviewed to determine the appropriateness and effectiveness of these PRN orders, with the objective of decreasing their use as much as possible.

B   4.   The organization's compliance with its own monitoring process is evaluated regularly.

---

* **Psychotropic medication** Any medication whose intended purpose is to alter perception, mental status, or behavior. These include, but are not limited to, those medications that produce drug dependence. Some examples of drug classes that are considered psychotropic medications include, but are not limited to, hypnotics, antipsychotics, long- and short-acting benzodiazepines, sedatives/anxiolytics, and antidepressants.

Standard MM.7.30 ▬▬▬▬▬▬▬▬▬▬▬▬▬▬▬▬▬▬▬▬▬▬▬

Not applicable

Standard MM.7.40 ▬▬▬▬▬▬▬▬▬▬▬▬▬▬▬▬▬▬▬▬▬▬▬

Investigational medications are safely controlled and administered.

Rationale for MM.7.40

The organization protects the safety of residents participating in investigational or clinical medication studies by ensuring that these activities are adequately controlled and supported. In addition, the organization should be sensitive to the use of particular populations for experimentation and research and review all investigational medications to evaluate safety (*see* standard RI.2.180).

Element of Performance for MM.7.40

B   1.   Procedures for the use of investigational medications, when used, are implemented and maintained, including the following:
- Having a written process for reviewing, approving, supervising, and monitoring investigational medications use
- Specifying that when an investigational medication protocol is being conducted independent of the organization, the organization will review and accommodate, as appropriate, the resident's continued participation in the protocol (*see* standard RI.2.180)
- Specifying that when pharmacy services are provided, the pharmacy controls the storage, dispensing, labeling, and distribution of the investigational medication

Evaluation

Standard MM.8.10 ▬▬▬▬▬▬▬▬▬▬▬▬▬▬▬▬▬▬▬▬▬▬▬

The organization evaluates its medication management system.

Elements of Performance for MM.8.10

B   1.   The organization evaluates its medication management system for risk points and identifies areas to improve safety.

B   2.   The organization routinely evaluates the literature for new technologies or successful practices that have been demonstrated to enhance safety in other organizations to determine if it can improve its own medication management system.

B   3.   The organization should also review internally generated reports to identify trends or issues in its own system (*see* standards PI.2.10 and PI.2.20).

B   4.   The pharmacy and long term care facility collaborate to determine whether the medication management system is effective.

B   5.   When a pharmacy is the primary provider of pharmaceutical services to a long term care facility, the pharmacy collaborates with the long term care facility to implement a medication management system to control all medications.

B   6.   When a pharmacy is the primary provider of pharmaceutical services to a long term care facility or consultant pharmacist services are provided, the pharmacy or pharmacist participates in educating the long term care facility about the following:
- The collection and use of performance measures for medication management
- Techniques to reduce medication errors and minimize waste of medications

MM

MM

Surveillance, Prevention, and Control of Infection

Overview

Prevention of health care–associated infections (HAIs) represents one of the major safety initiatives that a long term care organization can undertake. The Centers for Disease Control and Prevention (CDC)* estimates that each year approximately 2 million patients admitted to acute care hospitals in the United States acquire infections that were not related to the condition for which they were hospitalized. Residents of long term care facilities are often transferred to and from hospital settings, making infection prevention and control a priority. Older adults may not present with the typical signs and symptoms of infection, making identification of these residents with infections more challenging.

The design and scope of the long term care organization's infection prevention and control program (hereafter referred to as the "IC program") are based on the risk(s) that the organization faces for the transmission of infectious disease. Therefore, the organization assesses its risk and designs the IC program based on this assessment. Once the organization has designed its IC program, the program must be monitored to ensure that the infection prevention and control activities are implemented.

The goal of an effective IC program is to reduce the risk of acquisition and transmission of HAIs. Long term care organizations must do the following to achieve this goal:
- The organization incorporates its infection program as a major component of its safety and performance improvement programs
- The organization performs an ongoing assessment to identify its risks for the acquisition and transmission of infectious agents
- The organization uses an epidemiological approach that consists of surveillance, data collection, and trend identification
- The organization effectively implements infection prevention and control processes
- The organization educates and collaborates with leaders across the organization to effectively participate in the design and implementation of the IC program
- The organization integrates its efforts with health care and community leaders to the extent practicable, recognizing that infection prevention and control is a communitywide effort
- The organization plans for responding to infections that may potentially overwhelm its resources

A program with aims of such broad scope and depth requires the direct involvement of organization leaders. Only with the ongoing attention and direction of

---

* Monitoring hospital-acquired infections to promote patient safety—United States, 1990–1999. *MMWR Morb Mortal Wkly Rep* 49:149–153, Mar. 10, 2000.

organization leadership can the appropriate scope of the program be determined and adequately resourced.

The standards in this chapter, which focus on development and implementation of plans to prevent and control infections, are supported by standards in other chapters, such as "Management of the Environment of Care," "Management of Human Resources," "Improving Organization Performance," and "Leadership," to produce a comprehensive approach to infection control.

IC

Standards

The following is a list of all standards for this function. They are presented here for your convenience without footnotes or other explanatory text. If you have a question about a term used here, please check the Glossary.

Note: *A revised standard numbering system is being used with the reformatted standards. The revised numbering system will allow for more flexibility to add standards while maintaining the current label for each standard.*

The IC Program and Its Components

IC.1.10   The risk of development of a health care–associated infection is minimized through an organizationwide infection control program.

IC.2.10   The infection control program identifies risks for the acquisition and transmission of infectious agents on an ongoing basis.

IC.3.10   Based on risks, the organization establishes priorities and sets goals for preventing the development of health care–associated infections within the organization.

IC.4.10   Once the organization has prioritized its goals, strategies must be implemented to achieve those goals.

IC.5.10   The infection control program evaluates the effectiveness of the infection control interventions and, as necessary, redesigns the infection control interventions.

IC.6.10   As part of emergency management activities, the organization prepares to respond to an influx, or the risk of an influx, of infectious residents.

Structure and Resources for the IC Program

IC.7.10   The infection control program is managed effectively.

IC.8.10   Representatives from relevant components/functions within the organization collaborate to implement the infection control program.

IC.9.10   Organization leaders allocate adequate resources for the infection control program.

IC

Understanding the Parts of This Chapter

To help you navigate this reformatted standards chapter, it may be helpful to think of its parts this way:

- The **standard** is the "goal"
- The **rationale** explains why it's important to achieve this goal
- The **elements of performance** identify the step(s) needed to achieve this goal

These parts are defined as follows.

Standard A statement that defines the performance expectations and/or structures or processes that must be in place for an organization to provide safe, high-quality care, treatment, and services. An organization is either "compliant" or "not compliant" with a standard.

Accreditation decisions are based on simple counts of the standards that are determined to be "not compliant."

Rationale A statement that provides background, justification, or additional information about a standard. A standard's rationale is not scored. In some instances, the rationale for a standard is self-evident. Therefore, not every standard has a written rationale.

Elements of performance (EPs) The specific performance expectations and/or structures or processes that must be in place for an organization to provide safe, high-quality care, treatment, and services. The scoring of EP compliance determines an organization's overall compliance with a standard. EPs are evaluated on the following scale:

> **0** Insufficient compliance
> **1** Partial compliance
> **2** Satisfactory compliance
> **NA** Not applicable

You will find a **measure of success** icon—Ⓜ—next to some EPs. Measures of success (MOS) need to be developed for certain EPs when a standard is judged to be out of compliance through either the Periodic Performance Review (PPR) or the onsite survey. An MOS is defined as a quantifiable measure, usually related to an audit, that can be used to determine whether an action has been effective and is being sustained.*

Assessing Your Compliance

Once you are familiar with the parts of this chapter, you can begin to assess your compliance with its requirements. The scoring category designations are provided next to each EP for your convenience. If you would like to assess your organization's performance, mark your scores for the EPs and standards by following the simple steps described below.

---

* For more information about MOS, *see* "The New Joint Commission Accreditation Process" chapter in this book.

Two components are scored for each EP: (1) compliance with the requirement itself **and** (2) compliance with the track record* for that requirement. Scoring has been simplified and track record achievements (which have always been part of the scoring) have been appropriately modified.

Note: *Some standards and EPs do not apply to a particular type of organization; these standards and EPs are marked "not applicable" and the related text is not included. Your organization is not expected to comply with standards and EPs marked "not applicable."*

In addition, some standards and EPs that do apply to organizations may not apply to the specific care, treatment, and services that your individual organization provides. Although these standards and EPs are included in the book, you are not expected to comply with them. If you are unsure about the standards or EPs that apply to your organization, please contact the Joint Commission's Standards Interpretation Group at 630/792-5900.

Step 1: Score Your Compliance with Each Element of Performance

Before you can determine your compliance with the standards, you must score your compliance with each EP. There are three scoring criterion categories: A, B, and C (described below). Please note that for each EP scoring criterion category, your organization must meet the performance requirement itself and the track record achievements (*see* "Track Record Achievements").

Category A

These EPs relate to the presence or absence of the requirement(s) and are scored either yes (2) or no (0); however, score 1 for partial compliance is also possible based on track record achievements.

If an A EP has multiple components designated by bullets, your organization must be compliant with all the bullets to receive a score of 2. If your organization does not meet one or more requirements in the bullets, you will receive a score of 0.

Category B

Category B EPs are scored in two steps:
1. As with category A EPs, category B EPs relate to the presence or absence of the requirement(s). If your organization *does not meet* the requirement(s), the EP is scored 0; there is no need to assess your compliance with the principles of good process design.
2. If your organization *does meet* the requirement(s), but there is concern about the quality or comprehensiveness of the effort, then and only then should you assess the qualitative aspect of the EP. That is, review the applicable principles of good process design and ask how the principles were applied in the situation under discussion. Good process design has the following characteristics:

---

* **Track record** The amount of time that an organization has been in compliance with a standard, EP, or other requirement.

- Is consistent with your organization's mission, values, and goals
- Meets the needs of patients
- Reflects the use of currently accepted practices (doing the right thing, using resources responsibly, using practice guidelines)
- Incorporates current safety information and knowledge such as sentinel event data and National Patient Safety Goals
- Incorporates relevant performance improvement results

This two-part evaluation applies to both simple and bulleted B EPs. First, the EPs are assessed to determine whether the requirements are present. If the EP has multiple components designated by bullets, as with the category A EPs, your organization must meet the requirements in *all* the bulleted items to get a score of 2. If your organization meets *none* of the requirements in the bullets, it receives a score of 0. If your organization meets *at least one, but not all,* of the bulleted requirements, it receives a score of 1 for the EPs.

Use the following rules to determine your EP score:
- Your EP score is 0 if your organization does not meet the requirement(s); you *do not* need to assess your compliance with the preceding applicable principles of good process design
- Your EP score is 1 if your organization does meet the requirement(s) but considered only *some* of the preceding applicable principles of good process design
- Your EP score is 2 if your organization does meet the requirement(s) *and* considered *all* the preceding principles of good process design

IC

Category C

C EPs are scored 0, 1, or 2 based on the number of times your organization does not meet the EP. These EPs are frequency based and require totaling the number of occurrences (that is, results of performance or nonperformance) related to a particular EP. Each situation discovered by a surveyor(s) will be counted as a separate occurrence.

Note: *Multiple events of the same type related to a single resident and single practitioner/staff member are counted as* one occurrence only.

Use the following rules to determine your EP score:
- Your EP score is 2 if you find one or fewer occurrences of noncompliance with the EP
- Your EP score is 1 if you find two occurrences of noncompliance with the EP
- Your EP score is 0 if you find three or more occurrences of noncompliance with the EP

If an EP in the C category has multiple requirements designated by bullets, the following scoring guidelines apply:
- If there are fewer than two findings in all bullets, the EP is scored 2
- If there are three or more findings in all bullets, the EP is scored 0
- In all other combinations of findings, the EP is scored 1

Track Record Achievements

In addition to meeting the requirement(s) in each EP, regardless of category, your organization must also meet the following track record achievements:

Score	Initial Survey	Full Survey
2	4 months or more	12 months or more
1	2 to 3 months	6 to 11 months
0	Fewer than 2 months	Fewer than 6 months

Sample Sizes

If during an onsite survey, your organization has been found to be not compliant with one or more standards, you must demonstrate Evidence of Standards Compliance (ESC) for each standard that is not compliant. The ESC must address compliance at the EP level; when an EP within a noncompliant standard requires an MOS, your organization must demonstrate achievement with the MOS when completing the ESC.

Note: *Not every EP requires an MOS. EPs that do require an MOS are clearly marked in this chapter. Organizations are required to demonstrate achievement with an MOS only for EPs within a noncompliant standard that require an MOS. Organizations do not need to demonstrate achievement with an MOS for any EP within a compliant standard.*

When demonstrating achievement with an MOS during the ESC process, your organization is **required** to use the following sample sizes, which were established because of their statistical significance, their relative simplicity in application, and their sensitivity to an organization's population size:

- For a population size of fewer than 30 cases,* sample 100% of available cases
- For a population size of 30 to 100 cases, sample 30 cases
- For a population size of 101 to 500 cases, sample 50 cases
- For a population size greater than 500 cases, sample 70 cases

Note: *Organizations are* encouraged, but not required, *to follow this sample size when demonstrating achievement with an MOS for an EP within a noncompliant standard after conducting a full, Option 1, or Option 2 PPR.*

When conducting PPR (optional use) or demonstrating an ESC (mandatory use), use the following percentages to determine your EP score: 90% through 100% of your sample size is in compliance = score 2; 80% through 89% of your sample size is in compliance = score 1; less than 80% of your sample size is in compliance = score 0.

In addition, the following information should govern your organization's selection of samples:

- The appropriate sample size should be determined by the specific population related to the survey findings

---

* *Case* refers to a single instance in which a situation related to a survey finding occurs. For example, if a survey finding was related to **pain assessment**, then a case would be any resident record. If a survey finding was related to **pain management**, a case would be any resident record for residents receiving pain management.

IC

- The sampling approach should involve either systematic random sampling (for example, your organization selects every second or third case for review) or simple random sampling (for example, your organization uses a series of random numbers generated by a computer to identify the cases to be reviewed)
- If your organization chooses not to use these sample sizes while conducting PPR options 1 or 2, you should make sure that your sample size is sufficiently large enough to ensure statistical significance
- When submitting a clarifying ESC, if your organization selects records as part of its sample, the records should be from a period of no more than three months before the last date of the survey
- Assessment of MOS compliance is conducted for a four-month period following the date of ESC approval. Your organization should select records as a part of your sample following the date of ESC approval and use the required sample sizes. MOS percentage compliance rates are derived from the average of all four months.

Step 2: Use Your EP Scores to Gauge Your Compliance with the Standards

Now that you have evaluated and scored each EP for a particular standard, use these simple rules to determine your compliance with the standard itself:

- Your organization is not in compliance (that is, "not compliant") with the standard if any EP is scored 0
- Otherwise, your organization is in compliance with a standard if 65% or more of its EPs are scored 2

IC

Standards, Rationales, Elements of Performance, and Scoring

The IC Program and Its Components

Standard IC.1.10

The risk of development of a health care–associated infection is minimized through an organizationwide infection control program.

Rationale for IC.1.10

The risk of HAIs exists throughout the organization. An effective IC program that can systematically identify risks and respond appropriately must involve all relevant programs and settings within the organization.

Elements of Performance for IC.1.10

B   1.   An organizationwide IC program is implemented.

B   2.   Individuals and/or positions with the authority to take steps to prevent or control the acquisition and transmission of infectious agents are identified.

B   3.   All applicable organizational components and functions are integrated into the IC program.

B   4.   Systems are in place to communicate with licensed independent practitioners; staff; students/trainees; volunteers; and, as appropriate, visitors, residents, and families about infection prevention and control issues, including their responsibilities in preventing the spread of infection within the organization.

B   5.   The organization has systems for reporting infection surveillance, prevention, and control information to the following:
   ● The appropriate staff within the organization
   ● Federal, state, and local public health authorities in accordance with law and regulation
   ● Accrediting bodies (see Sentinel Event Reporting, page SE-5)
   ● The referring or receiving organization when a resident was transferred or referred and the presence of an HAI was not known at the time of transfer or referral

B   6.   Systems for the investigation of outbreaks of infectious diseases are in place.

B   7.   Applicable policies and procedures are in place throughout the organization.

IC

B   8.   Written policies and procedures include at least the following departments' participation in infection prevention and control activities: clinical services, food services, housekeeping, maintenance, and laundry
services, hotel service (for example, beauty shops), resident activities,
and staff health.

B   9.   The organization has a written IC plan* that includes the following:
   - A description of prioritized risks
   - A statement of the goals of the IC program
   - A description of the organization's strategies to minimize, reduce, or
     eliminate the prioritized risks
   - A description of how the strategies will be evaluated

Standard IC.2.10

The infection control program identifies risks for the acquisition and transmission
of infectious agents on an ongoing basis.

Rationale for IC.2.10

An organization's risks of infection will vary based on the organization's geographic
location, the community environment, the types of programs/services provided, and
the characteristics and behaviors of the population served. As these risks change
over time—sometimes rapidly—risk assessment must be an ongoing process.

IC

Elements of Performance for IC.2.10

B   1.   The organization identifies risks for the transmission and acquisition of
infectious agents throughout the organization based on the following
factors:
   - The geographic location and community environment of the organi-
     zation, program/services provided, and the characteristics of the
     population served
   - The results of the analysis of the organization's infection prevention
     and control data
   - The care, treatment, and services provided

A   2.   The risk analysis is formally reviewed at least annually and whenever
significant changes occur in any of the preceding factors.

B   3.   Surveillance activities, including data collection and analysis, are used to
identify infection prevention and control risks pertaining to the following:
   - Residents
   - Licensed independent practitioners, staff, volunteers, and
     student/trainees
   - Visitors and families, as warranted

---

* **Written plan** A succinct, useful document, formulated beforehand, that identifies needs, lists strategies to
meet those needs, and sets goals and objectives. The format of the "plan" may include narratives, policies and
procedures, protocols, practice guidelines, clinical paths, care maps, or a combination of these.

Standard IC.3.10

Based on risks, the organization establishes priorities and sets goals for preventing the development of health care–associated infections within the organization.

Rationale for IC.3.10

The risks of HAIs within an organization are many while resources are limited. An effective IC program requires a thoughtful prioritization of the most important risks to be addressed. Priorities and goals related to the identified risks guide the choice and design of strategies for infection prevention and control in an organization. These priorities and goals provide a framework for evaluating the strategies.

Elements of Performance for IC.3.10

B　1.　Priorities are established and goals related to preventing the acquisition and transmission of potentially infectious agents are developed based on the risks identified.

These goals include, but are not limited to, the following:

A　2.　Limiting unprotected exposure to pathogens throughout the organization

A　3.　Enhancing hand hygiene

　　4.　Not applicable

A　5.　Minimizing the risk of transmitting infections associated with the use of procedures, medical equipment, and medical devices

IC

Standard IC.4.10

Once the organization has prioritized its goals, strategies must be implemented to achieve those goals.

Rationale for IC.4.10

The organization plans and implements interventions to address the IC issues that it finds important based on prioritized risks and associated surveillance data.

Elements of Performance for IC.4.10

B　1.　Interventions are designed to incorporate relevant guidelines* for infection prevention and control activities.

Interventions are implemented which include the following (EPs 2–3):

A　2.　An organizationwide hand hygiene program that complies with current Centers for Disease Control and Prevention (CDC) hand hygiene guidelines (National Patient Safety Goal 7, requirement 7.a)[†]

---

* Examples of guidelines include those offered by the CDC, Healthcare Infection Control Practices Advisory Committee (HICPAC), and National Quality Forum (NQF).

[†] Organizations are required to comply with all 1A, 1B, and 1C CDC recommendations.

B   3.   Methods to reduce the risks associated with procedures, medical equipment,* and medical devices, including the following:
- Appropriate storage, cleaning, disinfection, sterilization, and/or disposal of supplies and equipment
- Reuse of equipment designated by the manufacturer as disposable in a manner that is consistent with regulatory and professional standards
- The appropriate use of personal protective equipment

B   4.   Implementation of applicable precautions, as appropriate, is based on the following:
- The potential for transmission
- The mechanism of transmission
- The care, treatment, and services setting
- The emergence and reemergence of pathogens in the community that could affect the organization

Interventions are implemented which include the following (EPs 5–8):

C Ⓜ   5.   Screening for exposure and/or immunity to infectious diseases that licensed independent practitioners, staff, student/trainees, and volunteers may come in contact with in their work is available as warranted

C Ⓜ   6.   Referral for assessment, potential testing, immunization and/or prophylaxis/treatment, and counseling as appropriate of licensed independent practitioners, staff, students/trainees, and volunteers who are identified as potentially having an infectious disease or risk of infectious disease that may put the population they serve at risk

C Ⓜ   7.   Referral for assessment, potential testing, immunization and/or prophylaxis/treatment, and counseling as appropriate of residents, students/trainees, and volunteers who have been exposed to infectious disease(s) at the organization and licensed independent practitioners

B   8.   Reduction of risks associated with animals brought into the organization

Standard IC.5.10

The infection control program evaluates the effectiveness of the infection control interventions and, as necessary, redesigns the infection control interventions.

Rationale for IC.5.10

The evaluation of the effectiveness of interventions helps to identify which activities of the IC program are effective and which activities need to be changed to improve outcomes.

---

* **Medical equipment** Fixed and portable equipment used for the diagnosis, treatment, monitoring, and direct care of individuals.

Elements of Performance for IC.5.10

A   1.   The organization formally evaluates and revises the goals and program (or portions of the program) at least annually and whenever risks significantly change.

B   2.   The evaluation addresses changes in the scope of the IC program (for example, resulting from the introduction of new services or new sites of care).

B   3.   The evaluation addresses changes in the results of the IC program risk analysis.

B   4.   The evaluation addresses emerging and reemerging problems in the health care community that potentially affect the organization (for example, highly infectious agents).

B   5.   The evaluation addresses the assessment of the success or failure of interventions for preventing and controlling infection.

B   6.   The evaluation addresses responses to concerns raised by leadership and others within the organization.

B   7.   The evaluation addresses the evolution of relevant infection prevention and control guidelines that are based on evidence or, in the absence of evidence, expert consensus.

IC

Standard IC.6.10

As part of emergency management activities, the organization prepares to respond to an influx, or the risk of an influx, of infectious residents.

Rationale for IC.6.10

The health care organization is an important resource for the continued functioning of a community. An organization's ability to deliver care, treatment, or services is threatened when it is ill-prepared to respond to an epidemic or infections likely to require expanded or extended care capabilities over a prolonged period. Therefore, it is important for an organization to plan how to prevent the introduction of the infection into the organization, how to quickly recognize that this type of infection has been introduced, and/or how to contain the spread of the infection if it is introduced.

This planned response may include a broad range of options, including the temporary halting of services and/or admissions, delaying transfer or discharge, limiting visitors within an organization, or fully activating the organization's emergency management plan. The actual response depends upon issues such as the extent to which the community is affected by the spread of the infection, the types of services offered, and the organization's capabilities.

The concepts included in these standards are supported by standards found elsewhere in the book, including standard EC.4.10.

Elements of Performance for IC.6.10

B   1.   The organization plans its response to an influx or risk of an influx of infectious residents.

B   2.   The organization has a plan for managing an ongoing influx of potentially infectious residents over an extended period.

B   3.   The organization does the following:
- Determines how it will keep abreast of current information about the emergence of epidemics or new infections which may result in the organization activating its response
- Determines how it will disseminate critical information to staff and other key practitioners
- Identifies resources in the community (through local, state, and/or federal public health systems) for obtaining additional information

Structure and Resources for the IC Program

Standard IC.7.10

The infection control program is managed effectively.

IC

Rationale for IC.7.10

The IC program requires management by an individual (or individuals) with knowledge that is appropriate to the risks identified by the organization, as well as knowledge of the analysis of infection risks, principles of infection prevention and control, and data analysis. This individual may be employed by the organization or the organization may contract with this individual. The number of individuals and their qualifications are based on the organization's size, complexity, and needs.

Elements of Performance for IC.7.10

A   1.   The organization assigns responsibility for managing IC program activities to one or more individuals whose number, competency, and skill mix are determined by the goals and objectives of the IC activities.

B   2.   Qualifications of the individual(s) responsible for managing the IC program are determined by the risks entailed in the care, treatment, and services provided, the organization's resident population(s), and the complexity of the activities that will be carried out.

       Note: *Qualifications may be met through ongoing education, training, experience, and/or certification (such as that offered by the Certification Board for Infection Control [CBIC]) in the prevention and control of infections).*

B   3.   This individual(s) coordinates all infection prevention and control activities within the organization.

B   4.   This individual(s) facilitates ongoing monitoring of the effectiveness of prevention and/or control activities and interventions.

Standard IC.8.10

Representatives from relevant components/functions within the organization collaborate to implement the infection control program.

Rationale for IC.8.10

The successful creation of an organizationwide IC program requires collaboration with all relevant components/functions. This collaboration is vital to successful data gathering and interpretation, design of interventions, and effective implementation of interventions. Individuals within the organization who have the power to implement plans and make decisions about interventions related to infection prevention and control participate in the IC program. While a formal committee consisting of leadership and other components is not required as evidence of this collaboration, the organization may want to consider this option.

Elements of Performance for IC.8.10

B   1.   Organization leaders, with licensed independent practitioners, and other direct and indirect resident care staff, including, when applicable, administration, building maintenance/engineering, food services, housekeeping, and pharmacy

B   2.   These representatives participate in the following:
- Development of strategies for each components/functions role in the IC program
- Assessment of the adequacy of the human, information, physical, and financial resources allocated to support infection prevention and control activities
- Assessment of the overall failure or success of key processes for preventing and controlling infection
- The review and revision of the IC program as warranted to improve outcomes

IC

Standard IC.9.10

Organization leaders allocate adequate resources for the infection control program.

Rationale for IC.9.10

Adequate resources are needed to effectively plan and successfully implement a program of this scope.

Elements of Performance for IC.9.10

A   1.   The effectiveness of the organization's infection prevention and control activities is reviewed on an ongoing basis, and findings are reported to the integrated resident safety program at least annually.

B   2.   Adequate systems to access information are provided to support infection prevention and control activities.

B   3.   When applicable, adequate laboratory support is provided to support infection prevention and control activities.

B   4.   Adequate equipment and supplies are provided to support infection prevention and control activities.

IC

Improving Organization Performance

Overview

Performance improvement (PI) is a continuous process. It involves measuring the functioning of important processes and services, and, when indicated, identifying changes that enhance performance. These changes are incorporated into new or existing work processes, products or services, and performance is monitored to ensure that the improvements are sustained.

PI focuses on outcomes of care, treatment, and services. Leaders establish a planned, systematic, and organizationwide approach(es) to PI. They set priorities for PI and ensure that the disciplines representing the scope of care, treatment, and services across the organization work collaboratively to plan and implement improvement activities. The leaders' responsibilities are described in the "Leadership" chapter (standards LD.4.10 through LD.4.70) of this book.

An important aspect of improving organization performance is effectively reducing factors that contribute to unanticipated adverse events and/or outcomes. Unanticipated adverse events and/or outcomes may be caused by poorly designed systems, system failures, or errors. Reducing unanticipated adverse events and/or unanticipated outcomes requires an environment in which residents, their families, and organization staff and leaders can identify and manage actual and potential risks to safety. Such an environment encourages the following:

- Recognizing and acknowledging risks and unanticipated adverse events
- Initiating actions to reduce these risks and unanticipated adverse events
- Reporting internally on risk reduction initiatives and their effectiveness
- Focusing on processes and systems
- Minimizing individual blame or retribution for involvement in an unanticipated adverse event
- Investigating factors that contribute to unanticipated adverse events and sharing that acquired knowledge both internally and with other organizations

The leaders are responsible for fostering such an environment through their personal example and by supporting effective responses to actual occurrences of unanticipated adverse events; ongoing proactive reduction of safety risks to residents; and integration of safety priorities into the design and redesign of all relevant organization processes, functions, and services. (*See* standard LD.4.50.)

This chapter focuses on the following fundamental components of PI:

- Measuring performance through data collection
- Assessing current performance
- Improving performance

Standards

The following is a list of all standards for this function. They are presented here for your convenience without footnotes or other explanatory text. If you have a question about a term used here, please check the Glossary.

Note: *A revised standard numbering system is being used with the reformatted standards. This revised numbering system will allow for more flexibility to add standards while maintaining the current label for each standard.*

PI.1.10   The organization collects data to monitor its performance.

PI.1.20   Not applicable

PI.2.10   Data are systematically aggregated and analyzed.

PI.2.20   Undesirable patterns or trends in performance are analyzed.

PI.2.30   Processes for identifying and managing sentinel events are defined and implemented.

PI.3.10   Information from data analysis is used to make changes that improve performance and resident safety and reduce the risk of sentinel events.

PI.3.20   An ongoing, proactive program for identifying and reducing unanticipated adverse events and safety risks to residents is defined and implemented.

PI

Understanding the Parts of This Chapter

To help you navigate this reformatted standards chapter, it may be helpful to think of its parts this way:

- The **standard** is the "goal"
- The **rationale** explains why it's important to achieve this goal
- The **elements of performance** identify the step(s) needed to achieve this goal

These parts are defined as follows.

Standard A statement that defines the performance expectations and/or structures or processes that must be in place for an organization to provide safe, high-quality care, treatment, and services. An organization is either "compliant" or "not compliant" with a standard.

Accreditation decisions are based on simple counts of the standards that are determined to be "not compliant."

Rationale A statement that provides background, justification, or additional information about a standard. A standard's rationale is not scored. In some instances, the rationale for a standard is self-evident. Therefore, not every standard has a written rationale.

Elements of performance (EPs) The specific performance expectations and/or structures or processes that must be in place for an organization to provide safe, high-quality care, treatment, and services. The scoring of EP compliance determines an organization's overall compliance with a standard. EPs are evaluated on the following scale:

0	Insufficient compliance
1	Partial compliance
2	Satisfactory compliance
NA	Not applicable

You will find a **measure of success** icon—**Ⓜ**—next to some EPs. Measures of success (MOS) need to be developed for certain EPs when a standard is judged to be out of compliance through either the Periodic Performance Review (PPR) or the onsite survey. An MOS is defined as a quantifiable measure, usually related to an audit, that can be used to determine whether an action has been effective and is being sustained.*

Assessing Your Compliance

Once you are familiar with the parts of this chapter, you can begin to assess your compliance with its requirements. The scoring category designations are provided next to each EP for your convenience. If you would like to assess your organization's performance, mark your scores for the EPs and standards by following the simple steps described below.

---

* For more information about MOS, *see* "The New Joint Commission Accreditation Process" chapter in this book.

Two components are scored for each EP: (1) compliance with the requirement itself **and** (2) compliance with the track record* for that requirement. Scoring has been simplified and track record achievements (which have always been part of the scoring) have been appropriately modified.

Note: *Some standards and EPs do not apply to a particular type of organization; these standards and EPs are marked "not applicable" and the related text is not included. Your organization is not expected to comply with standards and EPs marked "not applicable."*

In addition, some standards and EPs that do apply to organizations may not apply to the specific care, treatment, and services that your individual organization provides. Although these standards and EPs are included in the book, you are not expected to comply with them. If you are unsure about the standards or EPs that apply to your organization, please contact the Joint Commission's Standards Interpretation Group at 630/792-5900.

Step 1: Score Your Compliance with Each Element of Performance

Before you can determine your compliance with the standards, you must score your compliance with each EP. There are three scoring criterion categories: A, B, and C (described below). Please note that for each EP scoring criterion category, your organization must meet the performance requirement itself and the track record achievements (*see* "Track Record Achievements").

Category A

These EPs relate to the presence or absence of the requirement(s) and are scored either yes (2) or no (0); however, score 1 for partial compliance is also possible based on track record achievements.

If an A EP has multiple components designated by bullets, your organization must be compliant with all the bullets to receive a score of 2. If your organization does not meet one or more requirements in the bullets, you will receive a score of 0.

Category B

Category B EPs are scored in two steps:
1. As with category A EPs, category B EPs relate to the presence or absence of the requirement(s). If your organization *does not meet* the requirement(s), the EP is scored 0; there is no need to assess your compliance with the principles of good process design.
2. If your organization *does meet* the requirement(s), but there is concern about the quality or comprehensiveness of the effort, then and only then should you assess the qualitative aspect of the EP. That is, review the applicable principles of good process design and ask how the principles were applied in the situation under discussion. Good process design has the following characteristics:

---

* **Track record** The amount of time that an organization has been in compliance with a standard, EP, or other requirement.

- Is consistent with your organization's mission, values, and goals
- Meets the needs of patients
- Reflects the use of currently accepted practices (doing the right thing, using resources responsibly, using practice guidelines)
- Incorporates current safety information and knowledge such as sentinel event data and National Patient Safety Goals
- Incorporates relevant performance improvement results

This two-part evaluation applies to both simple and bulleted B EPs. First, the EPs are assessed to determine whether the requirements are present. If the EP has multiple components designated by bullets, as with the category A EPs, your organization must meet the requirements in *all* the bulleted items to get a score of 2. If your organization meets *none* of the requirements in the bullets, it receives a score of 0. If your organization meets *at least one, but not all,* of the bulleted requirements, it receives a score of 1 for the EPs.

Use the following rules to determine your EP score:
- Your EP score is 0 if your organization does not meet the requirement(s); you *do not* need to assess your compliance with the preceding applicable principles of good process design
- Your EP score is 1 if your organization does meet the requirement(s) but considered only *some* of the preceding applicable principles of good process design
- Your EP score is 2 if your organization does meet the requirement(s) *and* considered *all* the preceding principles of good process design

Category C

C EPs are scored 0, 1, or 2 based on the number of times your organization does not meet the EP. These EPs are frequency based and require totaling the number of occurrences (that is, results of performance or nonperformance) related to a particular EP. Each situation discovered by a surveyor(s) will be counted as a separate occurrence.

Note: *Multiple events of the same type related to a single resident and single practitioner/staff member are counted as* one occurrence only.

Use the following rules to determine your EP score:
- Your EP score is 2 if you find one or fewer occurrences of noncompliance with the EP
- Your EP score is 1 if you find two occurrences of noncompliance with the EP
- Your EP score is 0 if you find three or more occurrences of noncompliance with the EP

If an EP in the C category has multiple requirements designated by bullets, the following scoring guidelines apply:
- If there are fewer than two findings in all bullets, the EP is scored 2
- If there are three or more findings in all bullets, the EP is scored 0
- In all other combinations of findings, the EP is scored 1

PI

Track Record Achievements

In addition to meeting the requirement(s) in each EP, regardless of category, your organization must also meet the following track record achievements:

Score	Initial Survey	Full Survey
2	4 months or more	12 months or more
1	2 to 3 months	6 to 11 months
0	Fewer than 2 months	Fewer than 6 months

Sample Sizes

If during an onsite survey, your organization has been found to be not compliant with one or more standards, you must demonstrate Evidence of Standards Compliance (ESC) for each standard that is not compliant. The ESC must address compliance at the EP level; when an EP within a noncompliant standard requires an MOS, your organization must demonstrate achievement with the MOS when completing the ESC.

Note: *Not every EP requires an MOS. EPs that do require an MOS are clearly marked in this chapter. Organizations are required to demonstrate achievement with an MOS only for EPs within a noncompliant standard that require an MOS. Organizations do not need to demonstrate achievement with an MOS for any EP within a compliant standard.*

When demonstrating achievement with an MOS during the ESC process, your organization is **required** to use the following sample sizes, which were established because of their statistical significance, their relative simplicity in application, and their sensitivity to an organization's population size:

- For a population size of fewer than 30 cases,* sample 100% of available cases
- For a population size of 30 to 100 cases, sample 30 cases
- For a population size of 101 to 500 cases, sample 50 cases
- For a population size greater than 500 cases, sample 70 cases

Note: *Organizations are* encouraged, but not required, *to follow this sample size when demonstrating achievement with an MOS for an EP within a noncompliant standard after conducting a full, Option 1, or Option 2 PPR.*

When conducting PPR (optional use) or demonstrating an ESC (mandatory use), use the following percentages to determine your EP score: 90% through 100% of your sample size is in compliance = score 2; 80% through 89% of your sample size is in compliance = score 1; less than 80% of your sample size is in compliance = score 0.

In addition, the following information should govern your organization's selection of samples:

- The appropriate sample size should be determined by the specific population related to the survey findings

---

* *Case* refers to a single instance in which a situation related to a survey finding occurs. For example, if a survey finding was related to **pain assessment**, then a case would be any resident record. If a survey finding was related to **pain management**, a case would be any resident record for residents receiving pain management.

- The sampling approach should involve either systematic random sampling (for example, your organization selects every second or third case for review) or simple random sampling (for example, your organization uses a series of random numbers generated by a computer to identify the cases to be reviewed)
- If your organization chooses not to use these sample sizes while conducting PPR options 1 or 2, you should make sure that your sample size is sufficiently large enough to ensure statistical significance
- When submitting a clarifying ESC, if your organization selects records as part of its sample, the records should be from a period of no more than three months before the last date of the survey
- Assessment of MOS compliance is conducted for a four-month period following the date of ESC approval. Your organization should select records as a part of your sample following the date of ESC approval and use the required sample sizes. MOS percentage compliance rates are derived from the average of all four months.

Step 2: Use Your EP Scores to Gauge Your Compliance with the Standards

Now that you have evaluated and scored each EP for a particular standard, use these simple rules to determine your compliance with the standard itself:

- Your organization is not in compliance (that is, "not compliant") with the standard if any EP is scored 0
- Otherwise, your organization is in compliance with a standard if 65% or more of its EPs are scored 2

PI

Standards, Rationales, Elements of Performance, and Scoring

Standard PI.1.10

The organization collects data to monitor its performance.

Rationale for PI.1.10

Data help determine performance improvement priorities. The data collected for high priority and required areas are used to monitor the stability of existing processes, identify opportunities for improvement, identify changes that lead to improvement, or sustain improvement. Data collection helps identify specific areas that require further study. These areas are determined by considering the information provided by the data about process stability, risks, sentinel events, and priorities set by the leaders. In addition, the organization identifies those areas needing improvement and identifies desired changes. Performance measures are used to determine whether the changes result in desired outcomes. The organization identifies the frequency and detail of data collection.

Note: *The organization also collects data on the following areas that will be scored in their respective chapters:*
- *Evaluation and improvement of conditions in the environment (see "Management of the Environment of Care" chapter)*
- *Staffing effectiveness (see "Management of Human Resources" chapter)*

Note: *For long term care organizations that serve residents with dementia, the organization may measure performance in the following areas: psychotropic drugs, incidents, acute behavioral events, family involvement, do-not-resuscitate orders, appropriate use of services, transfers, programs that meet resident needs, infection control, environmental adaptations, and safety.*

Elements of Performance for PI.1.10

B   1.   The organization collects data for priorities identified by leaders (*see* standard LD.4.50).

A   2.   The organization considers collecting data in the following areas:
- Staff opinions and needs
- Staff perceptions of risks to individuals and suggestions for improving resident safety
- Staff willingness to report unanticipated adverse events

---

* The Joint Commission is moving from the phrase *satisfaction with care, treatment, and services* toward the more inclusive phrase *perception of care, treatment, and services* to better measure the performance of organizations meeting the needs, expectations and concerns of residents. By using this term, the organization will be prompted to assess not only residents' and/or families' satisfaction with care, treatment, or services, but also whether the organization meets their needs and expectations.

B   3.   The organization collects data on the perceptions of care, treatment, and services* of residents, including the following:
- Their specific needs and expectations
- How well the organization meets these needs and expectations
- How the organization can improve resident safety
- The effectiveness of pain management, when applicable

The organization collects data that measure the performance of each of the following potentially high-risk processes, when provided:

A   4.   Medication management

A   5.   Blood and blood product use

A   6.   Restraint use

       7.   Not applicable

A   8.   Behavior management and treatment

       9. Through 12.   Not applicable

Relevant information developed from the following activities is integrated into performance improvement initiatives. This occurs in a way consistent with any organization policies or procedures intended to preserve any confidentiality or privilege of information established by applicable law.

B   13. Risk management

B   14. Utilization management

B   15. Quality control

B   16. Infection control surveillance and reporting

B   17. Research, as applicable

PI

Standard PI.1.20

Not applicable

Standard PI.2.10

Data are systematically aggregated and analyzed.

Rationale for PI.2.10

Aggregating and analyzing data means transforming data into information. Aggregating data at points in time enables the organization to judge a particular process's stability or a particular outcome's predictability in relation to performance expectations. Accumulated data are analyzed in such a way that current performance levels, patterns, or trends can be identified.

Elements of Performance for PI.2.10

B   1.   Collected data are aggregated and analyzed.

B   2.   Data are aggregated at the frequency appropriate to the activity or process being studied.

B   3.   Statistical tools and techniques are used to analyze and display data.

B   4.   Data are analyzed and compared internally over time and externally* with other sources of information when available.

B   5.   Comparative data are used to determine if there is excessive variability or unacceptable levels of performance when available.

Standard PI.2.20

Undesirable patterns or trends in performance are analyzed.

Elements of Performance for PI.2.20

B   1.   Analysis is performed when data comparisons indicate that levels of performance, patterns, or trends vary substantially from those expected.

B   2.   Analysis occurs for those topics chosen by leaders as performance improvement priorities.

B   3.   Analysis is performed when undesirable variation occurs which changes priorities.

PI

An analysis is performed for the following:

A   4.   All confirmed transfusion reactions, if applicable to the organization

A   5.   All serious adverse drug events, if applicable and as defined by the organization

A   6.   All significant medication errors, if applicable and as defined by the organization

       7.   Not applicable

       8.   Not applicable

A   9.   Hazardous conditions

A   10. Staffing effectiveness issues

Standard PI.2.30

Processes for identifying and managing sentinel events are defined and implemented.

---

* External sources of information include recent scientific, clinical, and management literature, including sentinel event alerts; well-formulated practice guidelines or parameters; performance measures; reference databases; other organizations with similar processes; and standards that are periodically reviewed and revised.

Rationale for PI.2.30

Identifying, reporting, analyzing, and managing sentinel events can help the organization to prevent such incidents. Leaders define and implement such a program as part of the process to measure, assess, and improve the organization's performance.

Elements of Performance for PI.2.30

Processes for identifying and managing sentinel events include the following:

A 1. Defining "sentinel event" and communicating this definition throughout the organization. (At a minimum, the organization's definition includes those events subject to review under the Joint Commission's Sentinel Event Policy as published in this manual and may include any process variation that does not affect the outcome or result in an adverse event, but for which a recurrence carries significant chance of a serious adverse outcome or result in an adverse event, often referred to as a "near miss.")

A 2. Reporting sentinel events through established channels in the organization and, as appropriate, to external agencies in accordance with law and regulation

B 3. Conducting thorough and credible root cause analyses that focus on process and system factors

B 4. Creating, documenting, and implementing a risk-reduction strategy and action plan that includes measuring the effectiveness of process and system improvements to reduce risk

B 5. The processes are implemented.

PI

Standard PI.3.10 ▬▬▬▬▬▬

Information from data analysis is used to make changes that improve performance and resident safety and reduce the risk of sentinel events.

Elements of Performance for PI.3.10

B 1. The organization uses the information from data analysis to identify and implement changes that will improve the quality of care, treatment, and services.

B 2. The organization identifies and implements changes that will reduce the risk of sentinel events.

B 3. The organization uses the information from data analysis to identify changes that will improve resident safety.

B 4. Changes made to improve processes or outcomes are evaluated to ensure that they achieve the expected results.

B 5. Appropriate actions are undertaken when planned improvements are not achieved or sustained.

Standard PI.3.20

An ongoing, proactive program for identifying and reducing unanticipated adverse events and safety risks to residents is defined and implemented.

Rationale for PI.3.20

Organizations should proactively seek to identify and reduce risks to the safety of residents. Such initiatives have the obvious advantage of *preventing* adverse events rather than simply *reacting* when they occur. This approach also avoids the barriers to understanding created by hindsight bias and the fear of disclosure, embarrassment, blame, and punishment that can happen after an event.

Elements of Performance for PI.3.20

The following proactive activities to reduce risks to residents are conducted:

A   1.   Selecting a high-risk process* to be analyzed (at least one high-risk process is chosen annually—the choice should be based in part on information published periodically by the Joint Commission about the most frequent sentinel events and risks)

B   2.   Describing the chosen process (for example, through the use of a flowchart)

B   3.   Identifying the ways in which the process could break down[†] or fail to perform its desired function

B   4.   Identifying the possible effects that a breakdown or failure of the process could have on residents and the seriousness of the possible effects

B   5.   Prioritizing the potential process breakdowns or failures

B   6.   Determining why the prioritized breakdowns or failures could occur, which may include performing a hypothetical root cause analysis

B   7.   Redesigning the process and/or underlying systems to minimize the risk of the effects on residents

B   8.   Testing and implementing the redesigned process

B   9.   Monitoring the effectiveness of the redesigned process

---

* **High-risk process** A process that, if not planned and/or implemented correctly, has a significant potential for impacting the safety of the resident.

[†] The ways in which processes could break down or fail to perform its desired function are many times referred to as "the failure modes."

Leadership

Overview

An organization's leaders provide the framework for planning, directing, coordinating, providing, and improving care, treatment, and services to respond to community and resident needs and improve health care outcomes.

Effective leadership depends on the following processes:

- **Governance.** The governance of an organization sets the framework for supporting quality resident care, treatment, and services.
- **Management.** Leaders create an environment that enables an organization to fulfill its mission and meet or exceed its goals. They provide for a well-managed organization with clear lines of responsibility and accountability.
- **Planning, designing, and providing services.** Leaders develop a mission that is reflected in long-range, strategic, and operational plans; service design; resource allocation; and organizational policies. They provide organization, direction, and staffing for care, treatment, and services. Leaders also communicate objectives and coordinate efforts to integrate care, treatment, and services throughout the organization.
- **Improving safety and quality of care.** Leaders plan and implement a safety management program. They are ultimately responsible for the safety of all residents and staff. Leaders also establish expectations, plans, and priorities and manage the performance improvement process. They ensure that a process is in place to measure, assess, and improve the organization's governance, management, clinical, and support functions.
- **Teaching and coaching staff.** To realize the organization's vision and values, leaders are involved in teaching and coaching staff; thus, staff education is an essential leadership function.

Standards

The following is a list of all standards for this function. They are presented here for your convenience without footnotes or other explanatory text. If you have a question about a term used here, please check the Glossary.

Note: *A revised standard numbering system is being used with the reformatted standards. This revised numbering system will allow for more flexibility to add standards while maintaining the current label for each standard.*

LD.1.10   The organization identifies how it is governed.

LD.1.20   Governance responsibilities are defined in writing, as applicable.

LD.1.30   The organization complies with applicable law and regulation.

LD.2.10   An individual(s) or designee(s) is responsible for operating the organization according to the authority conferred by governance.

LD.2.20   Each organizational program, service, site, or department has effective leadership.

LD.2.30   A full-time registered nurse directs nursing services.

LD.2.40   The medical director's duties and responsibilities are defined.

LD.2.50   The leaders develop and monitor an annual operating budget and, as appropriate, a long-term capital expenditure plan.

LD.2.60 Through LD.2.200   Not applicable

LD.3.10   The leaders engage in both short-term and long-term planning.

LD.3.15   Not applicable

LD.3.20   Residents with comparable needs receive the same standard of care, treatment, and services throughout the organization.

LD.3.30   Not applicable

LD.3.40   Not applicable

LD.3.50   Services provided by consultation, contractual arrangements, or other agreements are provided safely and effectively.

LD.3.60   Communication is effective throughout the organization.

LD.3.70   The leaders define the required qualifications and competence of those staff who provide care, treatment, and services and recommend a sufficient number of qualified and competent staff to provide care, treatment, and services.

LD.3.80   The leaders provide for adequate space, equipment, and other resources.

LD.3.90   The leaders develop and implement policies and procedures for care, treatment, and services.

LD.3.100   Not applicable

LD.3.110   Not applicable

LD.3.120   The leaders plan for and support the provision and coordination of resident education activities.

LD.3.130   Academic education is arranged for children and youth, when appropriate.

LD.3.140   Not applicable

LD.3.150   Not applicable

LD.4.10   The leaders set expectations, plan, and manage processes to measure, assess, and improve the organization's governance, management, clinical, and support activities.

LD.4.20   New or modified services or processes are designed well.

LD.4.30   Not applicable

LD.4.40   The leaders ensure that an integrated resident safety program is implemented throughout the organization.

LD.4.50   The leaders set performance improvement priorities and identify how the organization adjusts priorities in response to unusual or urgent events.

LD.4.60   The leaders allocate adequate resources for measuring, assessing, and improving the organization's performance and improving resident safety.

LD

LD.4.70 The leaders measure and assess the effectiveness of the performance improvement and safety improvement activities.

LD

Understanding the Parts of This Chapter

To help you navigate this reformatted standards chapter, it may be helpful to think of its parts this way:

- The **standard** is the "goal"
- The **rationale** explains why it's important to achieve this goal
- The **elements of performance** identify the step(s) needed to achieve this goal

These parts are defined as follows.

Standard A statement that defines the performance expectations and/or structures or processes that must be in place for an organization to provide safe, high-quality care, treatment, and services. An organization is either "compliant" or "not compliant" with a standard.

Accreditation decisions are based on simple counts of the standards that are determined to be "not compliant."

Rationale A statement that provides background, justification, or additional information about a standard. A standard's rationale is not scored. In some instances, the rationale for a standard is self-evident. Therefore, not every standard has a written rationale.

Elements of performance (EPs) The specific performance expectations and/or structures or processes that must be in place for an organization to provide safe, high-quality care, treatment, and services. The scoring of EP compliance determines an organization's overall compliance with a standard. EPs are evaluated on the following scale:

> **0** Insufficient compliance
> **1** Partial compliance
> **2** Satisfactory compliance
> **NA** Not applicable

LD

You will find a **measure of success** icon—**ⓜ**—next to some EPs. Measures of success (MOS) need to be developed for certain EPs when a standard is judged to be out of compliance through either the Periodic Performance Review (PPR) or the onsite survey. An MOS is defined as a quantifiable measure, usually related to an audit, that can be used to determine whether an action has been effective and is being sustained.*

Assessing Your Compliance

Once you are familiar with the parts of this chapter, you can begin to assess your compliance with its requirements. The scoring category designations are provided next to each EP for your convenience. If you would like to assess your organization's performance, mark your scores for the EPs and standards by following the simple steps described below.

---

* For more information about MOS, *see* "The New Joint Commission Accreditation Process" chapter in this book.

Two components are scored for each EP: (1) compliance with the requirement itself **and** (2) compliance with the track record* for that requirement. Scoring has been simplified and track record achievements (which have always been part of the scoring) have been appropriately modified.

Note: *Some standards and EPs do not apply to a particular type of organization; these standards and EPs are marked "not applicable" and the related text is not included. Your organization is not expected to comply with standards and EPs marked "not applicable."*

In addition, some standards and EPs that do apply to organizations may not apply to the specific care, treatment, and services that your individual organization provides. Although these standards and EPs are included in the book, you are not expected to comply with them. If you are unsure about the standards or EPs that apply to your organization, please contact the Joint Commission's Standards Interpretation Group at 630/792-5900.

Step 1: Score Your Compliance with Each Element of Performance

Before you can determine your compliance with the standards, you must score your compliance with each EP. There are three scoring criterion categories: A, B, and C (described below). Please note that for each EP scoring criterion category, your organization must meet the performance requirement itself and the track record achievements (*see* "Track Record Achievements").

Category A

These EPs relate to the presence or absence of the requirement(s) and are scored either yes (2) or no (0); however, score 1 for partial compliance is also possible based on track record achievements.

If an A EP has multiple components designated by bullets, your organization must be compliant with all the bullets to receive a score of 2. If your organization does not meet one or more requirements in the bullets, you will receive a score of 0.

Category B

Category B EPs are scored in two steps:
1. As with category A EPs, category B EPs relate to the presence or absence of the requirement(s). If your organization *does not meet* the requirement(s), the EP is scored 0; there is no need to assess your compliance with the principles of good process design.
2. If your organization *does meet* the requirement(s), but there is concern about the quality or comprehensiveness of the effort, then and only then should you assess the qualitative aspect of the EP. That is, review the applicable principles of good process design and ask how the principles were applied in the situation under discussion. Good process design has the following characteristics:

---

* **Track record** The amount of time that an organization has been in compliance with a standard, EP, or other requirement.

- Is consistent with your organization's mission, values, and goals
- Meets the needs of patients
- Reflects the use of currently accepted practices (doing the right thing, using resources responsibly, using practice guidelines)
- Incorporates current safety information and knowledge such as sentinel event data and National Patient Safety Goals
- Incorporates relevant performance improvement results

This two-part evaluation applies to both simple and bulleted B EPs. First, the EPs are assessed to determine whether the requirements are present. If the EP has multiple components designated by bullets, as with the category A EPs, your organization must meet the requirements in *all* the bulleted items to get a score of 2. If your organization meets *none* of the requirements in the bullets, it receives a score of 0. If your organization meets *at least one, but not all,* of the bulleted requirements, it receives a score of 1 for the EPs.

Use the following rules to determine your EP score:

- Your EP score is 0 if your organization does not meet the requirement(s); you *do not* need to assess your compliance with the preceding applicable principles of good process design
- Your EP score is 1 if your organization does meet the requirement(s) but considered only *some* of the preceding applicable principles of good process design
- Your EP score is 2 if your organization does meet the requirement(s) *and* considered *all* the preceding principles of good process design

Category C

C EPs are scored 0, 1, or 2 based on the number of times your organization does not meet the EP. These EPs are frequency based and require totaling the number of occurrences (that is, results of performance or nonperformance) related to a particular EP. Each situation discovered by a surveyor(s) will be counted as a separate occurrence.

LD

Note: *Multiple events of the same type related to a single resident and single practitioner/staff member are counted as* one occurrence only.

Use the following rules to determine your EP score:

- Your EP score is 2 if you find one or fewer occurrences of noncompliance with the EP
- Your EP score is 1 if you find two occurrences of noncompliance with the EP
- Your EP score is 0 if you find three or more occurrences of noncompliance with the EP

If an EP in the C category has multiple requirements designated by bullets, the following scoring guidelines apply:

- If there are fewer than two findings in all bullets, the EP is scored 2
- If there are three or more findings in all bullets, the EP is scored 0
- In all other combinations of findings, the EP is scored 1

Track Record Achievements

In addition to meeting the requirement(s) in each EP, regardless of category, your organization must also meet the following track record achievements:

Score	Initial Survey	Full Survey
2	4 months or more	12 months or more
1	2 to 3 months	6 to 11 months
0	Fewer than 2 months	Fewer than 6 months

Sample Sizes

If during an onsite survey, your organization has been found to be not compliant with one or more standards, you must demonstrate Evidence of Standards Compliance (ESC) for each standard that is not compliant. The ESC must address compliance at the EP level; when an EP within a noncompliant standard requires an MOS, your organization must demonstrate achievement with the MOS when completing the ESC.

Note: *Not every EP requires an MOS. EPs that do require an MOS are clearly marked in this chapter. Organizations are required to demonstrate achievement with an MOS only for EPs within a noncompliant standard that require an MOS. Organizations do not need to demonstrate achievement with an MOS for any EP within a compliant standard.*

When demonstrating achievement with an MOS during the ESC process, your organization is **required** to use the following sample sizes, which were established because of their statistical significance, their relative simplicity in application, and their sensitivity to an organization's population size:

- For a population size of fewer than 30 cases,* sample 100% of available cases
- For a population size of 30 to 100 cases, sample 30 cases
- For a population size of 101 to 500 cases, sample 50 cases
- For a population size greater than 500 cases, sample 70 cases

Note: *Organizations are encouraged, but not required, to follow this sample size when demonstrating achievement with an MOS for an EP within a noncompliant standard after conducting a full, Option 1, or Option 2 PPR.*

When conducting PPR (optional use) or demonstrating an ESC (mandatory use), use the following percentages to determine your EP score: 90% through 100% of your sample size is in compliance = score 2; 80% through 89% of your sample size is in compliance = score 1; less than 80% of your sample size is in compliance = score 0.

In addition, the following information should govern your organization's selection of samples:

- The appropriate sample size should be determined by the specific population related to the survey findings

---

* *Case* refers to a single instance in which a situation related to a survey finding occurs. For example, if a survey finding was related to **pain assessment**, then a case would be any resident record. If a survey finding was related to **pain management**, a case would be any resident record for residents receiving pain management.

- The sampling approach should involve either systematic random sampling (for example, your organization selects every second or third case for review) or simple random sampling (for example, your organization uses a series of random numbers generated by a computer to identify the cases to be reviewed)
- If your organization chooses not to use these sample sizes while conducting PPR options 1 or 2, you should make sure that your sample size is sufficiently large enough to ensure statistical significance
- When submitting a clarifying ESC, if your organization selects records as part of its sample, the records should be from a period of no more than three months before the last date of the survey
- Assessment of MOS compliance is conducted for a four-month period following the date of ESC approval. Your organization should select records as a part of your sample following the date of ESC approval and use the required sample sizes. MOS percentage compliance rates are derived from the average of all four months.

Step 2: Use Your EP Scores to Gauge Your Compliance with the Standards

Now that you have evaluated and scored each EP for a particular standard, use these simple rules to determine your compliance with the standard itself:

- Your organization is not in compliance (that is, "not compliant") with the standard if any EP is scored 0
- Otherwise, your organization is in compliance with a standard if 65% or more of its EPs are scored 2

LD

Standards, Rationales, Elements of Performance, and Scoring

Standard LD.1.10

The organization identifies how it is governed.

Rationale for LD.1.10

The organization has governance with ultimate responsibility and legal authority for the safety and quality of care, treatment, and services. Governance establishes policy, promotes performance improvement, and provides for organizational management and planning.

Elements of Performance for LD.1.10

A 1. The organization identifies how it is governed.

A 2. The organization identifies lines of authority for key planning, management, and operations activities.

A 3. The organization identifies those responsible for governance.

Standard LD.1.20

Governance responsibilities are defined in writing, as applicable.

Elements of Performance for LD.1.20

A 1. Governance defines its responsibilities in writing, as applicable.

A 2. If the organization is part of a larger corporate structure, the scope and degree of leaders' involvement, authority, and responsibility in corporate policy decisions are described in writing.

B 3. Governance provides for organizational management and planning.

A 4. The organization's scope of services is defined in writing and approved by the governance.

A 5. Governance either selects the individual(s) responsible for operating the organization or approves one selected by corporate management or another group.

B 6. Governance provides for coordination and integration among the organization's leaders to establish policy, maintain quality care and resident safety, and provide for necessary resources.

A 7. Governance annually evaluates the organization's performance in relation to its vision, mission, and goals.

A 8. If the organization has an organized medical staff, the governance approves the medical staff's bylaws and rules and regulations.

Standard LD.1.30

The organization complies with applicable law and regulation.

Elements of Performance for LD.1.30

A   1.   The organization provides all care, treatment, and services in accordance with applicable licensure requirements, law, rules, and regulation.*

A   2.   The organization acts upon any reports and/or recommendations from authorized agencies, as appropriate.

A   3.   The organization possesses a license, certificate, or permit, as required by applicable law and regulation, to provide the health care services for which the organization is seeking accreditation.

Standard LD.2.10

An individual(s) or designee(s) is responsible for operating the organization according to the authority conferred by governance.

Elements of Performance for LD.2.10

B   1.   The individual(s) designated by governance is responsible for establishing internal controls to effectively operate the organization, including the following:
- Establishing and maintaining information and support systems
- Recruiting and retaining staff
- Conserving physical and financial assets

A   2.   When this individual(s) is absent from the organization, an appropriately qualified individual(s) is designated to perform the duties of that position.

A   3.   The individual with administrative authority is accessible to the organization on a full-time basis to address administrative issues as they arise in the organization and as required by law and regulation.

B   4.   As appropriate, reports are provided to governance.

Standard LD.2.20

Each organizational program, service, site, or department has effective leadership.

Rationale for LD.2.20

Effective leaders at the site or department level help create an environment or culture that enables an organization to fulfill its mission and meet or exceed its goals. They

---

* Applicable laws and regulations include, but are not limited to, individual and facility licensure; certification; Food and Drug Administration regulations; Drug Enforcement Agency regulations; Centers for Medicare & Medicaid Services regulations; Occupational Safety and Health Administration regulations; Department of Transportation regulations; Health Insurance Portability and Accountability Act; and other local, state, and federal laws and regulations.

support staff and instill in them a sense of ownership of their work processes. Although it may be appropriate for leaders to delegate work to qualified staff, the leaders are ultimately responsible for care, treatment, or services provided in their area.

Elements of Performance for LD.2.20

B   1. The program, service, site, or department leaders ensure that operations are effective and efficient.

B   2. Leaders hold staff accountable for their responsibilities.

B   3. Programs, services, sites, or departments providing resident care are directed by one or more qualified professionals with appropriate training and experience or by a qualified licensed independent practitioner with appropriate clinical privileges.

B   4. Responsibility for administrative and clinical direction of these programs, services, sites, or departments is defined in writing.

B   5. Leaders ensure that a process is in place to coordinate care, treatment, and services processes among programs, services, sites, or departments.

Standard LD.2.30

A full-time registered nurse directs nursing services.

Elements of Performance for LD.2.30

A   1. A full-time registered nurse directs nursing services.

A   2. When the director of nursing is responsible for more than one organization or specialty program, an appropriately qualified registered nurse is identified and responsible for the nursing staff activities in each setting.

A   3. When the director of nursing is absent, responsibility for continuity and supervision of nursing care is delegated to a registered nurse.

Standard LD.2.40

The medical director's duties and responsibilities are defined.

Elements of Performance for LD.2.40

A   1. The medical director is appointed by the administrator or designated by the organized medical staff.

A   2. The medical director's responsibilities are defined in a written agreement between the governing body and the medical director.

B   3. The medical director participates in the leadership of the organization by doing the following:
- Directing and coordinating medical care in the organization
- Participating in establishing policies, procedures, and guidelines for adequate, comprehensive services

LD

- Helping develop emergency treatment procedures for residents
- Helping develop resident transfer procedures
- Participating in the resident care management system
- Participating in in-service training programs

B   4.   The medical director provides advice and input to the administrator and to governance by doing the following:
- Making credentialing and privileging recommendations to the governance
- Consulting in the development and maintenance of an adequate medical record system
- Consulting with the organization's administrator and service directors about the organization's ability to meet residents' needs
- Advising the administrator about the adequacy and appropriateness of the organization's scope of services, medical equipment, and its professional and support staff
- Exploring the opportunities for and advising the administrator about future resident care programs
- Participating in managing the environment by reviewing and evaluating incident reports or summaries of incident reports, identifying hazards to health and safety, and making recommendations to the administrator
- Improving the performance of medical services as an integral part of improving organization performance
- Monitoring employees' health status and advising the administrator on employee health policies
- Working with other health care professionals to establish policies so that all health care professionals practice within the scope of their licenses

B   5.   The medical director serves as liaison on the organization's behalf by doing the following:
- Helping arrange and communicate to appropriate staff physician availability and coverage
- Communicating medical staff responsibilities and medical care policies, procedures, and guidelines to all licensed independent practitioners providing or ordering care
- If the organization has an organized medical staff, serving as a member, attending its meetings, and helping ensure adherence to its bylaws and rules and regulations
- If the organization has an organized medical staff, cooperating with it and the administrator to formulate the bylaws and rules and regulations needed for self-governance and to fulfill its responsibilities
- When there is no medical staff, being responsible for written rules and regulations for all licensed independent practitioners who attend residents in the organization

LD

- Being familiar with policies and programs of public health agencies that may affect resident care programs
- Acting as the organization's medical representative in the community

Note: *These EPs do not require the creation of a medical staff where one does not exist. That is entirely the long term care organization's decision.*

B   6.   When the organization's medical director does not have expertise in the full scope of services and programs provided, he or she seeks appropriate consultation.

A   7.   If the facility's medical director does not have the expertise to direct specialty programs, another physician with appropriate expertise is identified to direct the medical care provided, and the relationship between these two positions is clearly defined.

Standard LD.2.50

The leaders develop and monitor an annual operating budget and, as appropriate, a long-term capital expenditure plan.

Rationale for LD.2.50

Developing and monitoring an annual operating budget is essential to an organization's functioning. The budget describes the organization's goals and objectives in quantifiable terms. Operational or program budgets are developed in collaboration with appropriate staff and are consistent with the organization's budget. The following factors are considered during the budget process:

- The budget's underlying assumptions
- Information from the following:
  - Ongoing review of the system for determining resident care needs
  - Ongoing review of the organization's staffing plan
  - Performance improvement activities, including risk management and utilization review
  - Other sources addressing the adequacy of fiscal and other resource allocations for resident care
- Strategic planning information that indicates a need to revise fiscal allocations for providing resident care
- Measurement of performance relative to the approved budget, including methods for measuring and acting on identified and defined variances

Elements of Performance for LD.2.50

A   1.   An operating budget is developed annually and approved by the governance.

A   2.   The budget reflects the organization's goals and objectives and, at a minimum, meets applicable law and regulation.

B   3.   The leaders include staff input when developing the budget.

LD

A   4.   The governing body or authority approves a long-term capital expenditure plan, as appropriate.

A   5.   An independent public accountant conducts an annual audit of the organization's finances, unless otherwise provided by law.

    6.   Not applicable

B   7.   Implementation of the budget and, as appropriate, the long-term capital expenditure plan, is monitored.

Standards LD.2.60 Through LD.2.200
Not applicable

Standard LD.3.10
The leaders engage in both short-term and long-term planning.

Elements of Performance for LD.3.10
A   1.   Leaders create vision, mission, and goal statements.

A   2.   The organization's plan for services specifies which care, treatment, or services are provided directly and which through consultation, contract, or other agreement.

    3.   Not applicable

A   4.   **For subacute programs:** The organization has a statement outlining the program's philosophy and scope of services that clearly distinguishes the subacute patient from the traditional skilled resident based on the patient's needs and the organization's ability to meet those needs.

    5. Through 25. Not applicable

B   26.   Planning for care, treatment, and services addresses the following:
- The needs and expectations of residents and, as appropriate, families and referral sources
- Staff needs
- The scope of care, treatment, and services needed by residents at all of the organization's locations
- Resources (financial and human) for providing care and support services
- Recruitment, retention, development, and continuing education needs of all staff
- Data for measuring the performance of processes and outcomes of care

LD

Standard LD.3.15
Not applicable

Standard LD.3.20

Residents with comparable needs receive the same standard of care, treatment, and services throughout the organization.

Rationale for LD.3.20

Factors such as different individuals providing care, treatment, and services; different payment sources; or different settings of care do not intentionally negatively influence the outcome.

Elements of Performance for LD.3.20

B   1.   Residents with comparable needs receive the same standard of care, treatment, and services throughout the organization.

B   2.   The organization plans, designs, and monitors care, treatment, and services so they are consistent with the mission, vision, and goals.

Standard LD.3.30

Not applicable

Standard LD.3.40

Not applicable

Standard LD.3.50

Services provided by consultation, contractual arrangements, or other agreements are provided safely and effectively.

Elements of Performance for LD.3.50

A   1.   The leaders approve sources for the organization's services that are provided by consultation, contractual arrangements, or other agreements.

A   2.   The clinical leaders advise the organization's leaders on the sources of clinical services to be provided by consultation, contractual arrangements, or other agreements.

    3.   Not applicable

LD

A   4.   The nature and scope of services provided by consultation, contractual arrangements, or other agreements are defined in writing.*

B   5.   Services provided by consultation, contractual arrangements, or other agreements meet applicable Joint Commission standards.

B   6.   The organization evaluates the contracted care, treatment, and services to determine whether they are being provided according to the contract and the level of safety and quality that the organization expects.

A   7.   The organization retains overall responsibility and authority for services furnished under a contract.

A   8.   All reference and contract lab services† meet the applicable federal regulations for clinical laboratories and maintain evidence of the same.

Standard LD.3.60

Communication is effective throughout the organization.

Elements of Performance for LD.3.60

B   1.   The leaders ensure processes are in place for communicating relevant information throughout the organization in a timely manner.

B   2.   Effective communication occurs in the organization, among the organization's programs, among related organizations, with outside organizations, and with residents and families, as appropriate.

B   3.   The leaders communicate the organization's mission and appropriate policies, plans, and goals to all staff.

Standard LD.3.70

The leaders define the required qualifications and competence of those staff who provide care, treatment, and services and recommend a sufficient number of qualified and competent staff to provide care, treatment, and services.

LD

---

* When an organization contracts for resident care, treatment, and services rendered outside the organization but under the control of a Joint Commission–accredited organization, the primary organization can do the following:
- Specify in the contract that the contracting entity will ensure that all services provided by contracted individuals who are licensed independent practitioners will be within the scope of his or her privileges

or

- Verify that all contracted individuals who are licensed independent practitioners and who will be providing resident care, treatment, and services have appropriate privileges, for example, by obtaining a copy of the list of privileges

When an organization contracts for resident care, treatment, and services rendered outside the organization and under the control of a non–Joint Commission–accredited organization, all licensed independent practitioners who will be providing services are privileged by the Joint Commission–accredited organization through the process described in the "Management of Human Resources" chapter in this book.

† A written agreement (such as a formal contract) is not required for reference laboratories; however, it is required for a contract service where a major portion of laboratory testing is provided by an outside laboratory.

Rationale for LD.3.70

The determination of competence and qualifications of staff is based on the following:

- The organization's mission
- The organization's care, treatment, and services
- The complexity of care, treatment, and services needed by residents
- The technology used
- The health status of staff, as required by law and regulation

Element of Performance for LD.3.70

B   1.   The leaders provide for the allocation of competent qualified staff.

Standard LD.3.80

The leaders provide for adequate space, equipment, and other resources.

Elements of Performance for LD.3.80

B   1.   The leaders provide for the arrangement and allocation of space to facilitate efficient, effective delivery of care, treatment, and services.

B   2.   The leaders provide for the appropriateness of interior and exterior space for the care, treatment, and services offered and for the ages and other characteristics of the residents.

B   3.   The leaders provide for the safe use, maintenance, accessibility, and supervision of grounds, equipment, and special activity areas.

B   4.   The leaders provide for adequate equipment and other resources.

LD

Standard LD.3.90

The leaders develop and implement policies and procedures for care, treatment, and services.

Elements of Performance for LD.3.90

B   1.   The leaders develop policies and procedures that guide and support resident care, treatment, and services.

C Ⓜ   2.   Policies and procedures are consistently implemented.

Standard LD.3.100

Not applicable

Standard LD.3.110

Not applicable

Standard LD.3.120 ━━━━━━━━━━━━━━━━━━━━━━━━━━

The leaders plan for and support the provision and coordination of resident education activities.

Elements of Performance for LD.3.120

B   1.   The leaders plan and support resident education activities appropriate to the organization's mission and scope of services.

B   2.   The leaders identify and provide the resources necessary for achieving educational objectives.

Standard LD.3.130 ━━━━━━━━━━━━━━━━━━━━━━━━━━

Academic education is arranged for children and youth, when appropriate.

Rationale for LD.3.130

Educational resources are selected based on identified resident needs. The organization makes educational resources available that do the following:

- Help maintain the educational and intellectual development of residents
- Address opportunities to catch up for those residents who have fallen behind in their education because of their condition

Elements of Performance for LD.3.130

A   1.   Academic education is arranged for children and youth either through direct provision of services or community resources, such as tutors or attendance at classes in public schools, when appropriate.

B   2.   Educational resources are selected based on identified individual needs.

C   3.   The organization makes educational resources available that offer special education experiences for residents whose learning is hindered by their special needs.

Standard LD.3.140 ━━━━━━━━━━━━━━━━━━━━━━━━━━

Not applicable

Standard LD.3.150 ━━━━━━━━━━━━━━━━━━━━━━━━━━

Not applicable

Standard LD.4.10 ━━━━━━━━━━━━━━━━━━━━━━━━━━

The leaders set expectations, plan, and manage processes to measure, assess, and improve the organization's governance, management, clinical, and support activities.

Elements of Performance for LD.4.10

B   1.   The leaders set expectations for performance improvement.

B   2.   The leaders develop plans for performance improvement.

B   3.   The leaders manage processes to improve organization performance.

B   4.   The leaders participate in performance improvement activities.

B   5.   Appropriate individuals and professions from each relevant program, service, site, or department participate collaboratively in organizationwide performance improvement activities.

Standard LD.4.20 ━━━━━━━━━━━━━━━━━━━━━━━━━━━━━

New or modified services or processes are designed well.

Elements of Performance for LD.4.20

The design of new or modified services or processes incorporates the following:

B   1.   The needs and expectations of residents, staff, and others

B   2.   The results of performance improvement activities, when available

B   3.   Information about potential risks to residents, when available

B   4.   Current knowledge, when available and relevant (for example, practice guidelines, successful practices, information from relevant literature and clinical standards)

B   5.   Information about sentinel events, when available and relevant

B   6.   Testing and analysis to determine whether the proposed design or redesign is an improvement

B   7.   The leaders collaborate with staff and appropriate stakeholders to design services.

Standard LD.4.30 ━━━━━━━━━━━━━━━━━━━━━━━━━━━━━

Not applicable

Standard LD.4.40 ━━━━━━━━━━━━━━━━━━━━━━━━━━━━━

The leaders ensure that an integrated resident safety program is implemented throughout the organization.

Rationale for LD.4.40

The leaders should work to foster a safe environment throughout the organization by integrating safety priorities into all relevant organization processes, functions, and services. In pursuit of this effort, a resident safety program can work to improve safety by reducing the risk of system or process failures. As part of its responsibility to com-

LD

municate objectives and coordinate efforts to integrate resident care and support services throughout the organization and with contracted services, leadership takes the lead in developing, implementing, and overseeing a resident safety program.

The standard does not require the creation of new structures or "offices" in the organization; rather, the standard emphasizes the need to integrate all resident-safety activities, both existing and newly created, with the organization's leadership identified as accountable for this integration.

Elements of Performance for LD.4.40

The resident safety program includes the following:

A 1. One or more qualified individuals or an interdisciplinary group assigned to manage the organizationwide safety program

B 2. Definition of the scope of the program's oversight, typically ranging from no-harm, frequently occurring "slips" to sentinel events with serious adverse outcomes

B 3. Integration into and participation of all components of the organization into the organizationwide program

B 4. Procedures for immediately responding to system or process failures, including care, treatment, or services for the affected individual(s), containing risk to others, and preserving factual information for subsequent analysis

B 5. Clear systems for internal and external reporting of information about system or process failures

B 6. Defined responses to various types of unanticipated adverse events and processes for conducting proactive risk assessment/risk reduction activities

B 7. Defined support systems* for staff members who have been involved in a sentinel event

A 8. Reports, at least annually, to the organization's governance or authority on system or process failures and actions taken to improve safety, both proactively and in response to actual occurrences

Standard LD.4.50

The leaders set performance improvement priorities and identify how the organization adjusts priorities in response to unusual or urgent events.

---

* Support systems provide individuals with additional help and support as well as additional resources through the human resources function or an employee assistance program. Support systems recognize that conscientious health care workers who are involved in sentinel events are themselves victims of the event and require support. Support systems also focus on the process rather than blame the involved individuals.

Elements of Performance for LD.4.50

B 1. The leaders set priorities for performance improvement for organizationwide activities, staffing effectiveness, and resident health outcomes.

B 2. The leaders give high priority to high-volume, high-risk, or problem-prone processes.

B 3. Performance improvement activities are reprioritized in response to significant changes in the internal or external environment.

Standard LD.4.60

The leaders allocate adequate resources for measuring, assessing, and improving the organization's performance and improving resident safety.

Elements of Performance for LD.4.60

B 1. Sufficient staff is assigned to conduct activities for performance improvement and safety improvement.

B 2. Adequate time is provided for staff to participate in activities for performance improvement and safety improvement.

B 3. Adequate information systems are provided to support activities for performance improvement and safety improvement.

B 4. Staff is trained in performance improvement and safety improvement approaches and methods.

Standard LD.4.70

LD

The leaders measure and assess the effectiveness of the performance improvement and safety improvement activities.

Elements of Performance for LD.4.70

B 1. Leaders continually monitor the effectiveness of the performance improvement and safety improvement activities.

B 2. The leaders develop and implement improvements for these activities.

B 3. The leaders assess the adequacy of the human, information, physical, and financial resources allocated to support performance improvement and safety improvement activities.

Management of the Environment of Care

Overview

The **goal** of this function is to provide a safe, functional, supportive, and effective environment for residents, staff members, and other individuals in the organization. This is crucial to providing quality resident care, achieving good outcomes, and improving resident safety. Achieving this goal depends on performing the following processes:

- Performing strategic and ongoing master planning by organization leaders for the space, clear circulation of occupants, equipment, supportive environment, and resources needed to safely and effectively support the services provided. Planning and designing of the environment is consistent with the organization's mission and vision and the resident's physical condition/health, cultural background, age, and cognitive abilities.
- Educating staff about the role of the environment in safely, sensitively, and effectively supporting resident care. The organization educates staff about the physical characteristics necessary for attaining such an environment and the processes for monitoring, maintaining, and reporting on the organization's environment of care.
- Developing standards to measure staff and organization performance in managing and improving the environment of care.
- Implementing plans to create and manage the organization's environment of care. An Information Collection and Evaluation System (ICES) is developed and used to continuously measure, assess, and improve the status of the environment of care.

The "environment of care" consists of three basic components: building(s), equipment, and people. A variety of key elements and issues can contribute to creating the way the space feels and works for residents, families, staff, and others experiencing the health care delivery system. In addition, the key elements and issues can be significant in their ability to positively influence resident outcomes and satisfaction and improve resident safety. These elements include the following:

- Light (both natural and artificial)
- Privacy (visual and auditory)
- Space size and configuration that are appropriate and consistent with the clinical philosophy
- Security
- Orientation and access to nature and the outside
- Clarity of access (both exterior and interior circulation)
- Color
- Efficient layouts that support staffing and overall functional operation

EC

When appropriately designed into and managed as part of the physical environment, these elements create safe, welcoming, and comfortable environments that support and maintain resident dignity and personhood, allow ease of interaction, reduce stressors, and encourage family participation in the delivery of care.

Effective management of the environment of care includes using processes and activities to do the following:
- Reduce and control environmental hazards and risks
- Prevent accidents and injuries
- Maintain safe conditions for residents, staff, and others coming to the organization's facilities
- Maintain an environment that is sensitive to resident needs for comfort, social interaction, and positive distraction
- Maintain an environment that minimizes unnecessary environmental stresses for residents, staff, and others coming to the organization's facilities
The standards in this chapter focus on how everyone in the organization participates in the processes and activities that make the care environment safe and effective. They also address department leaders' responsibility for identifying and communicating the care environment needs to the organization and allocating appropriate space, equipment, and resources to safely and effectively support the organization's services.

Note 1: *The standards in this chapter do not prescribe any particular structure (such as a safety committee), specific individual (such as one employee hired to be a safety officer), or format for the required designs and planning activities.*

Note 2: *The standards do not require the Statement of Conditions™ compliance document to be completed by anyone other than an employee of the organization. This statement is the basis for corrective actions needed to make the environment compliant with the requirements of the* Life Safety Code® (LSC), *NFPA 101®.*

Note 3: *The standards in this chapter require each organization to develop a written plan for the following:*
- *Safety management (EC.1.10)*
- *Security management (EC.2.10)*
- *Hazardous materials and waste management (EC.3.10)*
- *Emergency management (EC.4.10)*
- *Fire safety (EC.5.10)*
- *Medical equipment management (EC.6.10)*
- *Utilities management (EC.7.10)*

If an organization has multiple sites, it may have separate management plans for each of its locations, or it may choose to have one comprehensive set of plans. In either case, the organization must address specific risks and the unique conditions at each of its sites.

EC

Standards

The following is a list of all standards for this function. They are presented here for your convenience without footnotes or other explanatory text. If you have a question about a term used here, please check the Glossary.

Note: *A revised standard numbering system is being used with the reformatted standards. The revised numbering system will allow for more flexibility to add standards while maintaining the current label for each standard.*

Planning and Implementation Activities

EC.1.10   The organization manages safety risks.

EC.1.20   The organization maintains a safe environment.

EC.1.25   Not applicable

EC.1.27   Not applicable

EC.1.30   The organization develops and implements a policy to prohibit smoking except in specified circumstances.

EC.2.10   The organization identifies and manages its security risks.

EC.3.10   The organization manages its hazardous materials and waste risks.

EC.4.10   The organization addresses emergency management.

EC.4.20   The organization conducts drills regularly to test emergency management.

EC.5.10   The organization manages fire safety risks.

EC.5.20   Newly constructed and existing environments are designed and maintained to comply with the *Life Safety Code*®.

EC.5.30   The organization conducts fire drills regularly.

EC.5.40   The organization maintains fire-safety equipment and building features.

EC.5.50   The organization develops and implements activities to protect occupants during periods when a building does not meet the applicable provisions of the *Life Safety Code*®.

EC.6.10   The organization manages medical equipment risks.

EC

EC.6.20   Medical equipment is maintained, tested, and inspected.

EC.7.10   The organization manages its utility risks.

EC.7.20   The organization provides a reliable emergency electrical power source.

EC.7.30   The organization maintains, tests, and inspects its utility systems.

EC.7.40   The organization maintains, tests, and inspects its emergency power systems.

EC.7.50   The organization maintains, tests, and inspects its medical gas and vacuum systems.

EC.8.10   The organization establishes and maintains an appropriate environment.

EC.8.20   The organization establishes and maintains an appropriate dining environment.

EC.8.30   The organization manages the design and building of the environment when it is renovated, altered, or newly created.

Measuring and Improving Activities

EC.9.10   The organization monitors conditions in the environment.

EC.9.20   The organization analyzes identified environment issues and develops recommendations for resolving them.

EC.9.30   The organization improves the environment.

EC

Understanding the Parts of This Chapter

To help you navigate this reformatted standards chapter, it may be helpful to think of its parts this way:

- The **standard** is the "goal"
- The **rationale** explains why it's important to achieve this goal
- The **elements of performance** identify the step(s) needed to achieve this goal

These parts are defined as follows.

Standard A statement that defines the performance expectations and/or structures or processes that must be in place for an organization to provide safe, high-quality care, treatment, and services. An organization is either "compliant" or "not compliant" with a standard.

Accreditation decisions are based on simple counts of the standards that are determined to be "not compliant."

Rationale A statement that provides background, justification, or additional information about a standard. A standard's rationale is not scored. In some instances, the rationale for a standard is self-evident. Therefore, not every standard has a written rationale.

Elements of performance (EPs) The specific performance expectations and/or structures or processes that must be in place for an organization to provide safe, high-quality care, treatment, and services. The scoring of EP compliance determines an organization's overall compliance with a standard. EPs are evaluated on the following scale:

> 0   Insufficient compliance
> 1   Partial compliance
> 2   Satisfactory compliance
> NA Not applicable

You will find a **measure of success** icon—Ⓜ—next to some EPs. Measures of success (MOS) need to be developed for certain EPs when a standard is judged to be out of compliance through either the Periodic Performance Review (PPR) or the onsite survey. An MOS is defined as a quantifiable measure, usually related to an audit, that can be used to determine whether an action has been effective and is being sustained.*

Assessing Your Compliance

Once you are familiar with the parts of this chapter, you can begin to assess your compliance with its requirements. The scoring category designations are provided next to each EP for your convenience. If you would like to assess your organization's performance, mark your scores for the EPs and standards by following the simple steps described below.

---

* For more information about MOS, *see* "The New Joint Commission Accreditation Process" chapter in this book.

Two components are scored for each EP: (1) compliance with the requirement itself **and** (2) compliance with the track record* for that requirement. Scoring has been simplified and track record achievements (which have always been part of the scoring) have been appropriately modified.

Note: *Some standards and EPs do not apply to a particular type of organization; these standards and EPs are marked "not applicable" and the related text is not included. Your organization is not expected to comply with standards and EPs marked "not applicable."*

In addition, some standards and EPs that do apply to organizations may not apply to the specific care, treatment, and services that your individual organization provides. Although these standards and EPs are included in the book, you are not expected to comply with them. If you are unsure about the standards or EPs that apply to your organization, please contact the Joint Commission's Standards Interpretation Group at 630/792-5900.

Step 1: Score Your Compliance with Each Element of Performance

Before you can determine your compliance with the standards, you must score your compliance with each EP. There are three scoring criterion categories: A, B, and C (described below). Please note that for each EP scoring criterion category, your organization must meet the performance requirement itself and the track record achievements (*see* "Track Record Achievements").

Category A

These EPs relate to the presence or absence of the requirement(s) and are scored either yes (2) or no (0); however, score 1 for partial compliance is also possible based on track record achievements.

If an A EP has multiple components designated by bullets, your organization must be compliant with all the bullets to receive a score of 2. If your organization does not meet one or more requirements in the bullets, you will receive a score of 0.

Category B

Category B EPs are scored in two steps:
1. As with category A EPs, category B EPs relate to the presence or absence of the requirement(s). If your organization *does not meet* the requirement(s), the EP is scored 0; there is no need to assess your compliance with the principles of good process design.
2. If your organization *does meet* the requirement(s), but there is concern about the quality or comprehensiveness of the effort, then and only then should you assess the qualitative aspect of the EP. That is, review the applicable principles of good process design and ask how the principles were applied in the situation under discussion. Good process design has the following characteristics:

---

* **Track record** The amount of time that an organization has been in compliance with a standard, EP, or other requirement.

- Is consistent with your organization's mission, values, and goals
- Meets the needs of patients
- Reflects the use of currently accepted practices (doing the right thing, using resources responsibly, using practice guidelines)
- Incorporates current safety information and knowledge such as sentinel event data and National Patient Safety Goals
- Incorporates relevant performance improvement results

This two-part evaluation applies to both simple and bulleted B EPs. First, the EPs are assessed to determine whether the requirements are present. If the EP has multiple components designated by bullets, as with the category A EPs, your organization must meet the requirements in *all* the bulleted items to get a score of 2. If your organization meets *none* of the requirements in the bullets, it receives a score of 0. If your organization meets *at least one, but not all,* of the bulleted requirements, it receives a score of 1 for the EPs.

Use the following rules to determine your EP score:
- Your EP score is 0 if your organization does not meet the requirement(s); you *do not* need to assess your compliance with the preceding applicable principles of good process design
- Your EP score is 1 if your organization does meet the requirement(s) but considered only *some* of the preceding applicable principles of good process design
- Your EP score is 2 if your organization does meet the requirement(s) *and* considered *all* the preceding principles of good process design

Category C
C EPs are scored 0, 1, or 2 based on the number of times your organization does not meet the EP. These EPs are frequency based and require totaling the number of occurrences (that is, results of performance or nonperformance) related to a particular EP. Each situation discovered by a surveyor(s) will be counted as a separate occurrence.

Note: *Multiple events of the same type related to a single resident and single practitioner/staff member are counted as* one occurrence only.

Use the following rules to determine your EP score:
- Your EP score is 2 if you find one or fewer occurrences of noncompliance with the EP
- Your EP score is 1 if you find two occurrences of noncompliance with the EP
- Your EP score is 0 if you find three or more occurrences of noncompliance with the EP

If an EP in the C category has multiple requirements designated by bullets, the following scoring guidelines apply:
- If there are fewer than two findings in all bullets, the EP is scored 2
- If there are three or more findings in all bullets, the EP is scored 0
- In all other combinations of findings, the EP is scored 1

EC

Track Record Achievements

In addition to meeting the requirement(s) in each EP, regardless of category, your organization must also meet the following track record achievements:

Score	Initial Survey	Full Survey
2	4 months or more	12 months or more
1	2 to 3 months	6 to 11 months
0	Fewer than 2 months	Fewer than 6 months

Sample Sizes

If during an onsite survey, your organization has been found to be not compliant with one or more standards, you must demonstrate Evidence of Standards Compliance (ESC) for each standard that is not compliant. The ESC must address compliance at the EP level; when an EP within a noncompliant standard requires an MOS, your organization must demonstrate achievement with the MOS when completing the ESC.

Note: *Not every EP requires an MOS. EPs that do require an MOS are clearly marked in this chapter. Organizations are required to demonstrate achievement with an MOS only for EPs within a noncompliant standard that require an MOS. Organizations do not need to demonstrate achievement with an MOS for any EP within a compliant standard.*

When demonstrating achievement with an MOS during the ESC process, your organization is **required** to use the following sample sizes, which were established because of their statistical significance, their relative simplicity in application, and their sensitivity to an organization's population size:

- For a population size of fewer than 30 cases,* sample 100% of available cases
- For a population size of 30 to 100 cases, sample 30 cases
- For a population size of 101 to 500 cases, sample 50 cases
- For a population size greater than 500 cases, sample 70 cases

EC

Note: *Organizations are* encouraged, but not required, *to follow this sample size when demonstrating achievement with an MOS for an EP within a noncompliant standard after conducting a full, Option 1, or Option 2 PPR.*

When conducting PPR (optional use) or demonstrating an ESC (mandatory use), use the following percentages to determine your EP score: 90% through 100% of your sample size is in compliance = score 2; 80% through 89% of your sample size is in compliance = score 1; less than 80% of your sample size is in compliance = score 0.

In addition, the following information should govern your organization's selection of samples:

- The appropriate sample size should be determined by the specific population related to the survey findings

---

* *Case* refers to a single instance in which a situation related to a survey finding occurs. For example, if a survey finding was related to **pain assessment**, then a case would be any resident record. If a survey finding was related to **pain management**, a case would be any resident record for residents receiving pain management.

- The sampling approach should involve either systematic random sampling (for example, your organization selects every second or third case for review) or simple random sampling (for example, your organization uses a series of random numbers generated by a computer to identify the cases to be reviewed)
- If your organization chooses not to use these sample sizes while conducting PPR options 1 or 2, you should make sure that your sample size is sufficiently large enough to ensure statistical significance
- When submitting a clarifying ESC, if your organization selects records as part of its sample, the records should be from a period of no more than three months before the last date of the survey
- Assessment of MOS compliance is conducted for a four-month period following the date of ESC approval. Your organization should select records as a part of your sample following the date of ESC approval and use the required sample sizes. MOS percentage compliance rates are derived from the average of all four months.

Step 2: Use Your EP Scores to Gauge Your Compliance with the Standards

Now that you have evaluated and scored each EP for a particular standard, use these simple rules to determine your compliance with the standard itself:

- Your organization is not in compliance (that is, "not compliant") with the standard if any EP is scored 0
- Otherwise, your organization is in compliance with a standard if 65% or more of its EPs are scored 2

EC

Standards, Rationales, Elements of Performance, and Scoring

Planning and Implementation Activities

No organization can ensure that residents, staff, and others coming to the organization's facilities will never suffer an accidental injury. However, organizations can minimize avoidable risks and injuries through sound planning, resource allocation (*see* "Leadership" chapter), effective training (*see* "Management of Human Resources" chapter), implementation, and ongoing monitoring and improvement of risk reduction activities. These activities can be accomplished through the management process, staff activities, and/or technology.

Standard EC.1.10 ━━━━━━━━━━━━━━━━━━━━━━━━━━━━━━━━

The organization manages safety risks.

Rationale for EC.1.10

Each organization has inherent safety risks associated with providing services for residents, the performance of daily activities by staff, and the physical environment in which services occur. It is important that each organization identifies these risks and plans and implements processes to minimize the likelihood of those risks causing incidents.

Elements of Performance for EC.1.10

B   1.   The organization develops and maintains a written management plan describing the processes it implements to effectively manage the environmental safety of residents, staff, and other people coming to the organization's facilities.

A   2.   The organization identifies a person(s), as designated by leadership, to coordinate the development, implementation, and monitoring of the safety management activities.

A   3.   The organization identifies a person(s) to intervene whenever conditions immediately threaten life or health or threaten damage to equipment or buildings.

B   4.   The organization conducts comprehensive, proactive risk assessments that evaluate the potential adverse impact of buildings, grounds, equipment, occupants, and internal physical systems on the safety and health of residents, staff, and other people coming to the organization's facilities.

C Ⓜ   5.   The organization uses the risks identified to select and implement procedures and controls to achieve the lowest potential for adverse impact

EC

on the safety and health of residents, staff, and other people coming to the organization's facilities.

C Ⓜ 6. The organization establishes safety policies and procedures that are practiced and reviewed as frequently as necessary, but at least every three years.

7. Not applicable

B 8. The organization ensures that a process exists for responding to product safety recalls by appropriate organization staff.

B 9. The organization ensures that all grounds and equipment are maintained appropriately.

Standard EC.1.20 ▬▬▬▬▬▬▬▬▬▬▬▬▬▬▬▬▬▬▬▬▬▬▬▬

The organization maintains a safe environment.

Rationale for EC.1.20

It is essential that the organization conduct periodic environmental tours to determine if its current processes for managing resident, public, and staff safety risks are being practiced correctly and are effective. These tours can also be used to assess staff knowledge and behaviors, identify new or altered risks in areas where construction or changes in services have occurred, and identify opportunities to improve the environment.

Elements of Performance for EC.1.20

B 1. The organization conducts environmental tours to identify environmental deficiencies, hazards, and unsafe practices.

C Ⓜ 2. The organization conducts environmental tours at least every six months in all areas where individuals are served.

C Ⓜ 3. The organization conducts environmental tours at least annually in areas where individuals are not served.

Standard EC.1.25 ▬▬▬▬▬▬▬▬▬▬▬▬▬▬▬▬▬▬▬▬▬▬▬▬

Not applicable

Standard EC.1.27 ▬▬▬▬▬▬▬▬▬▬▬▬▬▬▬▬▬▬▬▬▬▬▬▬

Not applicable

Standard EC.1.30 ▬▬▬▬▬▬▬▬▬▬▬▬▬▬▬▬▬▬▬▬▬▬▬▬

The organization develops and implements a policy to prohibit smoking except in specified circumstances.

EC

Rationale for EC.1.30

This standard is intended to reduce the following risks:

- To people who smoke, including possible adverse effects on care, treatment, and services
- Of passive smoking for others
- Of fire

The standard prohibits smoking in all areas of all building(s) under the organization's control, except for residents in circumstances specified in the elements of performance.

Elements of Performance for EC.1.30

B 1. The organization develops a policy regarding smoking in all areas of all building(s) under the organization's control.

B 2. The organization's policy prohibits smoking in all areas of all building(s) under the organization's control (no medical exceptions allowed) for the following:
- All children or youth residents

B 3. The organization's policy may permit residents to smoke in the organization's buildings under the following circumstance:
- A resident meets criteria developed and approved by the organization's leaders

B 4. When residents are permitted to smoke in the organization's buildings, they smoke only under the following circumstances:
- In designated locations environmentally separate from care, treatment, and services areas*
- After the organization has taken measures to minimize fire risks

C Ⓜ 5. Residents who do smoke in the organization's buildings are provided education, including information about options for smoking cessation.

B 6. The organization identifies and implements a process(es) for monitoring compliance with the policy.

B 7. The organization develops strategies to eliminate the incidence of policy violations when identified.

Standard EC.2.10

The organization identifies and manages its security risks.

---

* **Note:** *This does not require that a designated smoking area be a specific distance from care, treatment, and services areas. A physically separate, well-ventilated room (a designated area for authorized smoking by residents that is exhausted to the outside) is acceptable.*

Rationale for EC.2.10

It is essential that an organization manages the physical and personal security of residents, staff (including addressing the risks of violence in the workplace), and individuals coming to the organization's facilities. In addition, security of the established environment, equipment, supplies, and information is also important.

Elements of Performance for EC.2.10

B 1. The organization develops and maintains a written management plan describing the processes it implements to effectively manage the security of residents, staff, and other people coming to the organization's facilities.

A 2. The organization identifies a person(s), as designated by leadership, to coordinate the development, implementation, and monitoring of the security management activities.

B 3. The organization conducts proactive risk assessments that evaluate the potential adverse impact of the external environment and the services provided on the security of residents, staff, and other people coming to the organization's facilities.*

C Ⓜ 4. The organization uses the risks identified to select and implement procedures and controls to achieve the lowest potential for adverse impact on security.

B 5. The organization identifies, as appropriate, residents, staff, and other people entering the organization's facilities.

C Ⓜ 6. The organization controls access to and egress from security-sensitive areas, as determined by the organization.

B 7. The organization identifies and implements security procedures that address actions taken in the event of a security incident.

  8. Not applicable

B 9. The organization identifies and implements security procedures that address handling of situations involving VIPs or the media.

EC

Standard EC.3.10

The organization manages its hazardous materials and waste[†] risks.

---

* The potential for workplace violence and for resident elopement or wandering is considered during the risk assessment.

† **Hazardous materials (HAZMAT) and waste** Materials whose handling, use, and storage are guided or regulated by local, state, or federal regulation. Examples include the Occupational Safety and Health Administration Regulations for Bloodborne Pathogens (regarding blood, other infectious materials, contaminated items that would release blood or other infectious materials, or contaminated sharps); the Nuclear Regulatory Commission regulations for handling and disposal of radioactive waste; management of hazardous vapors (such as glutaraldehyde, ethylene oxide, and nitrous oxide); chemicals regulated by the Environmental Protection Agency; Department of Transportation requirements; and hazardous energy sources (for example, ionizing or nonionizing radiation, lasers, microwaves, and ultrasound).

Rationale for EC.3.10

Organizations must identify materials they use that need special handling and implement processes to minimize the risks of their unsafe use and improper disposal.

Elements of Performance for EC.3.10

B 1. The organization develops and maintains a written management plan describing the processes it implements to effectively manage hazardous materials and waste.

B 2. The organization creates and maintains an inventory that identifies hazardous materials and waste used, stored, or generated using criteria consistent with applicable law and regulation (for example, the EPA and OSHA).

The organization establishes and implements processes for selecting, handling, storing, transporting, using, and disposing of hazardous materials and waste from receipt or generation through use and/or final disposal, including managing the following (EPs 3–6):

C Ⓜ 3. Chemicals

A 4. Chemotherapeutic materials

A 5. Radioactive materials

C Ⓜ 6. Infectious and regulated medical wastes, including sharps

B 7. The organization provides adequate and appropriate space and equipment for safely handling and storing hazardous materials and waste.

    8. Not applicable

B 9. The organization identifies and implements emergency procedures that include the specific precautions, procedures, and protective equipment used during hazardous materials and waste spills or exposures.

A 10. The organization maintains documentation, including required permits, licenses, and adherence to other regulations.

C Ⓜ 11. The organization maintains required manifests for handling hazardous materials and waste.

C Ⓜ 12. The organization properly labels hazardous materials and waste.

B 13. The organization effectively separates hazardous materials and waste storage and processing areas from other areas of the facility.

Standard EC.4.10

The organization addresses emergency management.

Rationale for EC.4.10

An emergency* in the organization or its community could suddenly and significantly affect the need for the organization's services or its ability to provide those services. Therefore, an organization needs to have an emergency management plan that comprehensively describes its approach to emergencies in the organization or in its community.

Elements of Performance for EC.4.10

A   1.   The organization conducts a hazard vulnerability analysis† to identify potential emergencies that could affect the need for its services or its ability to provide those services.

A   2.   The organization establishes the following with the community:
- Priorities among the potential emergencies identified in the hazard vulnerability analysis
- The organization's role in relation to a communitywide emergency management program
- An "all-hazards" command structure within the organization that links with the community's command structure

B   3.   The organization develops and maintains a written emergency management plan describing the process for disaster readiness and emergency management and implements it when appropriate.

A   4.   At a minimum, an emergency management plan is developed with the involvement of the organization's leaders, including the administrator, the medical director, the nursing leader, and other clinical leaders.

B   5.   The plan identifies specific procedures that describe mitigation,† preparedness,§ response, and recovery strategies, actions, and responsibilities for each priority emergency.

B   6.   The plan provides processes for initiating the response and recovery phases of the plan, including a description of how, when, and by whom the phases are to be activated.

EC

---

* **Emergency** A natural or manmade event that significantly disrupts the environment of care (for example, damage to the organization's building[s] and grounds due to severe winds, storms, or earthquakes); that significantly disrupts care, treatment, and services (for example, loss of utilities such as power, water, or telephones due to floods, civil disturbances, accidents, or emergencies within the organization or in its community); or that results in sudden, significantly changed, or increased demands for the organization's services (for example, bioterrorist attack, building collapse, plane crash in the organization's community). Some emergencies are called "disasters" or "potential injury creating events" (PICEs).

† **Hazard vulnerability analysis** The identification of potential emergencies and the direct and indirect effects these emergencies may have on the organization's operations and the demand for its services.

‡ **Mitigation activities** Those activities an organization undertakes in attempting to lessen the severity and impact of a potential emergency.

§ **Preparedness activities** Those activities an organization undertakes to build capacity and identify resources that may be used if an emergency occurs.

B 7. The plan provides processes for notifying staff when emergency response measures are initiated.

B 8. The plan provides processes for notifying external authorities of emergencies, including possible community emergencies identified by the organization.

B 9. The plan provides processes for identifying and assigning staff to cover all essential staff functions under emergency conditions.

B 10. The plan provides processes for managing the following under emergency conditions:
- Activities related to care, treatment, and services (for example, scheduling, modifying, or discontinuing services; controlling information about residents; referrals; transporting residents)
- Staff support activities (for example, housing, transportation, incident stress debriefing)
- Staff family support activities
- Logistics relating to critical supplies (for example, supplies, food, linen, water)
- Security (for example, access, crowd control, traffic control)
- Communication with the news media

11. Not applicable

B 12. The plan provides processes for evacuating the entire facility (both horizontally and, when applicable, vertically) when the environment cannot support adequate care, treatment, and services.

B 13. The plan provides processes for establishing an alternate care site(s) that has the capabilities to meet the needs of residents when the environment cannot support adequate care, treatment, and services, including processes for the following:
- Transporting residents, staff, and equipment to the alternative care site(s)
- Transferring to and from the alternative care site(s), the necessities of residents (for example, medications, medical records)
- Tracking of residents
- Interfacility communication between the organization and the alternative care site(s)

B 14. The plan provides processes for identifying care providers and other personnel during emergencies.

B 15. The plan provides processes for cooperative planning with health care organizations that together provide services to a contiguous geographic area (for example, among organizations serving a town or borough) to facilitate the timely sharing of information about the following:
- Essential elements of their command structures and control centers for emergency response

EC

- Names and roles of individuals in their command structures and command center telephone numbers
- Resources and assets that could potentially be shared in an emergency response
- Names of residents and deceased individuals brought to their organizations to facilitate identifying and locating victims of the emergency

16. Not applicable

17. Not applicable

B 18. The plan identifies backup internal and external communication systems in the event of failure during emergencies.

B 19. The plan identifies alternate roles and responsibilities of staff during emergencies, including to whom they report in the organization's command structure and, when activated, in the community's command structure.

B 20. The plan identifies an alternative means of meeting essential building utility needs when the organization is designated by its emergency management plan to provide continuous service during an emergency (for example, electricity, water, ventilation, fuel sources, medical gas/vacuum systems).

B 21. The plan identifies means for radioactive, biological, and chemical isolation and decontamination.

Standard EC.4.20

The organization conducts drills regularly to test emergency management.

Elements of Performance for EC.4.20

A 1. The organization tests the response phase of its emergency management plan twice a year, either in response to an actual emergency or in planned drills.*

   Note: *Tabletop exercises, though useful in planning or training, are only acceptable substitutes for communitywide practice drills.*

A 2. Drills are conducted at least four months apart and no more than eight months apart.

A 3. Organizations that offer emergency services or are community-designated disaster receiving stations must conduct at least one drill a year that includes an influx of volunteers or simulated residents.

A 4. The organization participates in at least one communitywide practice drill a year (where applicable) relevant to the priority emergencies identified

EC

---

* **Note:** *Drills that involve packages of information that simulate residents, their families, and the public are acceptable.*

in its hazard vulnerability analysis. The drill assesses the communication, coordination, and effectiveness of the organization's and community's command structures.

Note 1: *"Communitywide" may range from a contiguous geographic area served by the same health care providers, to a large borough, town, city, or region.*

Note 2: *Tests of EPs 3 and 4 may be separate, simultaneous, or combined.*

5. Not applicable

B 6. All drills are critiqued to identify deficiencies and opportunities for improvement.

Standard EC.5.10

The organization manages fire safety risks.

Rationale for EC.5.10

All facilities are designed, constructed, maintained, and operated to minimize the possibility of a fire emergency requiring the evacuation of occupants. Because the safety of occupants cannot be ensured adequately by dependence on evacuation of the building, their protection from fire shall be provided by appropriate arrangement of facilities; adequate, trained staff; and development of operating and maintenance procedures composed of the following:
- Design, construction, and compartmentation
- Provision for detection, alarm, and extinguishment
- Fire prevention and the planning, training, and drilling programs for the isolation of fire, transfer of occupants to areas of refuge, or evacuation of the building

Elements of Performance for EC.5.10

B 1. The organization develops and maintains a written management plan describing the processes it implements to effectively manage fire safety.

B 2. The organization identifies proactive processes for protecting residents, staff, and others coming to the organization's facilities, as well as protecting property from fire, smoke, and other products of combustion.

B 3. The organization identifies processes for regularly inspecting, testing, and maintaining fire protection and fire safety systems, equipment, and components.

B 4. The organization develops and implements a fire response plan that addresses the following:
- Facilitywide fire response
- Area-specific needs, including fire evacuation routes
- Specific roles and responsibilities of staff, licensed independent practitioners, and volunteers at a fire's point of origin

EC

- Specific roles and responsibilities of staff, licensed independent practitioners, and volunteers away from a fire's point of origin
- Specific roles and responsibilities of staff, licensed independent practitioners, and volunteers in preparing for building evacuation

B 5. The organization reviews proposed acquisitions of bedding, window draperies, and other curtains, furnishings, decorations, and other equipment for fire safety.

Standard EC.5.20

Newly constructed and existing environments are designed and maintained to comply with the *Life Safety Code*®.*

Rationale for EC.5.20

The *Life Safety Code*® (*LSC*) requires that a building is designed, constructed, and maintained with the capability of being fire safe. When undertaking the design of a newly remodeled building, the organization should also satisfy any requirements of others (local, state, or federal) that may be more stringent than the *LSC*.

Elements of Performance for EC.5.20

B 1. Each building in which residents are housed or receive care, treatment, and services complies with the *LSC*, NFPA 101® 2000;

or

Each building in which residents are housed or receive care, treatment, and services does not comply with the *LSC*, but the resolution of all deficiencies is evidenced through the following:
- An equivalency approved by the Joint Commission
or
- Continued progress in completing an acceptable Plan For Improvement (Statement of Conditions™ [SOC], Part 4)

A 2. A current, organizationwide SOC compliance document[†] has been prepared.

Note: *You can obtain a copy of the SOC from our Web site at http://www.jcaho.org or by calling Customer Service at 630/792-5800. You may make as many copies of the SOC as you wish. However, remember to keep the original blank for future copying.*

3. Not applicable

4. Not applicable

---

* *Life Safety Code*® is a registered trademark of the National Fire Protection Association, Quincy, Massachusetts.

[†] **Statement of Conditions™ (SOC) compliance document** A proactive document that helps an organization perform a critical self-assessment of its current level of compliance and describe how to resolve any *LSC* deficiencies. The SOC was created to be a living, ongoing management tool that should be used in a management process that continually identifies, assesses, and resolves *LSC* deficiencies.

EC

A   5.   The organization is making sufficient progress* toward the corrective actions described in a previously approved Statement of Conditions™.

Standard EC.5.30 ▬▬▬▬▬▬▬▬▬▬▬▬▬▬▬▬▬▬▬▬▬▬▬▬

The organization conducts fire drills regularly.

Rationale for EC.5.30

The development of a fire response plan is an important part of achieving a fire-safe environment (*see* standard EC.5.10). It is important that this plan be regularly evaluated during implementations (in drill scenarios or actual fire situations) for performance of the fire safety equipment and staff.

Implementation of the plan should be realistic and held at varied times. An implementation held at shift change may present an unrealistic picture as to the number of staff likely available any time a fire occurs. Actual evacuation of residents during the drills is not required.

Elements of Performance for EC.5.30

C Ⓜ   1.   Fire drills are conducted quarterly on all shifts in each buildings defined by the *LSC* as the following:
- Health care occupancy

2.   Not applicable

3.   Not applicable

C Ⓜ   4.   At least 50% of the required drills are unannounced.

B   5.   Staff in all areas of every building where residents are housed or treated participates in drills to the extent called for in the facility's fire plan. (*See* standard EC.5.10 for required content of fire response plan.)†

B   6.   All fire drills are critiqued to identify deficiencies and opportunities for improvement.

A   7.   The effectiveness of fire response training according to the fire plan is evaluated at least annually.

B   8.   During fire drills, staff knowledge is evaluated, including the following:
- When and how to sound fire alarms (where such alarms are available)
- When and how to transmit for offsite fire responders
- Containment of smoke and fire
- Transfer of residents to areas of refuge
- Fire extinguishment

---

* **Sufficient progress** Failure to make sufficient progress toward the corrective actions described in an approved SOC, Part 4, Plan For Improvement, would result in a recommendation of Conditional Accreditation.

† When drills are conducted between 9:00 P.M. and 6:00 A.M., a coded announcement will be permitted to be used instead of audible alarms.

- Specific fire response duties
- Preparation for building evacuation

Standard EC.5.40

The organization maintains fire-safety equipment and building features.

Note 1: *This standard does not require organizations to have the types of fire-safety equipment and building features discussed here. However, if these types of equipment or features exist within the organization, then the following maintenance, testing, and inspection requirements apply.*

Note 2: *Organizations that offer care, treatment, and services in leased facilities need to communicate maintenance expectations for building equipment not under their control to their landlord through contractual language, lease agreements, memos, and so forth. These organizations are not required to possess maintenance documentation but must only have access to such documentation as needed and during survey. It is also important that the landlord communicate to the organization any building equipment problems identified that could negatively affect the safety or health of residents, staff, and other people coming to the organization, as well as the landlord's plan to resolve such issues.*

Elements of Performance for EC.5.40

C Ⓜ 1. Initiating devices and fire detection and alarm equipment are tested as follows:*
- All supervisory signal devices (except valve tamper switches) are tested at least quarterly
- All valve tamper switches and water flow devices are tested at least semiannually
- All duct detectors, electromechanical releasing devices, heat detectors, manual fire alarm boxes, and smoke detectors are tested at least annually

C Ⓜ 2. Occupant alarm notification devices, including all audible devices, speakers, and visible devices, are tested at least annually.

A 3. Off-premises emergency services notification transmission equipment is tested at least quarterly.

C Ⓜ 4. For water-based automatic fire-extinguishing systems, all fire pumps are tested at least weekly under no-flow condition.†

C Ⓜ 5. For water-based automatic fire-extinguishing systems, all water-storage tank high- and low-water level alarms are tested at least semiannually.

EC

---

* For additional guidance, see NFPA 72-1999 edition (Table 7-3.2).

† For additional guidance, see NFPA 25-1998 edition.

C Ⓜ 6. For water-based automatic fire-extinguishing systems, all water-storage tank low-water temperature alarms (during cold weather only) are tested at least monthly.

C Ⓜ 7. For water-based automatic fire-extinguishing systems, main drain tests are conducted at least annually at all system risers.

C Ⓜ 8. For water-based automatic fire-extinguishing systems, all fire department connections are inspected quarterly.

A 9. For water-based automatic fire-extinguishing systems, all fire pumps are tested at least annually under flow.

A 10. Kitchen automatic fire-extinguishing systems are inspected for proper operation at least semiannually. (Actual discharge of the fire-extinguishing system is not required.)

C Ⓜ 11. Carbon dioxide and other gaseous automatic fire-extinguishing systems are tested for proper operation at least annually. (Actual discharge of the fire-extinguishing system is not required.)

C Ⓜ 12. All portable fire extinguishers* are clearly identified, inspected at least monthly, and maintained at least annually.

C Ⓜ 13. All standpipe occupant hoses are hydrostatically tested five years after installation and at least every three years thereafter,[†] and systems receive water-flow tests at least every five years.[‡]

C Ⓜ 14. All fire and smoke dampers are operated at least every four years (with fusible links removed where applicable) to verify that they fully close.[§]

A 15. All automatic smoke-detection shutdown devices for air-handling equipment are tested at least annually.[‖]

C Ⓜ 16. All horizontal and vertical sliding and rolling fire doors are tested for proper operation and full closure at least annually.[#]

EC

---

* For additional guidance, see NFPA 10-1998 edition (sections 1-6, 4-3, and 4-4).

[†] For additional guidance, see NFPA 1962-1998 edition (section 2-3).

[‡] For additional guidance, see NFPA 25-1998 edition.

[§] For additional guidance, see NFPA 90A-1999 edition (section 3-4.7).

[‖] For additional guidance, see NFPA 90A-1999 edition (section 4-4.1).

[#] For additional guidance, see NFPA 80-1999 edition (section 15-2.4).

Standard EC.5.50

The organization develops and implements activities to protect occupants during periods when a building does not meet the applicable provisions of the *Life Safety Code®*.

Note: *This standard does not apply to facilities classified as a business occupancy by the* LSC.

Rationale for EC.5.50

When building code deficiencies are identified and cannot be immediately corrected or during renovation or construction activities, the safety of residents, staff, and other people coming to the organization's facilities is diminished. Organizations need to proactively identify administrative actions (for example, additional training, additional inspections, additional fire drills, and so on) to be taken if these scenarios arise.

Elements of Performance for EC.5.50

B   1.   Each organization develops a policy for using interim life safety measures (ILSMs).

B   2.   The policy includes written criteria for evaluating various deficiencies and construction hazards to determine when and to what extent one or more of the following measures apply:
- Ensuring free and unobstructed exits. Staff receives additional information/communication when alternative exits are designated. Buildings or areas under construction must maintain escape routes for construction workers at all times, and the means of exiting construction areas are inspected daily.
- Ensuring free and unobstructed access to emergency services and for fire, police, and other emergency forces
- Ensuring that fire alarm, detection, and suppression systems are in good working order. A temporary but equivalent system must be provided when any fire system is impaired. Temporary systems must be inspected and tested monthly.*
- Ensuring that temporary construction partitions are smoke-tight and built of noncombustible or limited combustible materials that will not contribute to the development or spread of fire
- Providing additional fire-fighting equipment and training staff in its use
- Prohibiting smoking throughout the organization's buildings and in and near construction areas
- Developing and enforcing storage, housekeeping, and debris-removal practices that reduce the building's flammable and combustible fire load to the lowest feasible level
- Conducting a minimum of two fire drills per shift per quarter

EC

---

* The *LSC,* NFPA 101 - 2000 edition, requires that the municipal fire department is notified (or applicable emergency forces group) and a fire watch is provided whenever an approved fire alarm or automatic sprinkler system is out of service for more than 4 hours in a 24-hour period in an occupied building.

- Increasing surveillance of buildings, grounds, and equipment, with special attention to excavations, construction areas, construction storage, and field offices
- Training staff to compensate for impaired structural or compartmentalization* features of fire safet.
- Conducting organizationwide safety education programs to promote awareness of fire-safety building deficiencies, construction hazards, and ILSMs

A   3.   Each organization implements ILSMs as defined in its policy.

Standard EC.6.10

The organization manages medical equipment risks.

Rationale for EC.6.10

Medical equipment is a significant contributor to the quality of care. It is used in treatment, diagnostic activities, and monitoring of the resident. It is essential that the equipment is appropriate for the intended use; that staff, including licensed independent practitioners, be trained to use the equipment safely and effectively; and that the equipment is maintained appropriately by qualified individuals.

Elements of Performance for EC.6.10

B   1.   The organization develops and maintains a written management plan describing the processes it implements to manage the effective, safe, and reliable operation of medical equipment.

B   2.   The organization identifies and implements a process(es) for selecting and acquiring medical equipment.[†]

B   3.   The organization establishes and uses risk criteria[‡] for identifying, evaluating, and creating an inventory of equipment to be included in the medical equipment management plan before the equipment is used. These criteria address the following:
- Equipment function (diagnosis, care, treatment, life support, and monitoring)
- Physical risks associated with use
- Equipment incident history

---

* **Compartmentalization** The concept of using various building components (fire walls and doors, smoke barriers, fire rated floor slabs, and so forth) to prevent the spread of fire and the production's combustion and to provide a safe means of egress to an approved exit. The presence of these features varies depending upon the building occupancy classification.

[†] **Note:** *The acquisition process includes initially evaluating the condition and function of the equipment when received and evaluating the training of users before use on residents.*

[‡] **Note:** *The organization may choose not to use risk criteria to limit the types of equipment to be included in the medical equipment management plan, but rather include all medical equipment.*

EC

B   4.   The organization identifies appropriate inspection and maintenance strategies for all equipment on the inventory for achieving effective, safe, and reliable operation of all equipment in the inventory.*

B   5.   The organization defines intervals for inspecting, testing, and maintaining appropriate equipment on the inventory (that is, those pieces of equipment on the inventory benefiting from scheduled activities to minimize the clinical and physical risks) that are based upon criteria such as manufacturers' recommendations, risk levels, and current organization experience.

B   6.   The organization identifies and implements processes for monitoring and acting on equipment hazard notices and recalls.

B   7.   The organization identifies and implements processes for monitoring and reporting incidents in which a medical device is suspected or attributed to the death, serious injury, or serious illness of any individual, as required by the Safe Medical Devices Act of 1990.

A   8.   The organization identifies and implements processes for emergency procedures that address the following:
- What to do in the event of equipment disruption or failure
- When and how to perform emergency clinical interventions when medical equipment fails
- Availability of backup equipment
- How to obtain repair services

Standard EC.6.20 ▬▬▬▬▬▬▬▬▬▬
Medical equipment is maintained, tested, and inspected.

Elements of Performance for EC.6.20
C Ⓜ   1.   The organization documents a current, accurate, and separate inventory of all equipment identified in the medical equipment management plan, regardless of ownership.

A   2.   The organization documents performance and safety testing of all equipment identified in the medical equipment management program before initial use.

A   3.   The organization documents inspection and maintenance of equipment used for life support† that is consistent with maintenance strate-

EC

---

* **Note:** *Organizations may use different strategies for different items as appropriate. For example, strategies such as predictive maintenance, interval-based inspections, corrective maintenance, or metered maintenance may be selected to ensure reliable performance.*

† **Life support equipment** Those devices intended to sustain life and whose failure to perform its primary function, when used according to manufacturer's instructions and clinical protocol, is expected to result in imminent death in the absence of immediate intervention (examples include ventilators, anesthesia machines, and heart-lung bypass machines).

gies to minimize clinical and physical risks identified in the equipment management plan (*see* standard EC.6.10).

C Ⓜ 4. The organization documents inspection and maintenance of non–life support equipment on the inventory that is consistent with maintenance strategies to minimize clinical and physical risks identified in the equipment management plan (*see* standard EC.6.10).

5. Not applicable

A Ⓜ 6. The organization documents chemical and biological testing of water used in renal dialysis and other applicable tests based upon regulations, manufacturers' recommendations, and organization experience.

Standard EC.7.10

The organization manages its utility risks.

Rationale for EC.7.10

Utility systems* are essential to the proper operation of the environment of care and significantly contribute to effective, safe, and reliable provision of care to residents in health care organizations. It is important that health care organizations establish and maintain a utility systems management program to promote a safe, controlled, and comfortable environment that does the following:

- Ensures operational reliability of utility systems
- Reduces the potential for organization-acquired illness to be transmitted through the utility systems
- Assesses the reliability and minimizes potential risks of utility system failures

Elements of Performance for EC.7.10

1. Through 6. Not applicable

B 7. The organization develops and maintains a written management plan describing the processes it implements to manage the effective, safe, and reliable operation of utility systems.

B 8. The organization designs and installs utility systems that meet the resident care and operational needs of the services in the organization's buildings.

B 9. The organization establishes risk criteria† for identifying, evaluating, and creating an inventory of operating components of systems before the equipment is used.

---

* **Utility systems** May include electrical distribution; emergency power; vertical and horizontal transport; heating, ventilating, and air conditioning; plumbing, boiler, and steam; piped gases; vacuum systems; or communication systems, including data-exchange systems.

† **Note:** *The organization may choose not to use risk criteria to limit the types of utility systems to be included in the utility management plan, but rather include all utility systems.*

These criteria address the following:
- Life support
- Infection control
- Support of the environment
- Equipment support
- Communication

B   10. The organization develops appropriate strategies for all utility systems equipment on the inventory for ensuring effective, safe, and reliable operation of all equipment in the inventory.*

B   11. The organization defines intervals for inspecting, testing, and maintaining appropriate utility systems equipment on the inventory (that is, those pieces of equipment on the inventory benefiting from scheduled activities to minimize the clinical and physical risks) that are based upon criteria such as manufacturers' recommendations, risk levels, and current organization experience.

A   12. The organization identifies and implements emergency procedures for responding to utility system disruptions or failures that address the following:
- What to do if utility systems malfunction
- Identification of an alternative source of organization-defined essential utilities
- Shutting off the malfunctioning systems and notifying staff in affected areas
- How and when to perform emergency clinical interventions when utility systems fail
- Obtaining repair services

B   13. The organization maps the distribution of utility systems.

C Ⓜ   14. The organization labels controls for a partial or complete emergency shutdown.

B   15. The organization identifies and implements processes to minimize pathogenic biological agents in cooling towers, domestic hot/cold water systems, and other aerosolizing water systems.

A   16. The organization designs, installs, and maintains ventilation equipment to provide appropriate pressure relationships, air-exchange rates, and filtration efficiencies for ventilation systems serving areas specially designed† to control airborne contaminants (such as biological agents, gases, fumes, and dust).

EC

---

* **Note:** *Organizations may use different strategies as appropriate. For example, strategies such as predictive maintenance, interval-based inspections, corrective maintenance, or metered maintenance may be selected to ensure reliable performance.*

† **Areas specially designed** Include spaces such as rooms for residents diagnosed or suspected of having airborne communicable diseases (for example, pulmonary or laryngeal tuberculosis), residents in "protective isolation" rooms (for example, those receiving bone marrow transplants), laboratories, pharmacies, and sterile supply rooms.

Standard EC.7.20 ▬▬▬▬▬▬▬▬▬▬▬▬▬▬▬▬▬▬▬▬▬

The organization provides an emergency electrical power source.

Rationale for EC.7.20

The organization properly installs an emergency power source that is adequately sized, designed, and fueled, as required by the *LSC* occupancy requirements and the services provided.

Elements of Performance for EC.7.20

The organization provides a reliable emergency power system*, as required by the *LSC* occupancy requirements, that supplies electricity to the following areas when normal electricity is interrupted:

A   1.   Alarm systems

C Ⓜ 2.   Exit route illumination

A   3.   Emergency communication systems

C Ⓜ 4.   Illumination of exit signs

The organization provides a reliable emergency power system, as required by the services provided and residents served, that supplies electricity to the following areas when normal electricity is interrupted:

     5.   Not applicable

     6.   Not applicable

     7.   Not applicable

A   8.   Elevators (at least one for nonambulatory clients)

A   9.   Medical air compressors

A   10.   Medical and surgical vacuum systems

A   11.   Areas where electrically powered life-support equipment is used

Standard EC.7.30 ▬▬▬▬▬▬▬▬▬▬▬▬▬▬▬▬▬▬▬▬▬

The organization maintains, tests, and inspects its utility systems.

Note: *Organizations that offer care, treatment, and services in leased facilities need to communicate maintenance expectations for building equipment not under their control to their landlord through contractual language, lease agreements, memos, and so forth. These organizations are not required to possess maintenance documentation but must only have access to such documentation as needed and during survey. It is also important that the landlord communicate to the organization any building equipment problems identified that could negatively affect the safety or health of residents,*

---

* **Reliable emergency power system** For guidance in establishing a reliable emergency power system (that is, an Essential Electrical Distribution System), see NFPA 99-2002 edition (chapters 13 and 14).

staff, and other people coming to the organization, as well as the landlord's plan to resolve such issues.

Elements of Performance for EC.7.30

C Ⓜ 1. The organization maintains documentation of a current, accurate, and separate inventory of utility components identified in the utility management plan.

A 2. The organization maintains documentation of performance and safety testing of each critical component identified in the plan before initial use.

A 3. The organization maintains documentation of maintenance of critical components of life support utility systems/equipment consistent with maintenance strategies identified in the utility management plan (*see* standard EC.7.10).

A 4. The organization maintains documentation of maintenance of critical components of infection control utility systems/equipment for high-risk residents consistent with maintenance strategies identified in the utility management plan (*see* standard EC.7.10).

C Ⓜ 5. The organization maintains documentation of maintenance of critical components of non–life support utility systems/equipment on the inventory consistent with maintenance strategies identified in the utility management plan (*see* standard EC.7.10).

Standard EC.7.40

The organization maintains, tests, and inspects its emergency power systems.

Note: *This standard does not require organizations to have the types of emergency power systems discussed here. However, if an organization has these types of systems, then the following maintenance, testing, and inspection requirements apply.*

EC

Elements of Performance for EC.7.40

C Ⓜ 1. The organization tests each generator 12 times a year, with testing intervals not less than 20 days and not more than 40 days apart. These tests shall be conducted for at least 30 continuous minutes under a dynamic load that is at least 30% of the nameplate rating of the generator.

> **Note:** *Organizations may choose to test to less than 30% of the emergency generator's nameplate. However, these organizations shall (in addition to performing a test for 30 continuous minutes under operating temperature at the intervals described here) revise their existing documented management plan to conform to current NFPA 99 and NFPA 110 testing and maintenance activities. These activities shall include inspection procedures for assessing the prime movers' exhaust gas temperature against the minimum temperature recommended by the manufacturer.*

If diesel-powered generators do not meet the minimum exhaust gas temperatures as determined during these tests, they shall be exercised for 30 continuous minutes at the intervals described here with available Emergency Power Supply Systems (EPSS) load and exercised annually with supplemental loads of the following:

- *25% of nameplate rating for 30 minutes, followed by*
- *50% of nameplate rating for 30 minutes, followed by*
- *75% of nameplate rating for 60 minutes for a total of 2 continuous hours*

C Ⓜ 2. The organization tests all automatic transfer switches 12 times a year, with testing intervals not less than 20 days and not more than 40 days apart.

C Ⓜ 3. The organization tests all battery-powered lights required for egress. Testing includes (a) a functional test at 30-day intervals for a minimum of 30 seconds and (b) an annual test for a duration of 1.5 hours.

C Ⓜ 4. The organization tests Stored Emergency Power Supply Systems (SEPSS) whose malfunction may severely jeopardize the occupants' life and safety.* Testing includes (a) a quarterly functional test for 5 minutes or as specified for its class,† whichever is less and (b) an annual test at full load for 60% of the full duration of its class.

Standard EC.7.50

The organization maintains, tests, and inspects its medical gas and vacuum systems.

Note: *This standard does not require organizations to have the medical gas and vacuum systems discussed here. However, if an organization has these types of systems, then the following maintenance, testing, and inspection requirements apply.*

Elements of Performance for EC.7.50

A 1. The organization inspects, tests, and maintains critical components of piped medical gas systems, including master signal panels, area alarms, automatic pressure switches, shutoff valves, flexible connectors, and outlets.

A 2. The organization tests piped medical gas and vacuum systems when the systems are installed, modified, or repaired, including cross-connection testing, piping purity testing, and pressure testing.

---

* **Stored Emergency Power Supply Systems (SEPSS)** Are intended to automatically supply illumination or power to critical areas and equipment essential for safety to human life. Included are systems that supply emergency power for such functions as illumination for safe exiting, ventilation where it is essential to maintain life, fire detection and alarm systems, public safety communications systems, and processes where the current interruption would produce serious life safety or health hazards to residents, the public, or staff. **Note:** *Other non-SEPSS battery back-up emergency power systems that an organization has determined to be critical for operations during a power failure (for example, laboratory equipment, electronic medical records) should be properly tested and maintained in accordance with manufacturer's recommendations.*

† **Class** Defines the minimum time for which the SEPSS is designed to operate at its rated load without being recharged. (For additional guidance, see NFPA 111 [1996 edition] *Standard on Stored Electrical Energy Emergency and Standby Power Systems.*)

EC

A   3.   The organization maintains the main supply valve and area shut-off valves of piped medical gas and vacuum systems to be accessible and clearly labeled.

Standard EC.8.10

The organization establishes and maintains an appropriate environment.

Rationale for EC.8.10

It is important that the physical environment is functional and promotes caring. It should contribute to relieving loneliness, boredom, and hopelessness.* The environment should also encourage independence and promote quality of life.

Elements of Performance for EC.8.10

B   1.   Interior spaces should be the following:
- Appropriate to the care, treatment, and services provided and the needs of the residents related to age and other characteristics
- Include closet and drawer space provided for storing personal property and other items provided for use by residents. Lockers, drawers, or closet space is provided for residents who are in charge of their own personal grooming and who wear street clothes (for example, behavioral health care clients who wear street clothes and are expected to meet their personal grooming needs).
- Allow for good recreational interchange, consider personal preferences when feasible, and accommodate equipment, such as wheelchairs, that are necessary to activities of daily living
- Have equipment for rehabilitation and activities adequate to accomplish goals without compromising the environment's safety

B   2.   Furnishings and equipment should do the following:
- Be maintained to be safe and in good repair
- Reflect the resident's level of ability and needs

B   3.   Outside areas are the following:
- Appropriate and safe considering the care, treatment, and services provided and the needs of the residents related to age and other characteristics
- Used during appropriate seasons

C Ⓜ   4.   Areas used by the residents are safe, clean, functional, and comfortable.

B   5.   Lighting is suitable for care, treatment, and services and the specific activities being conducted.

    6.   Not applicable

EC

---

* A powerful tool for improving the quality of life for the elderly is "**The Eden Alternative**™". Part of its mission statement is to relieve loneliness, boredom, and hopelessness. Additional information about its concepts can be found at http://www.edenalt.com.

B   7.   Ventilation provides for acceptable levels of temperature and humidity and eliminates odors.

      8.   Not applicable

      9.   Not applicable

    10.   Not applicable

A   11.   Door locks and other structural restraints used are consistent with the needs of residents, program policy, law, and regulation.

A   12.   Emergency access provision is provided to all locked and occupied spaces.

    13.   Not applicable

    14.   Not applicable

B   15.   Spaces are accessible for safe wandering and exploring.

B   16.   **For long term care subacute services only:** The physical environment may need special modifications to accommodate the complex services offered to subacute care residents. Lighting levels, electrical outlets and load, and emergency generator capacity meet the scope of services offered for subacute care.

Standard EC.8.20 ▬▬▬▬▬▬▬▬▬▬▬▬▬▬▬▬▬▬▬▬▬▬▬

The organization establishes and maintains an appropriate dining environment.

Elements of Performance for EC.8.20

C Ⓜ   1.   The dining environment encourages eating and socialization, for instance, by providing minor distractions and small group settings.

C Ⓜ   2.   Dining areas are free from loud and distracting noises according to the residents' needs.

      3.   Not applicable

      4.   Not applicable

      5.   Not applicable

C Ⓜ   6.   Dining areas have adequate space for residents with equipment such as ventilators and cardiac monitors.

C Ⓜ   7.   Dining areas have the following characteristics:
- Offer residents a selection of seating
- Include tables with height(s) to facilitate independent eating
- Have staff that help residents sit in a regular dining chair, when possible

EC

Standard EC.8.30

The organization manages the design and building of the environment when it is renovated, altered, or newly created (*see also* standard EC.5.50).

Elements of Performance for EC.8.30

B   1.   When planning for the size, configuration, and equipping of the space of renovated, altered, or new construction, the organization uses one of the following: applicable state rules and regulations; *Guidelines for Design and Construction of Hospitals and Health Care Facilities*, 2001 edition, published by the American Institute of Architects; or standards or guidelines that provide design criteria.

B   2.   When planning demolition, construction, or renovation, the organization conducts a proactive risk assessment using risk criteria to identify hazards that could potentially compromise care, treatment, and services in occupied areas of the organization's buildings. The scope and nature of the activities should determine the extent of risk assessment.

B   3.   When planning demolition, construction, or renovation, the organization uses risk criteria that address the impact of demolition, renovation, or new construction on air quality requirements, infection control, utility requirements, noise, vibration, and emergency procedures.

B   4.   When planning demolition, construction, or renovation, the organization selects and implements proper controls, as required, to reduce risk and minimize impact of these activities.

Measuring and Improving Activities

EC

Standard EC.9.10

The organization monitors conditions in the environment.

Elements of Performance for EC.9.10

B   1.   The organization establishes and implements process(es) for reporting and investigating the following:*

- Injuries to residents or others coming to the organization's facilities, as well as incidents of property damage
- Occupational illnesses and injuries to staff
- Security incidents involving residents, staff, or others coming to the organization's facilities or property
- Hazardous materials and waste spills, exposures, and other related incidents

---

* Organizations have the flexibility to develop a single reporting method that addresses one or more of the items listed.

- Fire-safety management problems, deficiencies, and failures
- Equipment-management problems, failures, and user errors
- Utility systems management problems, failures, or user errors

B   2. The organization's leaders assign a person(s) (hereafter referred to as the "assigned person[s]") to monitor and respond to conditions in the organization's environment. The assigned individual performs the following tasks:
   - Coordinates the ongoing, organizationwide collection of information about deficiencies and opportunities for improvement in the environment of care
   - Coordinates the ongoing collection and dissemination of other sources of information, such as published hazard notices or recall reports
   - Coordinates the preparation of summaries of deficiencies, problems, failures, and user errors related to managing the environment of care*
   - Coordinates the preparation of summaries on findings, recommendations, actions taken, and results of performance improvement (PI) activities
   - Participates in hazard surveillance and incident reporting
   - Participates in developing safety policies and procedures

B   3. The organization establishes and implements a process(es) for ongoing monitoring of performance regarding actual or potential risk(s) in each of the environment of care management plans.†

A   4. Each of the environment of care management plans is evaluated at least annually.

B   5. The objectives, scope, performance, and effectiveness of each of the environment of care management plans are evaluated at least annually.

6. Through 9. Not applicable

B   10. Environmental safety monitoring and response activities are communicated to the resident safety program required in the "Leadership" chapter of this book.

EC

Standard EC.9.20

The organization analyzes identified environment issues and develops recommendations for resolving them.

---

* **Notes:** *Incidents involving residents may be reported to appropriate staff such as staff in quality assessment, improvement, or other functions. However, at least a summary of incidents is shared with the person designated to coordinate safety management activities (see standard EC.1.10). Review of incident reports often requires that various legal processes be followed to preserve confidentiality. Opportunities to improve care, treatment, and services or to prevent future similar incidents are not lost as a result of the legal process followed.*

† The environment of care plans are for managing safety, security, hazardous materials and waste, emergency management, fire safety, medical equipment, and utilities.

Elements of Performance for EC.9.20

B 1. The organization establishes an ongoing process for resolving environment of care issues that involves representatives from clinical, administrative, and support services.

C ⓜ 2. A multidisciplinary improvement team meets at least bimonthly to address environment of care issues.*

B 3. The organization analyzes environment of care issues in a timely manner.

B 4. Recommendations are developed and approved as appropriate.

B 5. Appropriate staff establishes measurement guidelines.

B 6. Environment of care issues are communicated to the organization's leaders and person(s) responsible for PI activities.

7. Not applicable

A 8. A recommendation for one or more PI activities is communicated at least annually to the organization's leaders based on the ongoing performance monitoring of the environment of care management plans.

B 9. Recommendations for resolving environmental safety issues are communicated, when appropriate, to those responsible for managing the resident safety program required in the "Leadership" chapter of this book.

Standard EC.9.30 ▬▬▬▬▬▬▬

The organization improves the environment.

Elements of Performance for EC.9.30

B 1. Appropriate staff participates in implementing recommendations.

B 2. Appropriate staff monitors the effectiveness of the recommendation's implementation.

B 3. Monitoring results are reported through appropriate channels, including the organization's leaders.

B 4. Monitoring results are reported to the multidisciplinary improvement team responsible for resolving environment of care issues.

B 5. Results of monitoring are reported (when appropriate) to those responsible for managing the resident safety program required in the "Leadership" chapter of this book.

EC

---

* **Note:** *Meetings held less frequently than bimonthly are acceptable when supported by current organization experience and the multidisciplinary improvement team's approval. Ongoing justification of meeting frequency depends on a satisfactory annual evaluation of performance as required by standard EC.9.10.*

EC

Management of Human Resources

Overview

The goal of the human resources function is to ensure that the organization determines the qualifications and competencies for all staff positions (individuals such as employees, contractors, or temporary agency personnel who provide services in the organization) based on its mission; population(s); and care, treatment, and services. Organizations must also provide the right number of competent staff to meet residents' needs. To meet this goal, the organization carries out the following processes and activities:

- **Providing an adequate number of staff.** The organization determines the appropriate level of staffing to fulfill its mission and meet the needs of the population(s) served. There is a sufficient number of staff based on the organization's determination of the appropriate level of staffing.
- **Providing competent staff.** The organization provides for competent staff either through traditional employer-employee arrangements or through contractual arrangements with other entities or persons. An initial review of credentials and qualifications is performed. Experience, education, and abilities are confirmed during orientation.
- **Orienting, training, and educating staff.** The organization provides ongoing in-service and other education and training to increase staff knowledge of specific work-related issues.
- **Assessing, maintaining, and improving staff competence.** Ongoing, periodic competence assessment evaluates staff members' continuing abilities to perform throughout their association with the organization.

HR

Standards

The following is a list of all standards for this function. They are presented here for your convenience without footnotes or other explanatory text. If you have a question about a term used here, please check the Glossary.

Note: *A revised standard numbering system is being used with the reformatted standards. The revised numbering system will allow for more flexibility to add standards while maintaining the current label for each standard.*

Planning

HR.1.10   The organization provides an adequate number and mix of staff and licensed independent practitioners that are consistent with the organization's staffing plan.

HR.1.20   The organization has a process to ensure that a person's qualifications are consistent with his or her job responsibilities.

HR.1.30   The organization uses data on clinical/service screening indicators in combination with human resource screening indicators to assess staffing effectiveness.

Orientation, Training, and Education

HR.2.10   Orientation provides initial job training and information.

HR.2.20   Staff members, licensed independent practitioners, students, and volunteers, as appropriate, can describe or demonstrate their roles and responsibilities, based on specific job duties or responsibilities, relative to safety.

HR.2.30   Ongoing education, including in-services, training, and other activities, maintains and improves competence.

Assessing Competence

HR.3.10   Competence to perform job responsibilities is assessed, demonstrated, and maintained.

HR.3.20   The organization periodically conducts performance evaluations.

HR.3.30 Through HR.3.60   Not applicable

HR

Credentialing and Granting of Privileges of Licensed Independent Practitioners

HR.4.10   There is a process for ensuring the competence of all practitioners permitted by law and the organization to practice independently.

HR.4.20   Practitioners permitted by law and the organization to practice independently are granted clinical privileges.

HR.4.30   The organization has a process for granting temporary clinical privileges, when appropriate.

HR.4.40   There are mechanisms, including a fair hearing and appeal process, for addressing adverse decisions regarding reappointment, denial, reduction, suspension, or revocation of clinical privileges that may relate to quality of care, treatment, and service issues.

HR.4.50   Clinical privileges and appointments/reappointments are reviewed and revised at least every two years.

HR

Understanding the Parts of This Chapter

To help you navigate this reformatted standards chapter, it may be helpful to think of its parts this way:

- The **standard** is the "goal"
- The **rationale** explains why it's important to achieve this goal
- The **elements of performance** identify the step(s) needed to achieve this goal

These parts are defined as follows.

Standard A statement that defines the performance expectations and/or structures or processes that must be in place for an organization to provide safe, high-quality care, treatment, and services. An organization is either "compliant" or "not compliant" with a standard.

Accreditation decisions are based on simple counts of the standards that are determined to be "not compliant."

Rationale A statement that provides background, justification, or additional information about a standard. A standard's rationale is not scored. In some instances, the rationale for a standard is self-evident. Therefore, not every standard has a written rationale.

Elements of performance (EPs) The specific performance expectations and/or structures or processes that must be in place for an organization to provide safe, high-quality care, treatment, and services. The scoring of EP compliance determines an organization's overall compliance with a standard. EPs are evaluated on the following scale:

> 0 Insufficient compliance
> 1 Partial compliance
> 2 Satisfactory compliance
> NA Not applicable

You will find a **measure of success** icon—**Ⓜ**—next to some EPs. Measures of success (MOS) need to be developed for certain EPs when a standard is judged to be out of compliance through either the Periodic Performance Review (PPR) or the onsite survey. An MOS is defined as a quantifiable measure, usually related to an audit, that can be used to determine whether an action has been effective and is being sustained.*

Assessing Your Compliance

Once you are familiar with the parts of this chapter, you can begin to assess your compliance with its requirements. The scoring category designations are provided next to each EP for your convenience. If you would like to assess your organization's performance, mark your scores for the EPs and standards by following the simple steps described below.

---

* For more information about MOS, *see* "The New Joint Commission Accreditation Process" chapter in this book.

Two components are scored for each EP: (1) compliance with the requirement itself **and** (2) compliance with the track record* for that requirement. Scoring has been simplified and track record achievements (which have always been part of the scoring) have been appropriately modified.

Note: *Some standards and EPs do not apply to a particular type of organization; these standards and EPs are marked "not applicable" and the related text is not included. Your organization is not expected to comply with standards and EPs marked "not applicable."*

In addition, some standards and EPs that do apply to organizations may not apply to the specific care, treatment, and services that your individual organization provides. Although these standards and EPs are included in the book, you are not expected to comply with them. If you are unsure about the standards or EPs that apply to your organization, please contact the Joint Commission's Standards Interpretation Group at 630/792-5900.

Step 1: Score Your Compliance with Each Element of Performance

Before you can determine your compliance with the standards, you must score your compliance with each EP. There are three scoring criterion categories: A, B, and C (described below). Please note that for each EP scoring criterion category, your organization must meet the performance requirement itself and the track record achievements (*see* "Track Record Achievements").

Category A

These EPs relate to the presence or absence of the requirement(s) and are scored either yes (2) or no (0); however, score 1 for partial compliance is also possible based on track record achievements.

If an A EP has multiple components designated by bullets, your organization must be compliant with all the bullets to receive a score of 2. If your organization does not meet one or more requirements in the bullets, you will receive a score of 0.

Category B

Category B EPs are scored in two steps:

1. As with category A EPs, category B EPs relate to the presence or absence of the requirement(s). If your organization *does not meet* the requirement(s), the EP is scored 0; there is no need to assess your compliance with the principles of good process design.
2. If your organization *does meet* the requirement(s), but there is concern about the quality or comprehensiveness of the effort, then and only then should you assess the qualitative aspect of the EP. That is, review the applicable principles of good process design and ask how the principles were applied in the situation under discussion. Good process design has the following characteristics:

HR

---

* **Track record** The amount of time that an organization has been in compliance with a standard, EP, or other requirement.

- Is consistent with your organization's mission, values, and goals
- Meets the needs of patients
- Reflects the use of currently accepted practices (doing the right thing, using resources responsibly, using practice guidelines)
- Incorporates current safety information and knowledge such as sentinel event data and National Patient Safety Goals
- Incorporates relevant performance improvement results

This two-part evaluation applies to both simple and bulleted B EPs. First, the EPs are assessed to determine whether the requirements are present. If the EP has multiple components designated by bullets, as with the category A EPs, your organization must meet the requirements in *all* the bulleted items to get a score of 2. If your organization meets *none* of the requirements in the bullets, it receives a score of 0. If your organization meets *at least one, but not all,* of the bulleted requirements, it receives a score of 1 for the EPs.

Use the following rules to determine your EP score:
- Your EP score is 0 if your organization does not meet the requirement(s); you *do not* need to assess your compliance with the preceding applicable principles of good process design
- Your EP score is 1 if your organization does meet the requirement(s) but considered only *some* of the preceding applicable principles of good process design
- Your EP score is 2 if your organization does meet the requirement(s) *and* considered *all* the preceding principles of good process design

Category C
C EPs are scored 0, 1, or 2 based on the number of times your organization does not meet the EP. These EPs are frequency based and require totaling the number of occurrences (that is, results of performance or nonperformance) related to a particular EP. Each situation discovered by a surveyor(s) will be counted as a separate occurrence.

Note: *Multiple events of the same type related to a single resident and single practitioner/staff member are counted as* one occurrence only.

Use the following rules to determine your EP score:
- Your EP score is 2 if you find one or fewer occurrences of noncompliance with the EP
- Your EP score is 1 if you find two occurrences of noncompliance with the EP
- Your EP score is 0 if you find three or more occurrences of noncompliance with the EP

If an EP in the C category has multiple requirements designated by bullets, the following scoring guidelines apply:
- If there are fewer than two findings in all bullets, the EP is scored 2
- If there are three or more findings in all bullets, the EP is scored 0
- In all other combinations of findings, the EP is scored 1

Track Record Achievements

In addition to meeting the requirement(s) in each EP, regardless of category, your organization must also meet the following track record achievements:

Score	Initial Survey	Full Survey
2	4 months or more	12 months or more
1	2 to 3 months	6 to 11 months
0	Fewer than 2 months	Fewer than 6 months

Sample Sizes

If during an onsite survey, your organization has been found to be not compliant with one or more standards, you must demonstrate Evidence of Standards Compliance (ESC) for each standard that is not compliant. The ESC must address compliance at the EP level; when an EP within a noncompliant standard requires an MOS, your organization must demonstrate achievement with the MOS when completing the ESC.

Note: *Not every EP requires an MOS. EPs that do require an MOS are clearly marked in this chapter. Organizations are required to demonstrate achievement with an MOS only for EPs within a noncompliant standard that require an MOS. Organizations do not need to demonstrate achievement with an MOS for any EP within a compliant standard.*

When demonstrating achievement with an MOS during the ESC process, your organization is **required** to use the following sample sizes, which were established because of their statistical significance, their relative simplicity in application, and their sensitivity to an organization's population size:

- For a population size of fewer than 30 cases,* sample 100% of available cases
- For a population size of 30 to 100 cases, sample 30 cases
- For a population size of 101 to 500 cases, sample 50 cases
- For a population size greater than 500 cases, sample 70 cases

Note: *Organizations are* encouraged, but not required, *to follow this sample size when demonstrating achievement with an MOS for an EP within a noncompliant standard after conducting a full, Option 1, or Option 2 PPR.*

HR

When conducting PPR (optional use) or demonstrating an ESC (mandatory use), use the following percentages to determine your EP score: 90% through 100% of your sample size is in compliance = score 2; 80% through 89% of your sample size is in compliance = score 1; less than 80% of your sample size is in compliance = score 0.

In addition, the following information should govern your organization's selection of samples:

- The appropriate sample size should be determined by the specific population related to the survey findings

---

* *Case* refers to a single instance in which a situation related to a survey finding occurs. For example, if a survey finding was related to **pain assessment**, then a case would be any resident record. If a survey finding was related to **pain management**, a case would be any resident record for residents receiving pain management.

- The sampling approach should involve either systematic random sampling (for example, your organization selects every second or third case for review) or simple random sampling (for example, your organization uses a series of random numbers generated by a computer to identify the cases to be reviewed)
- If your organization chooses not to use these sample sizes while conducting PPR options 1 or 2, you should make sure that your sample size is sufficiently large enough to ensure statistical significance
- When submitting a clarifying ESC, if your organization selects records as part of its sample, the records should be from a period of no more than three months before the last date of the survey
- Assessment of MOS compliance is conducted for a four-month period following the date of ESC approval. Your organization should select records as a part of your sample following the date of ESC approval and use the required sample sizes. MOS percentage compliance rates are derived from the average of all four months.

Step 2: Use Your EP Scores to Gauge Your Compliance with the Standards

Now that you have evaluated and scored each EP for a particular standard, use these simple rules to determine your compliance with the standard itself:

- Your organization is not in compliance (that is, "not compliant") with the standard if any EP is scored 0
- Otherwise, your organization is in compliance with a standard if 65% or more of its EPs are scored 2

HR

Standards, Rationales, Elements of Performance, and Scoring

Planning

Standard HR.1.10

The organization provides an adequate number and mix of staff and licensed independent practitioners are consistent with the organization's staffing plan.

Elements of Performance for HR.1.10

B 1. The organization has an adequate number and mix of staff and licensed independent practitioners to meet the care, treatment, and services needs of the residents.

A 2. Nursing care and services are provided 24 hours a day, 7 days a week, including relief personnel during vacation periods, sick leaves, emergencies, and holidays.

A 3. Except when waived by the state, a registered nurse supervises nursing care at least eight consecutive hours a day, seven days a week.

A 4. If any resident(s) requires a registered nurse's services, at least one registered nurse, who is currently licensed by the state in which he or she practices, is on duty* on each shift, seven days a week.[†]

Standard HR.1.20

The organization has a process to ensure that a person's qualifications are consistent with his or her job responsibilities.

Rationale for HR.1.20

HR

This requirement pertains to staff and students as well as volunteers who work in the same capacity as staff when they provide care, treatment, and services.

Elements of Performance for HR.1.20

B 1. The leaders define the required competence and qualifications of staff in all program(s) or service(s).

---

* The use of a registered nurse "on call" instead of "on duty" should be the exception and must not adversely affect resident care.

† If none of the residents requires a registered nurse's services, registered nurse coverage on each shift is optional; however, a licensed practical (vocational) nurse, who is currently licensed by the state in which he or she practices, is assigned to each shift seven days a week. Supervision is provided on all shifts.

    2. Not applicable

The organization verifies the following (EPs 3–6):

C Ⓜ 3. Current licensure, certification, or registration

C Ⓜ 4. Education, experience, and competence appropriate for assigned responsibilities

C Ⓜ 5. Information on criminal background

C Ⓜ 6. Compliance with applicable health screening requirements established by the organization*

C Ⓜ 7. Staff supervises students when they provide resident care, treatment, and services as part of their training.

    8. Through 17. Not applicable

A   18. Individuals who do not possess a license, registration, or certification do not provide or have not provided care, treatment, and services in the organization that would, under applicable law or regulation, require such a license, registration, or certification.

A   19. Individuals who do not possess a license, registration, or certification do not provide or have not provided care, treatment, and services in the organization that would, under applicable law or regulation, require such a license, registration, or certification and which would have placed the organization's residents at risk for a serious adverse outcome.

Standard HR.1.30

The organization uses data on clinical/service screening indicators[†] in combination with human resource screening indicators[‡] to assess staffing effectiveness.[§]

HR

---

* The Americans with Disabilities Act (ADA) bars certain discrimination based on physical or mental impairments. To prevent such discrimination, the act prohibits or mandates various activities. Organizations should examine their hiring and evaluation procedures for activities prohibited or mandated. For example, health care organizations need to determine whether the ADA applies to some or all applicants to their organization. If applicable, the ADA would prohibit an inquiry about the applicant's overall health status. The inquiry must be limited to dealing with the applicant's ability to perform essential job functions, perhaps defined by the privileges or position requirements sought. The Joint Commission has and will absolutely construe these standards to be consistent with the organization's effort to meet ADA compliance efforts.

[†] An example of a clinical/service screening indicator is adverse drug events.

[‡] Examples of human resource screening indicators are overtime and staff vacancy rate.

[§] **Staffing effectiveness** is defined as the number, competency, and skill mix of staff related to the provision of needed services.

Rationale for HR.1.30

Multiple screening indicators that relate to resident outcomes, including clinical/service and human resources screening indicators, may be indicative of staffing effectiveness.

Elements of Performance for HR.1.30

A   1.   The organization selects a minimum of four screening indicators: two clinical/service and two human resources indicators. The focus is on the relationship between human resource and clinical/service screening indicators, with the clear understanding that no one indicator, in and of itself, can directly demonstrate staffing effectiveness.

A   2.   The organization selects at least one of the human resource and one of the clinical/service screening indicators from a list of Joint Commission–identified screening indicators. The organization chooses additional screening indicators based on its unique characteristics, specialties, and services.

B   3.   The organization determines the rationale for screening indicator selection.

B   4.   The organization defines the direct and indirect caregivers included in the human resource screening indicators based on the impact, if any, the absence of such caregivers is expected to have on resident outcomes.

B   5.   The organization uses the data collected and analyzed from the selected screening indicators to identify potential staffing effectiveness issues when performance varies from expected targets (for example, ranges of desired performance, external comparisons, or improvement goals).

B   6.   The organization analyzes data over time per screening indicator (for example, identification of trends or patterns using a line graph, run chart, or control chart) to determine the stability of a process.

B   7.   The organization analyzes all screening indicator data in combination (for example, a table or matrix report, multiple line graphs, spider or radar diagrams, or scatter diagrams).

A   8.   The organization analyzes screening indicator data at the level in which staffing needs are planned in the organization and in collaboration with other areas in the organization, as needed.

B   9.   The organization reports at least annually to the leaders on the aggregation and analysis of data related to staffing effectiveness (*see* standards PI.1.10 and PI.2.20) and any actions taken to improve staffing.

B   10.   The organization can provide evidence of actions taken, as appropriate, in response to analyzed data.

HR

List of Joint Commission Screening Indicators for Long Term Care

1. Prevalence of pressure ulcers (Clinical/Service)
2. Resident satisfaction (Clinical/Service)
3. Family satisfaction (Clinical/Service)
4. Prevalence of falls (Clinical/Service)
5. Resident complaints (Clinical/Service)
6. Injuries to residents (Clinical/Service)
7. Family complaints (Clinical/Service)
8. Restraint use (Clinical/Service)
9. Prevalence of weight loss (Clinical/Service)
10. Elopements/wandering of residents (Clinical/Service)
11. Adverse drug events (Clinical/Service)
12. Prevalence of dehydration (Clinical/Service)
13. Pain assessment and management (that is, wait time to receive medications) (Clinical/Service)
14. Urinary tract infection rate (Clinical/Service)
15. Change in resident functioning (Clinical/Service)
16. Prevalence of malnutrition (Clinical/Service)
17. Activities of daily living (ADLs) met or unmet (Clinical/Service)
18. Prevalence of urinary catheter use (Clinical/Service)
19. Average time in activities (Clinical/Service)
20. Antibiotic use (Clinical/Service)
21. Unexpected hospital admissions or emergency department visits (Clinical/Service)
22. Prevalence of depression (Clinical/Service)
23. Prevalence of more than eight prescribed medications (Clinical/Service)
24. Pneumonia rate (Clinical/Service)
25. Antipsychotic medication usage (Clinical/Service)
26. Staff vacancy rate (Human Resource)
27. Staff turnover rate (Human Resource)
28. Staff satisfaction (Human Resource)
29. Use of overtime (Human Resource)
30. Staff injury rate (Human Resource)
31. Nursing hours per resident day (R.N., L.P.N., C.N.A.) compared to baseline such as actual versus planned or budgeted (Human Resource)
32. Staff training hours (Human Resource)
33. Agency usage/contract staff (Human Resource)
34. Understaffing as compared to organization's staffing plan (Human Resource)
35. Use of sick time (Human Resource)
36. Activity staff hours per resident day (Human Resource)
37. Number of dietary staff per resident (Human Resource)
38. Number of housekeeping staff per resident (Human Resource)
39. Average response time for consultation order (Human Resource)

HR

Orientation, Training, and Education

Standard HR.2.10

Orientation provides initial job training and information.

Rationale for HR.2.10

Staff members; licensed independent practitioners, if applicable; students; and volunteers are oriented to their jobs as appropriate and the work environment before providing care, treatment, and services.

Elements of Performance for HR.2.10

As appropriate, each staff member, licensed independent practitioner, student, and volunteer is oriented to the following (EPs 1-5):

C Ⓜ 1. The organization's mission and goals

C Ⓜ 2. Organizationwide policies and procedures (including safety and infection control) and relevant unit, setting, or program-specific policies and procedures

C Ⓜ 3. Specific job duties and responsibilities and service, setting, or program-specific job duties and responsibilities related to safety and infection control

4. Not applicable

C Ⓜ 5. Cultural diversity and sensitivity

C Ⓜ 6. Staff, students, and volunteers are educated about the rights of residents and ethical aspects of care, treatment, and services and the process used to address ethical issues.

C Ⓜ 7. Staff is oriented to the effects of psychotropic medications, as appropriate.

Standard HR.2.20

HR

Staff members, licensed independent practitioners, students, and volunteers, as appropriate, can describe or demonstrate their roles and responsibilities, based on specific job duties or responsibilities, relative to safety.

Rationale for HR.2.20

The human element is the most critical factor in any process, determining whether the right things are done correctly. The best policies and procedures for minimizing risks in the environment where care, treatment, and services are provided are meaningless if staff; licensed independent practitioners, if applicable; students; and volunteers do not know and understand them well enough to perform them properly.

It is important that everyday precautions identified by the health care organization for minimizing various risks, including those related to resident safety and environmental safety,* are properly implemented. It is also important that the appropriate emergency procedures be instituted should an incident or failure occur in the environment.

Elements of Performance for HR.2.20

Staff members, licensed independent practitioners, students, and volunteers, as appropriate, can describe or demonstrate the following:

C Ⓜ 1. Risks within the organization's environment

C Ⓜ 2. Actions to eliminate, minimize, or report risks

C Ⓜ 3. Procedures to follow in the event of an incident

C Ⓜ 4. Reporting processes for common problems, failures, and user errors

Standard HR.2.30 ▬▬▬▬▬▬▬▬▬▬▬▬▬▬▬▬▬▬▬▬

Ongoing education, including in-services, training, and other activities, maintains and improves competence.

Elements of Performance for HR.2.30

The following occurs for staff, students, and volunteers who work in the same capacity as staff providing care, treatment, and services:

B 1. Training occurs when job responsibilities or duties change

C Ⓜ 2. Participation in ongoing in-services, training, or other activities occurs to increase staff, student, or volunteer knowledge of work-related issues

C Ⓜ 3. Ongoing in-services and other education and training are appropriate to the needs of the population(s) served and comply with law and regulation

C Ⓜ 4. Ongoing in-services, training, or other activities emphasize specific job-related aspects of safety and infection prevention and control

C Ⓜ 5. Ongoing in-services, training, or other education incorporate methods of team training, when appropriate

C Ⓜ 6. Ongoing in-services, training, or other education reinforce the need and ways to report unanticipated adverse events

C Ⓜ 7. Ongoing in-services or other education are offered in response to learning needs identified through performance improvement findings and other data analysis (that is, data from staff surveys, performance evaluations, or other needs assessments)

C Ⓜ 8. Ongoing education is documented

---

* The "Management of the Environment of Care" chapter of this book identifies risks associated with the following categories: safety, security, hazardous materials and waste, emergency management, laboratory/medical equipment, and utility management.

B   9.   Not applicable

B   10.   Staff members are educated, as appropriate to their responsibilities, about psychotropic medications, including the following:
- The need for a medication in relation to the resident's documented diagnosis and condition
- The potential for drug-drug and drug-food interactions
- Adverse reactions to psychotropic medications
- The use of a medication for an appropriate duration
- The optimal dose
- Frequent monitoring of the medication's effectiveness
- Nonmedication interventions and alternatives developed through interdisciplinary team assessment
- Reduction and discontinuation of a medication

Assessing Competence

Standard HR.3.10
Competence to perform job responsibilities is assessed, demonstrated, and maintained.

Rationale for HR.3.10
Competence assessment is systematic and allows for a measurable assessment of the person's ability to perform required activities. Information used as part of competence assessment may include data from performance evaluations, performance improvement, and aggregate data on competence, as well as the assessment of learning needs.

Elements of Performance for HR.3.10
The competence assessment process for staff, students, and volunteers who work in the same capacity as staff providing care, treatment, and services is based on the following (EPs 1–7):

HR

B   1.   Populations served

B   2.   Defined competencies to be required

B   3.   Defined competencies to be assessed during orientation

B   4.   Defined competencies that need to be assessed and reassessed on an ongoing basis, based on techniques, procedures, technology, equipment, or skills needed to provide care, treatment, and services

B   5.   A defined time frame for how often competence assessments are performed for each person, minimally, once in the three-year accreditation cycle and in accordance with law and regulation

B   6.   Assessment methods (appropriate to determine the skill being assessed)

B   7.   The use of qualified individuals to assess competence

C ⓜ 8.   The organization assesses and documents each person's ability to carry out assigned responsibilities safely, competently, and in a timely manner upon completion of orientation.

C ⓜ 9.   The organization assesses each person according to its competence assessment process.

B   10.   When improvement activities lead to a determination that a person with performance problems is unable or unwilling to improve, the organization modifies the person's job assignment or takes other appropriate action.

Standard HR.3.20

The organization periodically conducts performance evaluations.

Rationale for HR.3.20

Performance is evaluated as an ongoing process for providing positive and negative feedback to staff and students as well as volunteers who work in the same capacity as staff providing care, treatment, and services. Formal performance evaluations can be conducted concurrently with competence assessments or can be completed at a separate time.

Elements of Performance for HR.3.20

C ⓜ 1.   The organization conducts performance evaluations periodically at time frames identified by the organization (at a minimum, at least once in the three-year accreditation cycle).

C ⓜ 2.   Performance is evaluated based on the performance expectations described in job descriptions or through the privileging process.

      3.   Not applicable

C ⓜ 4.   Performance evaluations are documented.

HR

Credentialing and Granting of Privileges of Licensed Independent Practitioners

Standard HR.4.10

There is a process for ensuring the competence of all practitioners permitted by law and the organization to practice independently.

Rationale for HR.4.10

Appropriate leaders of the organization formally approve the process for appointment and reappointment. The description of the process is sufficiently detailed to permit tracking of the steps involved when examining credential files.

Credentialing criteria specify requirements for practitioner membership in the organization. These criteria are designed to help establish an applicant's background and current competence. Moreover, they help assure the organization and its residents that the residents will receive quality care. The core criteria are the following:

- Current licensure
- Relevant education, training, or experience
- Current competence
- Ability to perform requested privileges

Each organization develops its own criteria for determining an applicant's ability to provide care, treatment, and services within the scope of clinical privileges requested. Criteria for renewing or revising clinical privileges include procedure outcomes and other results of performance improvement activities.

The organization may add other reasonable criteria, such as current evidence of adequate professional liability insurance or evidence of continuing medical education.

The following principles summarize key concepts as they relate to privileging:

- The organization administrator may substitute for the governing body.
- An organized medical staff and bylaws are not required.
- The medical director is comparable to the Medical Executive Committee (MEC) in settings where no organized medical staff exists.
- In organizations without an organized medical staff, procedures for appointment; reappointment; and granting, renewal, or revision of clinical privileges are established by the medical director and approved by the governing body.
- Privileges may be delineated by category and should address cognitive and technical skills.
- Each organization defines its scope of care in such a way that practitioners can request privileges consistent with the scope of care.
- In hospital-based long term care units, the long term care medical director reviews the credentials file and makes recommendations to the appropriate group or individual.
- The organization's general credentialing process can be applied to determine credentials, but the privileges granted must be program- and category-specific.

Current licensure. Licensure is verified with the primary source at the time of appointment and initial granting of clinical privileges by a letter or secure electronic communication obtained from the appropriate state licensing board, if in a federal service. Verification of current licensure through the primary source through a secure electronic communication or by telephone is acceptable, if this verification is documented.

At the time of reappointment and renewal or revision of clinical privileges, current licensure is confirmed with the primary source or by viewing the applicant's current license or registration.

Relevant training and experience. *At the time of appointment and initial grant-ing of clinical privileges, the organization verifies relevant training or experience from the primary source(s), whenever feasible. Verification includes letters from profes-sional schools, internships, residency, or postdoctoral programs. Relevant training and experience may be obtained by contacting the primary source via a secure elec-tronic communication or by telephone, if this verification is documented. For appli-cants who have just completed training in an approved residency or postdoctoral program, a letter from the program director is enough.*

An external organization (for example, a credentials verification organization [CVO] or a Joint Commission–accredited health care organization functioning as a CVO) may be used to collect information from primary sources.

Note 1: *An organization may choose to use the credentialing information of a health care organization accredited by the Joint Commission (as long as it has determined that the organization meets the 10 CVO guidelines in Note 3 on page HR-19). The National Practitioner Data Bank must still be queried in this instance.*

The organization may choose to rely on a Joint Commission–accredited health care organization's credentialing information for some practitioners while conducting the process itself for others.

Regardless of the source of credentialing information, leadership is responsible for reviewing the information on the licensed independent practitioner and making deci-sions regarding the assigning and renewal/revision of clinical responsibilities.

Note 2: *It may not always be feasible to obtain information from the primary source. In rare or occasional instances, a primary source such as an educational institution no longer exists, or the applicant's records have been lost or destroyed. Applicants may have received education, training, and experience partially or wholly in a for-eign country, and for political or other reasons, information regarding their profes-sional background is not accessible. When undue delay occurs in deriving information from a primary source, granting of clinical privileges is withheld pending receipt of this information. Under these circumstances, the applicant may be given temporary privileges for a limited time in accordance with rules and regulations or policies and procedures, as well as state and federal regulations. Designated equiva-lent sources or other reliable secondary sources may also be used if there has been a documented attempt to contact the primary source.*

Designated equivalent sources are selected agencies that have been determined to maintain a specific item(s) of credential information identical to information at the primary source. Their designated equivalent sources are the following:
- *The American Medical Association (AMA) Physician Masterfile for verification of a physician's medical school graduation and residency completion*
- *The American Board of Medical Specialties (ABMS) for verification of a physician's board certification*
- *The Education Commission for Foreign Medical Graduates (ECFMG) for verifica-tion of a physician's foreign medical school graduation*
- *The American Osteopathic Association (AOA) Physician Database for predoctoral*

HR

education accredited by the AOA Bureau of Professional education; postdoctoral education approved by the AOA Council on Postdoctoral Training; and the Osteopathic Specialty Board Certification

- The Federation of State Medical Boards (FSMB) for all actions against a physician's medical license

These designated equivalent sources may be used by the organization or by a CVO used by the organization. There may be other designated equivalent sources for certain applicants, such as for licensure verification of an applicant in the federal service. The organization should communicate with the Joint Commission to determine whether a specific agency qualifies as a designated equivalent source under such special circumstances. The physician profiles from the AMA Physician Masterfile also include other primary source-reported information that is similar to primary source-verified information provided by a CVO. Use of this additional information is subject to the guidelines set forth in Note 3.

A primary source of verified information may designate to an agency the role of communicating credentials information. The delegated agency then becomes acceptable to be used as a primary source.

Note 3: *Any organization that bases its decisions in part on information obtained from a CVO should have confidence in the completeness, accuracy, and timeliness of that information. To achieve this level of confidence, the organization should evaluate the agency providing the information initially and then periodically as appropriate. The principles that guide such an evaluation include the following:*

- The agency makes known to the user the data and information it can provide
- The agency provides documentation to the user describing how its data collection, information development, and verification process(es) are performed
- The user is given sufficient, clear information on database functions, including any limitations of information available from the agency (practitioners not included in the database), the time frame for agency responses to requests for information, and a summary overview of quality control processes related to data integrity, security, transmission accuracy, and technical specifications
- The user and agency agree on the format for transmitting credentials information about an individual from the CVO
- The user can easily discern what information transmitted by the CVO is from a primary source and what is not
- For information transmitted by the agency that can go out of date (licensure, board certification), the date the information was last updated from the primary source is provided by the CVO
- The CVO certifies that the information transmitted to the user accurately presents the information obtained by it
- The user can discern whether the information transmitted by the CVO from a primary source is all the primary source information in the CVO's possession pertinent to a given item or, if not, where additional information can be obtained
- The user can engage the CVO's quality control processes when necessary to resolve concerns about transmission errors, inconsistencies, or other data issues that may be identified from time to time

HR

- *The user has a formal arrangement with the CVO for communicating changes in credentialing information*

Current competence. *Current competence at the time of appointment and initial granting of clinical privileges cannot be determined by board certification or admissibility alone. Instead, it is verified in writing by individuals personally acquainted with the applicant's professional and clinical performance, either in teaching facilities or in other organizations. Letters from authoritative sources provide the organization with information directly from the primary source(s). Such letters contain informed opinions about the applicant's scope and level of performance. The organization defines the number of reference letters required. Acceptable letters are those that describe the following:*

- *The applicant's actual clinical performance in general terms*
- *The applicant's satisfactory discharge of professional obligations as a licensed independent practitioner*
- *The applicant's acceptable ethical performance*

Ideally, letters also address at least two aspects of current competence: the types and outcomes of medical conditions managed by the applicant as the responsible licensed independent practitioner and the applicant's clinical judgment and technical skills.

At the time of reappointment, current competence is determined by the results of performance improvement activities; peer recommendations; and/or the evaluation of the individual's professional performance, clinical judgment, and technical skills. Peer recommendations come from appropriate practitioners in the same professional specialty and preferably the same discipline as the applicant. If no peers on staff are knowledgeable about the applicant, a peer recommendation may be obtained from outside the organization. Peer recommendations refer, as appropriate, to relevant training or experience, current competence, and how well the applicant fulfilled organization-specific obligations. Sources for peer recommendations may include the following:

- *A performance improvement committee, the majority of whose members are the applicant's peers*
- *A reference letter(s) or documented telephone conversation about the applicant from a peer(s) who is knowledgeable about the applicant's competence*
- *A department or major clinical service chair who is a peer*

Ability to perform requested privileges. *The applicant's ability to perform clinical privileges must be evaluated, and this evaluation is documented in the applicant's credentials file. Documentation may include the applicant's statement that no health problems exist that could affect his or her practice; this statement must be confirmed. Applicants applying for appointment or for initial clinical privileges need this statement confirmed by the director of a training program, by staff at another organization at which the applicant holds privileges, or by an individual the organization designates.*

Applicants applying for reappointment or renewed or revised clinical privileges must have their health status confirmed by at least a countersignature on the applicant's statement by a licensed independent practitioner knowledgeable of the applicant's health status.

HR

Elements of Performance for HR.4.10

1. Through 9. Not applicable

B   10. The organization has a defined process approved by the leaders for appointing and reappointing licensed independent practitioners.

A   11. The following occur at the time of appointment and initial granting of clinical privileges:
- Current licensure, including all actions against the license, is verified with the primary source and documented
- Relevant training and experience are verified from the primary source
- Current competence is verified from a knowledgeable source
- The applicant's ability to perform the clinical privileges* requested is evaluated

A   12. In addition to the above criteria, the organization collects and evaluates information on restriction of privileges at other health care organizations.

B   13. The NPDB is queried in a timely manner and before finalizing appointments and granting initial privileges for information on adverse privilege actions taken by a health care organization.†

A   14. Leaders review all credentials information and decide whether to appoint the licensed independent practitioner to provide care, treatment, and services.

C Ⓜ   15. The licensed independent practitioner is notified in writing of the governing body's decision.

B   16. Each credentials file demonstrates that the credentialing criteria are uniformly applied.

A   17. Individuals who do not possess a license, registration, or certification do not provide or have not provided health care services in the organization that would, under applicable law or regulation, require such a license, registration, or certification.

HR

---

* The ADA bars certain discrimination based on physical or mental impairment. To prevent such discrimination, the act prohibits or mandates various activities. Health care organizations need to determine the applicability of the ADA to their licensed independent practitioners. If applicable, the organization should examine its privileging or credentialing procedures as to how and when it ascertains and confirms an applicant's health status. For example, the act may prohibit inquiry as to an applicant's physical or mental health status before making an offer of membership and privileges but may not prohibit such inquiry after an offer is extended (without specific reference to health matters) to perform the specific privileges requested. Thus, the inquiry may be made and confirmed as a component of the application process. The Joint Commission cannot provide legal advice to organizations. However, the Joint Commission has and will absolutely construe this standard in such a manner as to be consistent with organization efforts to comply with the ADA.

† Additional information received from the NPDB query that the organization may choose to use includes medical malpractice payments, licensure disciplinary actions, adverse actions affecting professional society membership, sanctions for Medicare and Medicaid, and adverse professional review actions taken by health care organizations against health care practitioners other than physicians and dentists.

A 18. An individual who does not possess a license, registration, or certification does not provide or has not provided health care services in the organization that would, under applicable law or regulation, require such a license, registration, or certification and which could place the organization's residents at risk for a serious adverse outcome.

Standard HR.4.20

Individuals permitted by law and the organization to practice independently are granted clinical privileges.

Elements of Performance for HR.4.20

B 1. Criteria for determining the licensed independent practitioner's clinical privileges are specified in writing and uniformly applied to all applicants.

C Ⓜ 2. Clinical privileges for licensed independent practitioners are delineated according to organization policy and based on the licensed independent practitioner's current credentials and competence, as well as the population(s) served and the types of care, treatment, and services provided in the organization.

A 3. Individuals with clinical privileges practice within the scope of their privileges.

Standard HR.4.30

The organization has a process for granting temporary clinical privileges, when appropriate.

Rationale for HR.4.30

Privileges for licensed independent practitioners can be issued to meet the important needs of residents for a limited period, as defined by policies and procedures or rules and regulations. Privileges can also be issued for new applicants for a period not to exceed 120 days.

Elements of Performance for HR.4.30

B 1. Policies and procedures, rules, or regulations describe the process for assigning granting temporary privileges for meeting the important needs of residents or for new applicants.

A 2. To grant temporary clinical responsibilities privileges to meet the important needs of residents, there must be verification (which can be done by telephone) of current licensure and current competence.

A 3. To grant temporary privileges for new applicants, there must be verification (which may be done by telephone) of the following:
- Current licensure
- Relevant education training or experience

HR

- Current competence
- Ability to perform the privileges requested

A   4. To grant temporary privileges for new applicants, the results of the NPDB query have been obtained and evaluated.

A   5. To grant temporary privileges for new applicants, the applicant has the following:
- A complete application
- No current or previously successful challenge to licensure or registration
- Not been subject to involuntary termination of professional or medical staff membership at another organization, when applicable to the discipline
- Not been subject to involuntary limitation, reduction, denial, or loss of privileges, when applicable to the discipline

A   6. The administrator or designee grants temporary privileges for meeting important resident needs and for new applicants upon recommendation of clinical leadership or the medical director.

Standard HR.4.40

There are mechanisms, including a fair hearing and appeals process, for addressing adverse decisions regarding reappointment, denial, reduction, suspension, or revocation of clinical privileges that may relate to quality of care, treatment, and service issues.

Rationale for HR.4.40

Mechanisms for fair hearing and appeals processes are designed to allow the affected individual a fair opportunity to defend herself or himself regarding the adverse decision to an unbiased hearing committee and an opportunity to appeal the decision of the committee to the governance function. The purpose of a fair hearing and appeal is to assure full consideration and reconsideration of quality and safety issues and, under the current structure of reporting to the NPDB, to allow practitioners an opportunity to defend themselves.

HR

Elements of Performance for HR.4.40

The organization has developed a fair hearing and appeals process that does the following:

B   1. Is designed to provide a uniform and fair process

B   2. Has a mechanism to schedule a hearing of such requests

B   3. Has identified the procedures for the hearings to follow

B   4. Identifies or defines the composition of the hearing committee

B   5.   Provides for a mechanism to appeal an adverse decision through the governance function

Standard HR.4.50

Clinical privileges and appointments/reappointments are reviewed and revised at least every two years.

Elements of Performance for HR.4.50

A   1.   Policies and procedures or rules and regulations specify a period of no more than two years between appointments and reappointments and between granting, renewing, and revising clinical privileges.

C Ⓜ 2.   Credential files for licensed independent practitioners contain substantive information and indicate that clinical privileges are reviewed or revised at least every two years and are revised as needed; in addition, appointments and reappointments are made for a period of no more than two years.

A   3.   A reappraisal is conducted at the time of reappointment or renewal or revision of clinical privileges.

A   4.   The reappraisal addresses current competence and includes the following:
- Confirmation of adherence to organization policies and procedures, rules, or regulations
- Relevant information from organization performance improvement activities when evaluating professional performance, judgment, and clinical or technical skills
- Any results of review of the individual's clinical performance
- Clinical performance in the organization that is outside acceptable standards
- Relevant education, training, and experience, if changed since initial privileging and appointment, when available
- Verification of current licensure, including all actions against the license
- A statement that the individual can perform the care, treatment, and services he or she has been providing
- Evaluation of restrictions on privileges at a hospital(s) or other health care organization(s)
- A query of the NPDB for information on adverse privilege actions taken by a health care entity, when appropriate to the discipline

B   5.   Credentials files contain clear evidence that the full range of privileges has been included in the reappraisal.

HR

Management of Information

Overview

The **goal** of the information management function is to support decision making to improve resident outcomes; improve health care documentation; assure resident safety; and improve performance in resident care, treatment, and services, governance, management, and support processes. While efficiency, effectiveness, resident safety, and the quality of resident care can be improved by computerization and other technologies, the principles of good information management apply to all methods, whether paper-based or electronic. The standards in this chapter are designed to be equally compatible with paper-based systems, electronic systems, or hybrid systems.

An organization's provision of care, treatment, and services is a complex endeavor that is highly dependent on information. This includes information about the science of care, treatment, and services; the individual resident; the care, treatment, and services provided; the results of care, treatment, and services; and the performance of the organization itself. Furthermore, because many individuals and areas within the organization are involved in the provision of care, treatment, and services, their work must be coordinated and integrated. As a result, organizations must treat information as an important resource to be managed effectively and efficiently. Managing information is an active, planned activity. The organization's leaders have overall responsibility for managing information, just as they do for managing the organization's human, material, and financial resources.

The quality of care, treatment, and services is affected by the many transitions in information management that are currently in progress in health care, such as the transition from handwriting and traditional paper-based documentation to electronic information management, as well as the transition from free text* to structured† and interactive text.‡

To achieve the goals of this function, the following processes are performed well:
- Identifying information needs
- Designing the structure of the information management system

IM

---

* **Free text** Free-flowing, nonstructured type of speaking, writing, or inputting of information.

† **Structured text** Process that requires authors to put specific information into specific fields with passive guidance by the information system. In paper-based systems, a form encourages a practitioner to fill in fields or boxes. Electronic systems use the same principle for templates or macros, which are guides used to create standardized information documentation. The purpose is to produce data of more consistent quality, make information more usable for decision support, make information more complete and more easily retrievable, and save documentation time.

‡ **Interactive text** A more complex version of structured text, as it interactively prompts and provides feedback to the person using it. Typically, it uses a higher level of computer intelligence that interacts with the person who records information.

- Capturing,* organizing, storing, retrieving, processing,† and analyzing‡ data and information
- Transmitting,§ reporting, displaying, integrating, and using data and information
- Safeguarding data# and information

The standards in this chapter focus on organizationwide information planning and management processes to meet the organization's internal and external information needs. They describe a vision for effectively and continuously improving information management in health care organizations. Achieving this vision involves the following:

- Ensuring timely and easy access to complete information throughout the organization
- Assuring data accuracy
- Balancing requirements of security‖ and ease of access
- Producing and using aggregate data to pursue opportunities for improvement
- Ensuring data comparability within and among organizations, where possible, by following national, state, and other recognized standards and guidelines on form and content
- Accessing and using external knowledge bases and comparative data to pursue opportunities for improvement
- Redesigning information-related processes to improve efficiency and effectiveness, as well as resident safety and quality of resident care, treatment, and services
- Increasing collaboration and information sharing to enhance resident care

IM

---

* **Capture** The process of recording representations of human thought, perceptions, or actions as well as device-generated data or information that is gathered and/or computed about a resident as part of a health care encounter or about other matters in an organization.

† **Processing** The process that manipulates data and information by editing and updating.

‡ **Analyzing** The process that interprets the data and transforms it into information.

§ **Transmission** The sending of data and information from one location to another.

Data Uninterpreted observations or facts.

‖ **Security** The protection of data from intentional or unintentional destruction, modification, or disclosure.

Standards

The following is a list of all standards for this function. They are presented here for your convenience without footnotes or other explanatory text. If you have a question about a term used here, please check the Glossary.

Note: *A revised standard numbering system is being used with the reformatted standards. This revised numbering system will allow for more flexibility to add standards while maintaining the current label for each standard.*

Information Management Planning

IM.1.10   The organization plans and designs information management processes to meet internal and external information needs.

Confidentiality and Security

IM.2.10   Information privacy and confidentiality are maintained.

IM.2.20   Information security, including data integrity, is maintained.

IM.2.30   The organization has a process for maintaining continuity of information.

Information Management Processes

IM.3.10   The organization has processes in place to effectively manage information, including the capturing, reporting, processing, storing, retrieving, disseminating, and displaying of clinical/service and non-clinical data and information.

Information-Based Decision Making

IM.4.10   The information management system provides information for use in decision making.

Knowledge-Based Information

IM.5.10   Knowledge-based information resources are readily available, current, and authoritative.

Resident-Specific Information

IM.6.10   The organization has a complete and accurate medical clinical record for every individual assessed, cared for, treated, or served.

IM.6.20   Records contain resident-specific information, as appropriate to the care, treatment, and services provided.

IM

IM.6.30   Not applicable

IM.6.40   Not applicable

IM.6.50   Designated qualified personnel accept and transcribe verbal orders from authorized individuals.

IM.6.60   The organization can provide access to all relevant information from a resident's record when needed for use in resident care, treatment, and services.

IM.6.70   Clinical record documentation includes the provision of and response to the activities program at least quarterly.

IM.6.80   Clinical record documentation includes the provision of and response to nutrition care services at least quarterly.

IM.6.90   Clinical record documentation includes the provision of and response to nursing care.

IM.6.100   Clinical record documentation includes the provision of and response to medical treatment and care.

IM.6.110   Clinical record documentation includes the provision of and response to rehabilitation services.

IM.6.120   Clinical record documentation includes the provision of and response to social service interventions.

IM.6.130   Clinical record documentation includes the provision of education and its effectiveness.

IM.6.140   Clinical record documentation includes significant changes in the resident's condition, care, and treatment.

IM.6.150   Treatment provided to the resident by off-site sources is documented in the clinical record.

IM.6.160   The effects of medications on residents, and associated pharmacist's evaluation and physician consultation, are documented.

IM.6.170   Discharge information provided to the resident or to the family, as appropriate and permissible, and/or to the receiving organization is documented.

Understanding the Parts of This Chapter

To help you navigate this reformatted standards chapter, it may be helpful to think of its parts this way:

- The **standard** is the "goal"
- The **rationale** explains why it's important to achieve this goal
- The **elements of performance** identify the step(s) needed to achieve this goal

These parts are defined as follows.

Standard A statement that defines the performance expectations and/or structures or processes that must be in place for an organization to provide safe, high-quality care, treatment, and services. An organization is either "compliant" or "not compliant" with a standard.

Accreditation decisions are based on simple counts of the standards that are determined to be "not compliant."

Rationale A statement that provides background, justification, or additional information about a standard. A standard's rationale is not scored. In some instances, the rationale for a standard is self-evident. Therefore, not every standard has a written rationale.

Elements of performance (EPs) The specific performance expectations and/or structures or processes that must be in place for an organization to provide safe, high-quality care, treatment, and services. The scoring of EP compliance determines an organization's overall compliance with a standard. EPs are evaluated on the following scale:

> 0   Insufficient compliance
> 1   Partial compliance
> 2   Satisfactory compliance
> NA   Not applicable

You will find a **measure of success** icon—**Ⓜ**—next to some EPs. Measures of success (MOS) need to be developed for certain EPs when a standard is judged to be out of compliance through either the Periodic Performance Review (PPR) or the onsite survey. An MOS is defined as a quantifiable measure, usually related to an audit, that can be used to determine whether an action has been effective and is being sustained.*

IM

Assessing Your Compliance

Once you are familiar with the parts of this chapter, you can begin to assess your compliance with its requirements. The scoring category designations are provided next to each EP for your convenience. If you would like to assess your organization's performance, mark your scores for the EPs and standards by following the simple steps described below.

---

* For more information about MOS, *see* "The New Joint Commission Accreditation Process" chapter in this book.

Two components are scored for each EP: (1) compliance with the requirement itself **and** (2) compliance with the track record* for that requirement. Scoring has been simplified and track record achievements (which have always been part of the scoring) have been appropriately modified.

Note: *Some standards and EPs do not apply to a particular type of organization; these standards and EPs are marked "not applicable" and the related text is not included. Your organization is not expected to comply with standards and EPs marked "not applicable."*

In addition, some standards and EPs that do apply to organizations may not apply to the specific care, treatment, and services that your individual organization provides. Although these standards and EPs are included in the book, you are not expected to comply with them. If you are unsure about the standards or EPs that apply to your organization, please contact the Joint Commission's Standards Interpretation Group at 630/792-5900.

Step 1: Score Your Compliance with Each Element of Performance

Before you can determine your compliance with the standards, you must score your compliance with each EP. There are three scoring criterion categories: A, B, and C (described below). Please note that for each EP scoring criterion category, your organization must meet the performance requirement itself and the track record achievements (*see* "Track Record Achievements").

Category A

These EPs relate to the presence or absence of the requirement(s) and are scored either yes (2) or no (0); however, score 1 for partial compliance is also possible based on track record achievements.

If an A EP has multiple components designated by bullets, your organization must be compliant with all the bullets to receive a score of 2. If your organization does not meet one or more requirements in the bullets, you will receive a score of 0.

Category B

Category B EPs are scored in two steps:

1. As with category A EPs, category B EPs relate to the presence or absence of the requirement(s). If your organization *does not meet* the requirement(s), the EP is scored 0; there is no need to assess your compliance with the principles of good process design.
2. If your organization *does meet* the requirement(s), but there is concern about the quality or comprehensiveness of the effort, then and only then should you assess the qualitative aspect of the EP. That is, review the applicable principles of good process design and ask how the principles were applied in the situation under discussion. Good process design has the following characteristics:

---

* **Track record** The amount of time that an organization has been in compliance with a standard, EP, or other requirement.

IM

- Is consistent with your organization's mission, values, and goals
- Meets the needs of patients
- Reflects the use of currently accepted practices (doing the right thing, using resources responsibly, using practice guidelines)
- Incorporates current safety information and knowledge such as sentinel event data and National Patient Safety Goals
- Incorporates relevant performance improvement results

This two-part evaluation applies to both simple and bulleted B EPs. First, the EPs are assessed to determine whether the requirements are present. If the EP has multiple components designated by bullets, as with the category A EPs, your organization must meet the requirements in *all* the bulleted items to get a score of 2. If your organization meets *none* of the requirements in the bullets, it receives a score of 0. If your organization meets *at least one, but not all,* of the bulleted requirements, it receives a score of 1 for the EPs.

Use the following rules to determine your EP score:
- Your EP score is 0 if your organization does not meet the requirement(s); you *do not* need to assess your compliance with the preceding applicable principles of good process design
- Your EP score is 1 if your organization does meet the requirement(s) but considered only *some* of the preceding applicable principles of good process design
- Your EP score is 2 if your organization does meet the requirement(s) *and* considered *all* the preceding principles of good process design

Category C

C EPs are scored 0, 1, or 2 based on the number of times your organization does not meet the EP. These EPs are frequency based and require totaling the number of occurrences (that is, results of performance or nonperformance) related to a particular EP. Each situation discovered by a surveyor(s) will be counted as a separate occurrence.

Note: *Multiple events of the same type related to a single resident and single practitioner/staff member are counted as* one occurrence only.

Use the following rules to determine your EP score:
- Your EP score is 2 if you find one or fewer occurrences of noncompliance with the EP
- Your EP score is 1 if you find two occurrences of noncompliance with the EP
- Your EP score is 0 if you find three or more occurrences of noncompliance with the EP

If an EP in the C category has multiple requirements designated by bullets, the following scoring guidelines apply:
- If there are fewer than two findings in all bullets, the EP is scored 2
- If there are three or more findings in all bullets, the EP is scored 0
- In all other combinations of findings, the EP is scored 1

IM

Track Record Achievements

In addition to meeting the requirement(s) in each EP, regardless of category, your organization must also meet the following track record achievements:

Score	Initial Survey	Full Survey
2	4 months or more	12 months or more
1	2 to 3 months	6 to 11 months
0	Fewer than 2 months	Fewer than 6 months

Sample Sizes

If during an onsite survey, your organization has been found to be not compliant with one or more standards, you must demonstrate Evidence of Standards Compliance (ESC) for each standard that is not compliant. The ESC must address compliance at the EP level; when an EP within a noncompliant standard requires an MOS, your organization must demonstrate achievement with the MOS when completing the ESC.

Note: *Not every EP requires an MOS. EPs that do require an MOS are clearly marked in this chapter. Organizations are required to demonstrate achievement with an MOS only for EPs within a noncompliant standard that require an MOS. Organizations do not need to demonstrate achievement with an MOS for any EP within a compliant standard.*

When demonstrating achievement with an MOS during the ESC process, your organization is **required** to use the following sample sizes, which were established because of their statistical significance, their relative simplicity in application, and their sensitivity to an organization's population size:

- For a population size of fewer than 30 cases,* sample 100% of available cases
- For a population size of 30 to 100 cases, sample 30 cases
- For a population size of 101 to 500 cases, sample 50 cases
- For a population size greater than 500 cases, sample 70 cases

Note: *Organizations are* encouraged, but not required, *to follow this sample size when demonstrating achievement with an MOS for an EP within a noncompliant standard after conducting a full, Option 1, or Option 2 PPR.*

When conducting PPR (optional use) or demonstrating an ESC (mandatory use), use the following percentages to determine your EP score: 90% through 100% of your sample size is in compliance = score 2; 80% through 89% of your sample size is in compliance = score 1; less than 80% of your sample size is in compliance = score 0.

In addition, the following information should govern your organization's selection of samples:

- The appropriate sample size should be determined by the specific population related to the survey findings

---

* *Case* refers to a single instance in which a situation related to a survey finding occurs. For example, if a survey finding was related to **pain assessment**, then a case would be any resident record. If a survey finding was related to **pain management**, a case would be any resident record for residents receiving pain management.

- The sampling approach should involve either systematic random sampling (for example, your organization selects every second or third case for review) or simple random sampling (for example, your organization uses a series of random numbers generated by a computer to identify the cases to be reviewed)
- If your organization chooses not to use these sample sizes while conducting PPR options 1 or 2, you should make sure that your sample size is sufficiently large enough to ensure statistical significance
- When submitting a clarifying ESC, if your organization selects records as part of its sample, the records should be from a period of no more than three months before the last date of the survey
- Assessment of MOS compliance is conducted for a four-month period following the date of ESC approval. Your organization should select records as a part of your sample following the date of ESC approval and use the required sample sizes. MOS percentage compliance rates are derived from the average of all four months.

Step 2: Use Your EP Scores to Gauge Your Compliance with the Standards

Now that you have evaluated and scored each EP for a particular standard, use these simple rules to determine your compliance with the standard itself:

- Your organization is not in compliance (that is, "not compliant") with the standard if any EP is scored 0
- Otherwise, your organization is in compliance with a standard if 65% or more of its EPs are scored 2

IM

Standards, Rationales, Elements of Performance, and Scoring

Information Management Planning

Standard IM.1.10

The organization plans and designs information management processes to meet internal and external information needs.

Rationale for IM.1.10

Organizations vary in size, complexity, governance, structure, decision-making processes, and resources. Information management systems and processes vary accordingly. Only by first identifying the information needs can one then evaluate the extent to which they are planned for and at what performance level the needs are being met. Planning for the management of information does not require a formal written information plan but does require evidence of a planned approach that identifies the organization's information needs and supports its goals and objectives.

Elements of Performance for IM.1.10

B   1.   The organization bases its information management processes on the following thorough analysis of internal and external information needs:
- The analysis ascertains the flow of information in an organization, including information storage and feedback mechanisms
- The analysis considers what data and information are needed: within and among departments, services, or programs; within and among the staff, the administration, and governance structure; to support relationships with outside services and contractors; with licensing, accrediting, and regulatory bodies; with purchasers, payers, and employers; and to participate in national research and databases

B   2.   To guide development of processes for managing information used internally and externally, the organization assesses its information management needs based on the following:
- Its mission
- Its goals
- Its services
- Personnel
- Resident safety considerations
- Quality of care, treatment, and services
- Mode(s) of service delivery
- Resources
- Access to affordable technology
- Identification of barriers to effective communication among caregivers

IM

B   3.   The organization bases management, staffing, and material resource allocations for information management on the scope and complexity of care, treatment, and services provided.

B   4.   Appropriate staff participates in assessment, selection, integration, and use of information management systems for clinical/service and organization information.

B   5.   The organization has an ongoing process to assess the needs of the organization, departments, and individuals for knowledge-based information and uses this assessment as a basis for planning.

Confidentiality and Security

Standard IM.2.10
Information privacy* and confidentiality† are maintained.

Rationale for IM.2.10
Confidentiality of data and information applies across all systems and automated, paper, and verbal communications, as well as to clinical/service, financial, and business records and employee-specific information. The capture, storage, and retrieval processes for data and information are designed to be performed on a timely‡ basis without compromising the data and information's confidentiality. Protecting privacy and confidentiality of information is the responsibility of the whole organization. In achieving this responsibility, the organization provides appropriate safeguards for resident privacy and the confidentiality of information. These safeguards are consistent with available technology and legitimate needs for accessibility of the information to authorized individuals for the delivery of care, treatment, and services and effective functioning of the organization, research, and education.

Elements of Performance for IM.2.10
B   1.   The organization has developed a written process (in one or more policies) based on and consistent with applicable law that addresses the privacy and confidentiality of information.

B   2.   The organization's policy, including significant changes to the policy, has been effectively communicated to applicable staff.

B   3.   The organization has a process to monitor compliance with its policy.

IM

---

* **Privacy** An individual's right to limit the disclosure of personal information.

† **Confidentiality** The safekeeping of data/information so as to restrict access to individuals who have need, reason, and permission for such access.

‡ Defined by organization policy and based on the intended use of the information.

B   4.   The organization improves privacy and confidentiality by monitoring information and developments in technology.

C Ⓜ 5.   Individuals about whom personally identifiable health data and information may be maintained or collected are made aware of what uses and disclosures of the information will be made.

B   6.   For uses and disclosures of health information, the removal of personal identifiers is encouraged to the extent possible, consistent with maintaining the usefulness of the information.

C Ⓜ 7.   Protected health information* is used for the purposes identified or as required by law and not further disclosed without resident authorization.

B   8.   The organization preserves the confidentiality of data and information identified as sensitive and requires extraordinary means to preserve resident privacy.

Standard IM.2.20
Information security, including data integrity†, is maintained.

Rationale for IM.2.20
Policies and procedures address security procedures to ensure that only authorized personnel gain access to data and information. These policies can range from access to the paper chart to the various security levels and distribution of passwords in an electronic system. The basic premise of the policies is to provide the appropriate level of security and protection for sensitive resident, employee, and other information while facilitating access to data by those who have a legitimate need. The capture, storage, and retrieval processes for data and information are designed to provide for timely access without compromising the data and information's security and integrity.

Elements of Performance for IM.2.20

B   1.   The organization has developed a written (in one or more policies) based on and consistent with applicable law that addresses information security, including data integrity.

B   2.   The organization's policy, including significant changes to the policy, has been effectively communicated to applicable staff.

C Ⓜ 3.   The organization has an effective process for enforcing the policy.

C Ⓜ 4.   The organization monitors compliance with its policy.

IM

---

* **Protected health information** Health information that contains information such that an individual person can be identified as the subject of that information.

† **Integrity** In the context of data security, data integrity means the protection of data from accidental or unauthorized intentional change.

IM – 12

C ⓜ 5. The organization uses monitoring of information and developments in technology to improve information security, including data integrity.

B 6. The organization develops controls to safeguard data and information, including the clinical record, against loss, destruction, and tampering. Controls include the following:
- Policies when the removal of records is permitted
- Data and information protection against unauthorized intrusion, corruption, or damage
- Prevention of falsification of data and information
- Guidelines to prevent the loss and destruction of records
- Guidelines for destroying copies of records
- Protection of records in a manner that minimizes the possibility of damage from fire and water

B 7. Policies and procedures, including plans for implementation, for electronic information systems address the following: data integrity, authentication,* nonrepudiation,† encryption‡ as warranted, and auditability,§ as appropriate to the system and types of information, for example, resident information and billing information.

Standard IM.2.30

The organization has a process for maintaining continuity of information.

Rationale for IM.2.30

The overall purpose of the information continuity plan is to provide an alternative means of processing data, provide for recovery of data, and return to normal operations as soon as possible.

Elements of Performance for IM.2.30

B 1. The organization has a business continuity/disaster recovery plan for information systems, which includes the identification of the most critical information functions for resident care, treatment, and services and business processes, and the impact on the organization if these systems were severely interrupted, as priority areas of the continuity/disaster recovery plan.

B 2. The plan is tested periodically to ensure that the business interruption backup techniques are effective.

IM

---

* **Authentication** The validation of correctness for both the information itself and the person who is the author or user of information.

† **Nonrepudiation** The inability to dispute a document's content or authorship.

‡ **Encryption** The process of transforming plain text (readable) into cipher text that is unreadable without a special software key.

§ **Auditability** The ability to do a methodical examination and verification of all information activities such as entering and accessing.

B   3. For electronic systems, the organization has a process for disaster recovery and business continuity, as they would impact the management of information, which includes the following:
- Plans for scheduled and unscheduled interruptions, which includes end-user training with the downtime procedures
- Contingency procedures for operations interruptions (hardware, software, or other systems failure)
- Plans for minimal interruptions as a result of scheduled downtime
- An emergency service plan
- A back-up system (electronic or manual)
- Data retrieval and what it will address, including retrieval from storage and information presently in the system, retrieval of data in the event of system interruption, and back- up of data

Introduction to Managing Information for Clinical/Service and Organization Decision Making

An organization's ability to make the best decisions about clinical/service and organization issues depends heavily on having ready access to reliable and accurate information. To support the decision-making process, the organization follows certain procedures to successfully capture, process, store, and retrieve the needed information. It then supplies the information to management and others involved in the decision-making process.

Standards IM.3.10 and IM.4.10 address the procedures involved in information management in support of clinical/service and organization decision making; as such, these procedures are critical to resident care and safety and the efficient management of the organization. The procedures also apply in all information management environments, whether paper-based, electronic, or a hybrid of both.

The standards themselves also address all information management environments and can be particularly helpful to organizations transitioning from a paper-based environment to an electronic environment. The first standard addresses the tasks of collecting, processing, storing, retrieving, reporting, and disseminating data and information. The second standard addresses the use of the information.

IM

Information Management Processes

Standard IM.3.10

The organization has processes in place to effectively manage information, including the capturing, reporting, processing, storing, retrieving, disseminating, and displaying of clinical/service and nonclinical data and information.

Rationale for IM.3.10

Records resulting from data capture and report generation* are used for communication and continuity of the resident's care or financial and business operations over time. Records are also used for other purposes, including litigation and risk management activities, reimbursement, and statistics. Improved data capture and report generation systems enhance the value of the records. Potential benefits include improved resident care quality and safety, improved efficiency effectiveness and reduced costs in resident care, and financial and business operations. To maximize the benefits of data capture and report generation, these processes exhibit the following characteristics: unique ID, accuracy, completeness, timeliness,[†] interoperability,[‡] retrievability,[§] authentication and accountability,[#] auditability, confidentiality, and security.

The processing, storage, and retrieval functions are integral to electronic, computerized, and paper-based information systems in organizations. Important considerations for these functions include data elements, data accuracy, data confidentiality, data security, data integrity, permanence of storage (the time a medium can safely store information), ease of retrievability, aggregation of information, interoperability, clinical/service practice considerations, performance improvement, and decision support processing.

A goal for information storage is to be linked or centrally organized and accessible. This could include the organization having an index identifying where the information is stored and how to access it; or, as the organization moves to electronic systems, the organization creates all information systems to be interoperable within the enterprise. As more organizations automate various processes and activities, it is important to share critical data among systems. As challenges of interoperability have arisen, standards organizations have stepped in to develop industry standards. It is important that the organization is aware of the standards development organizations and their recommendations.

Internally and externally generated data and information are accurately disseminated to users. Access to accurate information is required to deliver, improve, analyze, and advance resident care and the systems that support health care delivery. Information may be accessed and disseminated through electronic information systems or paper-based records and reports. The use of information should be considered in developing forms, screen displays, and standard or ad hoc reports.

---

* **Report generation** The process of analyzing, organizing, and presenting recorded information for authentication and inclusion in the resident's health care record or in financial or business records.

[†] **Timeliness** The time between the occurrence of an event and the availability of data about the event. Timeliness is related to the use of the data.

[‡] **Interoperability** Enables authorized users to capture, share, and report information from any system, whether paper- or electronic-based.

[§] **Retrievability** The capability of efficiently finding relevant information.

[#] **Accountability** All information is attributable to its source (person or device).

IM

Elements of Performance for IM.3.10

B   1. Uniform data definitions and data capture methods are used, as follows:
- Minimum data sets, terminology, definitions, classifications, vocabulary, and nomenclature are standardized as needed
- Industry standards are used whenever possible

A Ⓜ 2. Abbreviations, acronyms, and symbols are standardized throughout the organization and there is a list of abbreviations, acronyms, and symbols not to use.

B   3. Quality control systems are used to monitor data content and collection activities, as follows:
- The method used assures timely and economical data collection with the degree of accuracy, completeness, and discrimination necessary for their intended use
- The method used minimizes bias in the data and regularly assesses the data's reliability, validity, and accuracy
- Those responsible for collecting and reviewing the data are accountable for information accuracy and completeness

B   4. Storage and retrieval systems are designed to support organization needs for clinical/service and organization-specific information, as follows:
- Storage and retrieval systems are designed to balance the ability to retrieve data and information with the intended use for the data and information
- Storage and retrieval systems are designed to balance security and confidentiality issues with accessibilit.
- Systems for paper and electronic records are designed to reduce disruption or inaccessibility during such times as diminished staffing and scheduled and unscheduled downtimes of electronic information systems

A   5. Data and information are retained for sufficient time to comply with law and regulation.

B   6. Data and information are retained for quality of care and other organization needs.

B   7. The necessary expertise and tools are available for collecting, retrieving, and analyzing data and their transformation into information.

B   8. Data are organized and transformed into information in formats useful to decision makers.

B   9. Dissemination of data and information is timely and accurate.

B   10. Data and information are disseminated in standard formats and methods to meet user needs and provide for easy retrievability and interpretation.

B   11. Industry or organization standards are used whenever possible for data display and transmission.

Information-Based Decision Making

Standard IM.4.10

The information management system provides information for use in decision making.

Rationale for IM.4.10

Information management supports timely and effective decision making at all organization levels. The information management processes support managerial and operational decisions; performance improvement activities; and resident care, treatment, and services decisions. Clinical and strategic decision making depends on information from multiple sources, including the resident record, knowledge-based information, comparative data/information, and aggregate data/information.

Elements of Performance for IM.4.10

To support clinical decision making, information found in the resident record must include the following:

C Ⓜ 1. Readily accessible throughout the system

C Ⓜ 2. Accurately recorded

C Ⓜ 3. Complete

C Ⓜ 4. Organized for efficient retrieval of needed data

C Ⓜ 5. Timely

B   6. Comparative performance data and information are available for decision making, if applicable.

B   7. The organization has the ability to collect and aggregate data and information to support care, treatment, and services delivery and operations, including the following:
- Individual care, treatment, and services and care, treatment, and services delivery
- Decision making
- Management and operations
- Analysis of trends over time
- Performance comparisons over time within the organization and with other organizations
- Performance improvement
- Infection control
- Resident safety

IM

Knowledge-Based Information

Standard IM.5.10
Knowledge-based information* resources are readily available, current, and authoritative.

Rationale for IM.5.10
Organization practitioners and staff have access to knowledge-based information to do the following:
- Help them acquire and maintain the knowledge and skills needed to maintain and improve competence
- Help with clinical/service and management decision making
- Provide appropriate information and education to residents and families
- Support performance improvement and resident safety activities
- Support the institution's educational and research needs

Elements of Performance for IM.5.10

1. Not applicable

B   2. The organization provides access to information resources needed by staff in print, electronic, Internet, audio, and/or other appropriate form.†

B   3. Knowledge-based resources are available at all times to clinical/service staff, through electronic means, after-hours access to an in-house collection, or other methods.

B   4. The organization has a plan to provide for access to information during times when electronic systems are unavailable.

Resident-Specific Information

IM

Standard IM.6.10
The organization has a complete and accurate medical clinical record for every individual assessed, cared for, treated, or served.

---

* **Knowledge-based information** A collection of stored facts, models, and information that can be used for designing and redesigning processes and for problem solving. In the context of this manual, knowledge-based information is found in the clinical, scientific, and management literature.

† Forms of information include current texts, periodicals, indexes, abstracts, reports, documents, databases, directories, discussion lists, successful practices, standards, protocols, practice guidelines, clinical trials, and other resources.

Rationale for IM.6.10

Resident-specific data and information are contained in the medical clinical record, to facilitate resident care, treatment, and services; serve as a financial and legal record; aid in research; support decision analysis; and guide professional and organization performance improvement. This information may be maintained as a paper record or as electronic health information.*

Elements of Performance for IM.6.10

A   1.   Only authorized individuals make entries in the clinical record.

A   2.   The organization defines which entries made by nonindependent practitioners require countersigning consistent with law and regulation.

A   3.   Standardized formats are used for documenting all care, treatment, and services provided to residents.

C ⓜ 4.   Every clinical record entry[†] is dated, the author identified and, when necessary according to law or regulation and organization policy, is authenticated.

C ⓜ 5.   At a minimum, the following are authenticated either by written signature, electronic signature, or computer key or rubber stamp:[‡]
- The history and physical examination
- Medication orders
- Practitioner orders
- Discharge summary

C ⓜ 6.   The clinical record contains sufficient information to identify the resident; support the diagnosis/condition; justify the care, treatment, and services; document the course and results of care, treatment, and services; and promote continuity of care among providers.

   7.   Not applicable

B   8.   The organization has a policy and procedures on the timely entry of all significant information into the resident's clinical record.

---

* **Electronic health information** A computerized format of the health care information in paper records that is used for the same range of purposes as paper records, namely to familiarize readers with the resident's status; document care, treatment, and services; plan for discharge; document the need for care, treatment, and services; assess the quality of care, treatment, and services; determine reimbursement rates; justify reimbursement claims; pursue clinical or epidemiological research; and measure outcomes of the care, treatment, and services process.

† Signatures do not have to be dated if they occur in real time of the entry. For paper-based records, counter-signatures entered for purposes of authentication after transcription or for verbal orders are dated when required by state or federal law and regulations and organization policy. For electronic records, electronic signatures will be date-stamped.

‡ Authentication can be shown by written signatures or initials, rubber-stamp signatures, or computer key. Authorized users of signature stamps or computer keys sign a statement assuring that they alone will use the stamp or key.

IM

A   9. The organization defines a complete record and the timeframe within which the record must be completed not to exceed 30 days after discharge.

       10. Not applicable

       11. Not applicable

B   12. Clinical records are reviewed on an ongoing basis at the point of care.

B   13. The review of clinical records is based on organization-defined indicators that address the presence, timeliness, readability (whether handwritten or printed), quality, consistency, clarity, accuracy, completeness, and authentication of data and information contained within the record.

B   14. The retention time of clinical record information is determined by the organization based on law and regulation and on its use for resident care, treatment, and services; legal, research, and operational purposes; as well as educational activities.

A   15. Clinical records are retained for five years from the resident's discharge date when there is no requirement in state law.

A   16. Clinical records of minors are retained for three years after the resident reaches legal age under the law.

A   17. Original clinical records are not released unless the organization is responding appropriately to federal or state laws, court orders, or subpoenas.

       18. Not applicable

A   19. In the event of a change in the organization's ownership, all residents' clinical records remain the organization's property and are transferred to the new owner unless otherwise indicated by law.

Standard IM.6.20

Records contain resident-specific information, as appropriate to the care, treatment, and services provided.

Elements of Performance for IM.6.20

C Ⓜ 1. Each clinical record contains, as applicable, the following clinical/case information:
- Emergency care, treatment, and services provided to the resident before his or her arrival, if any
- Documentation and findings of assessments*
- The initial medical assessment and conclusions or impressions drawn from medical history and physical examination
- The diagnosis, diagnostic impression, or conditions

IM

- The reason(s) for admission or care, treatment, and services
- The goals of the treatment care and treatment care plan
- Orders for care, treatment, and services as required by law and regulation
- Diagnostic and therapeutic orders
- All diagnostic and therapeutic procedures, tests, and results
- Progress notes made by authorized individuals
- All reassessments and plan of care revisions, when indicated
- Relevant observations
- Consultation reports
- Allergies to foods and medicines
- Every medication ordered or prescribed
- Every dose of medication administered and any adverse drug reaction
- Every medication dispensed or prescribed on discharge
- All relevant diagnoses/conditions established during the course of care, treatment, and services

C Ⓜ 2. Each clinical record contains, as applicable, the following demographic information:
- The resident's name, address, date of birth, religion, marital status, Social Security number, gender, and the name of any legally authorized representative
- The resident's legal status, as appropriate

C Ⓜ 3. Each clinical record contains, as applicable, the following information:
- Evidence of known advance directives
- Evidence of informed consent when required by organization policy
- Any orders, renewal of orders, and documentation that resuscitative services are to be withheld or life-sustaining treatment withdrawn
- Discharge plan or the reason for lack of ongoing plan when discharge potential does not exist
- Referrals or communications made to external or internal care providers and community agencies
- The physician's summary and the resident's final diagnosis when the resident is admitted from either a hospital or another health care organization

IM

Standard IM.6.30
Not applicable

Standard IM.6.40
Not applicable

---

* See the "Provision of Care, Treatment, and Services" chapter in this book.

Standard IM.6.50

Designated qualified personnel accept and transcribe verbal orders from autho-rized individuals.

Rationale for IM.6.50

Processes for receiving, transcribing, and authenticating verbal orders are estab-lished to protect the quality of resident care, treatment, and services.

Elements of Performance for IM.6.50

A   1.   Qualified personnel are identified, as defined by organization policy and, as appropriate, in accordance with state and federal law, and authorized to receive and record verbal orders.

C Ⓜ 2.   Each verbal order is dated and identifies the names of the individuals who gave and received it, and the record indicates who implemented it.

A   3.   When required by state or federal law and regulation, verbal orders are authenticated within the specified time frame.

A   4.   Implement a process for taking verbal or telephone orders or receiv-ing critical test results that require a verification "read-back" of the complete order or test result by the person receiving the order or test result.

Standard IM.6.60

The organization can provide access to all relevant information from a resident's record when needed for use in resident care, treatment, and services.

Rationale for IM.6.60

To facilitate continuity of care, providers have access to information about all previ-ous care, treatment, and services provided to a resident by the organization.

Elements of Performance for IM.6.60

B   1.   There is a manual or automated mechanism to track the location of all components of the medical clinical record.

B   2.   The organization uses a system to assemble required information or make available a summary of information relative for resident care, treatment, and services when the resident is seen.

Standard IM.6.70

Clinical record documentation includes the provision of and response to the activi-ties program at least quarterly.

Elements of Performance for IM.6.70

C Ⓜ 1. The provision of and response to the activities program based on the interdisciplinary care plan are documented at least quarterly in the clinical record.

C Ⓜ 2. The activity providers document in the clinical record and report to the charge nurse any changes in the resident's response to the activity program.

Standard IM.6.80

Clinical record documentation includes the provision of and response to nutrition care services at least quarterly.

Elements of Performance for IM.6.80

C Ⓜ 1. The provision of and response to nutrition care services based on the interdisciplinary care plan is documented at least quarterly in the clinical record.

C Ⓜ 2. Documentation includes the current status and changes in the resident's nutritional status, including the following information:
- The resident's acceptance of any prescribed diets
- The resident's food and fluid consumption
- Significant weight loss or gain
- Hydration status
- The resident's ability to eat independently
- The resident's ability to use adaptive devices for eating
- The current status and changes in the resident's physical or behavioral condition, including symptoms
- Any education provided and its effectiveness
- A summary of the resident's condition, which includes the extent to which nutritional goals included in the interdisciplinary care plan are achieved

Standard IM.6.90

Clinical record documentation includes the provision of and response to nursing care.

IM

Elements of Performance for IM.6.90

C Ⓜ 1. The provision of nursing care that is based on the interdisciplinary care plan and the resident's response to this care are documented in the clinical record.

C Ⓜ 2. Documentation includes at least the following:
- The medications and treatment given and any untoward reactions
- The nursing care provided
- Any education provided and its effectiveness

- The current status and changes in the resident's physical or behavioral condition, including symptoms
- A summary by licensed nursing staff of the resident's condition, which includes the extent to which nursing goals included in the interdisciplinary care plan are achieved, at least quarterly or more often if the resident's condition warrants

C ⓜ 3. **For subacute services only:** Nursing summaries are documented according to the following time frames:
- Every two weeks for the first quarter
- Every month for the second quarter
- Quarterly thereafter or more frequently when indicated by a change in the resident's condition

Standard IM.6.100
Clinical record documentation includes the provision of and response to medical treatment and care.

Elements of Performance for IM.6.100

C ⓜ 1. The provision of medical treatment and care and the resident's response to medical treatment and care are documented in the clinical record.

C ⓜ 2. Documentation in the resident's clinical record includes, before or on admission, the submission of the following:
- Admitting diagnosis
- Current medical findings
- Diet prescribed
- The resident's functional status

C ⓜ 3. Documentation in the resident's clinical record includes medical observations and recommendations made after the initial medical assessment, as well as progress notes that are reported at the time of observation and that describe significant changes in the resident's condition.

C ⓜ 4. Documentation in the resident's clinical record includes progress notes recorded by the physician at each visit.

C ⓜ 5. Upon the resident's discharge, documentation in the resident's clinical record includes the completion of the transfer form, the discharge summary, and the resident's clinical record.

C ⓜ 6. If the resident expires in the organization, the course of events leading up to the resident's death is documented.

C ⓜ 7. Documentation in the resident's clinical record includes evidence that the attending physician has reviewed the consulting physician's orders for consistency with the overall care plan.

IM

Standard IM.6.110 ━━━━━━━━━━━━━━━━━━━━━━━━━━━━━━━

Clinical record documentation includes the provision of and response to rehabilitation services.

Elements of Performance for IM.6.110

C Ⓜ 1. The provision of rehabilitation services provided that are based on the interdisciplinary care plan and the resident's response to these services are documented in the clinical record.

C Ⓜ 2. Documentation describes at least the following:
- The resident's and family's perception of and involvement in rehabilitation services
- The reason for the referral to rehabilitation services or admission for the comprehensive subacute services
- The rehabilitation treatments, modalities, or procedures provided
- The resident's response to treatment
- The resident's involvement in rehabilitation services
- The resident's progress toward treatment goals

C Ⓜ 3. Assessment of rehabilitation achievement and estimates of further rehabilitation potential are entered at least weekly.

C Ⓜ 4. Documentation includes a progress report and reassessment, including the following:
- A summary of the resident's condition, which includes the extent to which rehabilitation goals included in the interdisciplinary care plan are achieved, every two weeks for the first quarter, every month for the second quarter, and quarterly thereafter or more frequently when indicated by a change in the resident's condition
- Estimates of the resident's further rehabilitation potential
- A discharge plan

Standard IM.6.120 ━━━━━━━━━━━━━━━━━━━━━━━━━━━━━━━

Clinical record documentation includes the provision of and response to social service interventions.

Elements of Performance for IM.6.120

C Ⓜ 1. The provision of and the resident's response to social service interventions are documented in the clinical record.

C Ⓜ 2. Documentation of social service interventions includes at least the following:
- Specified goals related to social services, including discharge planning, that are an integral part of the interdisciplinary care plan
- The services provided and their outcomes
- A summary of the resident's problems, services provided, goals, and condition, which includes the extent to which social services goals

IM

IM – 25

included in the interdisciplinary care plan are achieved, at least quarterly or more often if the resident's condition warrants
- Referrals to outside agencies, resources, or individuals, as well as any follow-up actions or recommendations of outside agencies, resources, or individuals

c Ⓜ 3. When the organization provides subacute services, the summary is documented according to the following time frames:
- Every two weeks for the first quarter
- Every month for the second quarter
- Quarterly thereafter or more frequently, when indicated by a change in the resident's condition

Standard IM.6.130

Clinical record documentation includes the provision of education and its effectiveness.

Element of Performance for IM.6.130
c Ⓜ 1. The provision of and the resident's response to education are documented in the clinical record.

Standard IM.6.140

Clinical record documentation includes significant changes in the resident's condition, care, and treatment.

Element of Performance for IM.6.140
c Ⓜ 1. Clinical record documentation includes significant changes in the resident's condition, care, and treatment.

Standard IM.6.150

Treatment provided to the resident by off-site sources is documented in the clinical record.

Element of Performance for IM.6.150
c Ⓜ 1. Clinical record documentation includes treatment provided to the resident by off-site sources.

Standard IM.6.160

The effects of medications on residents, and associated pharmacist evaluation and physician consultation, are documented.

IM

Element of Performance for IM.6.160

C Ⓜ 1. The clinical record includes documentation of the following:
- The resident's response to medications
- The pharmacist's evaluation and consultation with the physician
- The need for any additional laboratory monitoring

Note: *The documentation may be included in the resident's clinical record or in another location such as the pharmacist's report.*

Standard IM.6.170

Discharge information provided to the resident or to the family, as appropriate and permissible, and/or to the receiving organization is documented.

Elements of Performance for IM.6.170

C Ⓜ 1. Clinical record documentation includes discharge information provided to the resident and/or to the receiving organization.

C Ⓜ 2. Discharge information includes the following:
- Medical findings, diagnosis(es), and treatment orders
- A summary of the care, treatment, and services provided and progress toward achieving goals
- Diet orders and medication orders
- Behavioral status, ambulation status, nutrition status, and rehabilitation potential
- The resident's physical and psychosocial status
- Nursing information useful in resident care
- Advance directives
- Referrals provided to the resident
- The reason for transfer, discharge, or referral
- The physician's orders for the resident's immediate care
- Instructions given to the resident before discharge
- The referring physician's name
- The physician who has agreed to be responsible for the resident's medical care and treatment, if other than the referring physician

IM

IM

Medicare/Medicaid Certification–Based LTC Accreditation Standards

Overview

This chapter contains standards, rationales, and elements of performance (EPs) applicable to those long term care organizations seeking the Joint Commission's Medicare/Medicaid certification–based long term care accreditation. These requirements are pulled directly out of the functional chapters in this book.

This subset of Joint Commission long term care accreditation standards has been identified for on-site review under the Medicare/Medicaid Certification–Based LTC Accreditation option. These standards go beyond the Conditions of Participation for Skilled Nursing Facilities/Nursing Facilities and address areas that are typically not evaluated during the state agency certification survey. This path to long term care accreditation focuses on systems and processes that support organization safety, performance improvement, resident and family education, credentialing and privileging of licensed independent practitioners, pain management, and point-of-care testing (POCT).

An organization is eligible for the Medicare/Medicaid certification-based accreditation option if it is Medicare/Medicaid certified as a Skilled Nursing Facility (SNF) or Nursing Facility (NF). The on-site survey is usually one day (organizations with an average daily census >300 will be scheduled additional time), and the fee is significantly less than the traditional long term care accreditation fee. Certificates reflect that the accreditation award is substantially based on Medicare/Medicaid certification for long term care. For more information, please visit the Joint Commission's Web site at http://www.jcaho.org.

Accreditation Participation Requirements

This section includes specific requirements for participation in the accreditation process and for maintaining an accreditation award. These differ from survey eligibility criteria in that the accreditation process may be initiated even when all Accreditation Participation Requirements (APRs) have not yet been met.

For an organization seeking accreditation for the first time, compliance with the APRs is assessed during the initial survey. For the accredited organization, compliance with these requirements is assessed throughout the accreditation cycle through on-site surveys, Evidence of Standards Compliance (ESCs), and periodic updates of organization-specific data and information. Organizations are either compliant or not compliant with APRs. Some APRs are only applicable to the Medicare/Medicaid Certification–Based LTC Accreditation option (for example, APR 4, EP 1, and APR 15). When an organization does not comply with an APR, the organization is assigned a requirement for improvement in the same context that noncompliance with a standard or EP generates a requirement for improvement. However, refusal to permit performance of an unscheduled or unannounced for-cause survey (APR 3) or falsification of information (APR 10), will immediately lead to Preliminary Denial of Accreditation. All requirements for improvement can impact the accreditation decision and follow-up requirements, as determined by established accreditation decision rules. Failure to resolve a requirement for improvement can ultimately lead to loss of accreditation.

Application for Accreditation

APR 1
When requested, the organization provides the Joint Commission with all official records and reports of public or publicly recognized licensing (for example, a state license), examining, reviewing, or planning bodies.*

Element of Performance for APR 1
1. The organization provides the Joint Commission with all official records and reports of licensing, examining, reviewing, or planning bodies.

MC

APR 2
The organization immediately reports any changes in the information provided in the application for accreditation and any changes made between surveys.†

---

* *See also* page APP-19 in the "Accreditation Policies and Procedures" chapter.

† *See also* page APP-37.

Rationale for APR 2

An organization that experiences a significant change in ownership or control, location, capacity, or the categories of services offered must notify the Joint Commission in writing not more than 30 days after such changes. The Joint Commission may decide that the organization must be resurveyed when a significant merger or consolidation has taken place. The Joint Commission continues the organization's accreditation until it determines whether a resurvey is necessary. Failure to provide timely notification to the Joint Commission of ownership, merger or consolidation, and service changes may result in interruption or loss of accreditation.

Element of Performance for APR 2

1. The organization notifies the Joint Commission not more than 30 days before or after a significant change in ownership or control, location, capacity, or the categories of services offered.

Acceptance of Survey

APR 3

An organization permits the performance of an unscheduled or unannounced for-cause survey* at the discretion of the Joint Commission.

Rationale for APR 3

The Joint Commission may perform either an unscheduled or unannounced for-cause survey when it becomes aware of potentially serious resident care or safety issues in an organization. Either type of survey can take place at any point in an organization's three-year accreditation cycle. An unscheduled or unannounced survey can either include all of the organization's services or address only those areas where a serious concern may exist. In addition, the Joint Commission conducts unannounced surveys on a random sample of accredited organizations at 9 to 30 months following the accreditation date. An organization's failure to permit an unscheduled or unannounced survey is grounds for withdrawal of accreditation.

Elements of Performance for APR 3

1. The organization permits the performance of an unscheduled for-cause survey.

2. The organization permits the performance of an unannounced for-cause survey.

MC

---

* *See also* page APP-39 for an explanation of the difference between an unscheduled and unannounced for-cause survey. In addition, see the last paragraph of "Continuous Compliance" on page APP-36.

Performance Measurement*

APR 4 ▬▬▬▬▬▬▬▬▬▬▬▬▬▬▬▬▬▬▬▬▬▬▬▬▬▬▬▬▬▬▬

The organization selects and uses performance measures relevant to the services provided and populations served.

Rationale for APR 4

Each Medicare/Medicaid-certified Skilled Nursing Facility/Nursing Facility required to collect and submit minimum data set (MDS) data to a state agency per Centers for Medicare & Medicaid Services (CMS) regulation must share monthly Facility Quality Indicator (QI) Profiles, Quality Measure (QM) reports, CMS Form 2567 reports, plans of correction, and/or publicly reported Quality Measure reports, as appropriate, with Joint Commission surveyors at the time of survey and discuss how the data were used to identify and prioritize performance improvement activities.

A long term care organization not required to collect MDS data must participate in a performance measurement system accepted for use in the accreditation process and use accepted performance measures from the performance measurement system.

Elements of Performance for APR 4

1. For a Medicare/Medicaid–certified Skilled Nursing Facility/Nursing Facility only: If the organization is required to collect and submit MDS data to a state agency per CMS regulation, it shares monthly Facility QI Profiles, QM reports, CMS Form 2567 reports, plans of correction, and/or publicly reported Quality Measure reports, as appropriate, at the time of survey and discusses how the data were used to identify and prioritize performance improvement activities.

2. Not applicable

3. For long term care organizations not required to collect MDS data: The organization participates in a performance measurement system accepted for use in the accreditation process and uses accepted performance measures from the performance measurement system.

APR 5 ▬▬▬▬▬▬▬▬▬▬▬▬▬▬▬▬▬▬▬▬▬▬▬▬▬▬▬▬▬▬▬

MC

A non–Medicare/Medicaid certified long term care organization selects and uses accepted performance measures from at least one listed performance measurement system.

---

* For additional information on performance measurement, see the "Performance Measurement and the ORYX Initiative" chapter. Organizations are also encouraged to keep up to date on any changes in ORYX requirements by reviewing recent issues of *Joint Commission Perspectives*® or going to the Performance Measurement area on the Joint Commission's Web site at http://www.jcaho.org/pms/index.htm.

Rationale for APR 5

The organization identifies the appropriate number of clinical measures that meet Joint Commission requirements. The organization submits data for its measures to the performance measurement system(s) at least quarterly, and such submissions identify monthly data points. An organization applying for initial survey must notify the Joint Commission of its measure selection(s) no later than the time of survey. Each organization must also notify the Joint Commission of any subsequent additions or changes to its measure selections. An individual measure must be used for at least four consecutive quarters before it can be replaced. For purposes of reporting to the Joint Commission, an organization will be expected to do the following:

- Continue to use a measure if the data suggest an unstable pattern of performance or otherwise identify an opportunity for improvement
  or
- Change to a new measure if the data reflect continuing stable and satisfactory performance

Elements of Performance for APR 5

1. The organization has selected a sufficient number of performance measures to meet current ORYX requirements.

2. The organization notifies the Joint Commission of its performance measures selections by the date requested.

3. The organization notifies the Joint Commission of any changes in its performance measures selections.

4. Each individual performance measure is used for at least four consecutive quarters.

APR 6

A non–Medicare/Medicaid certified long term care organization ensures that aggregate data for the measures are submitted to the Joint Commission at least quarterly.

Rationale for APR 6

Organization-specific aggregate data, reported as monthly data points, must be submitted four times per year by established deadlines from the performance measurement system to the Joint Commission for use in the accreditation process, as required by the Joint Commission. The Joint Commission has defined the type and format of performance measurement data to be submitted in a fashion consistent with nationally recognized standards.

The submission of organization-specific data will be performed by the selected performance measurement system(s) and will include comparative data for other organizations in the same performance measurement system that have selected the same performance measures.

MC

Element of Performance for APR 6

1. The organization ensures that aggregate data for the selected performance measures are submitted four times a year in accordance with established timelines to the Joint Commission.

Public Information Interviews

APR 8 ▬▬▬▬▬▬▬▬▬▬▬▬▬▬▬▬▬▬▬▬▬▬▬▬▬▬▬▬▬▬▬

The organization provides notice of an upcoming full accreditation survey and of the opportunity for a Public Information Interview (PII).*

Rationale for APR 8

An organization must provide an opportunity for the public to participate in a PII during a full survey. The public includes the following:

- Residents and their families
- Resident advocates and advocacy groups
- Members of the community for whom services are provided
- Organization personnel and staff

The organization is responsible for making the PII process widely known and effective as a source of compliance information in the accreditation process. The Joint Commission requires an organization scheduled for a full survey to post announcements of the survey date, the opportunity for a PII, and how to request an interview. To maximize participation, postings must be made throughout the organization in the form provided by the Joint Commission (*see* Public Notice Form on page APP-23). Organizations should post notices in public eating areas, on bulletin boards near major entrances, and in treatment or residential areas. In addition, if all staff members are not likely to see such postings, the organization must provide each staff member with a written announcement of the survey.

The organization must also provide potential PII participants with sufficient advance notice. The Joint Commission requires organizations to post public notices at least 30 days before the scheduled survey date. Notices must remain posted until the survey is completed.

MC

The organization should also promptly initiate community advertising or other communications as soon as it receives notice of the survey date. Appropriate steps to take in notifying the community of the opportunity for PIIs include the following:

- Informing all advocacy groups (such as organized resident groups and unions) that have substantively communicated with the organization in the previous 12 months
- Reaching other members of the community, for example through a public service announcement on radio or television, a classified advertisement in a local newspaper, or a notice in a community newsletter or other publication

---

* *See also* pages APP-22–APP-25.

- Informing individuals who inquire about the survey of the survey date(s) and opportunity to participate

Element of Performance for APR 8
1. The organization provides notice of an upcoming full survey and of the opportunity for a PII.

APR 9
The organization notifies the Joint Commission of any requests for a PII.*

Rationale for APR 9
The organization must promptly forward to the Joint Commission all written requests to participate in a PII. Organizations receiving an oral request should instruct the individual(s) to make the request in writing and mail it to the Joint Commission. The organization should provide the individual(s) needing assistance in doing this with the necessary support. The organization is responsible for notifying the interviewee(s) of the exact date, time, and place of the PII.

Elements of Performance for APR 9
1. The organization notifies the Joint Commission of any requests for a PII.

2. The organization notifies any interviewee(s) of the exact date, time, and place of the PII.

Misrepresentation of Information

APR 10
The organization does not misrepresent information in the accreditation process.†

Rationale for APR 10
Information provided by the organization and used by the Joint Commission for the accreditation process must be accurate and truthful. Such information may be the following:
- Provided orally
- Obtained through direct observation by Joint Commission surveyors
- Derived from documents supplied by the organization to the Joint Commission

MC

---

* *See also* pages APP-22–APP-25.

† *See also* page APP-10.

- Involve data submitted electronically by the organization through the performance measurement system to the Joint Commission

The Joint Commission requires each organization seeking accreditation to engage in the accreditation process in good faith. Any organization that fails to participate in good faith by falsifying information presented in the accreditation process may have its accreditation denied or removed by the Joint Commission.

For the purpose of this requirement, falsification is defined as the fabrication, in whole or in part, and through commission or omission, of any information provided by an applicant or accredited organization to the Joint Commission. This includes any redrafting, reformatting, or content deletion of documents. However, the organization may submit additional material that summarizes or otherwise explains the original information submitted to the Joint Commission. These additional materials must be properly identified, dated, and accompanied by the original documents.

Element of Performance for APR 10
1. The organization provides accurate and truthful information throughout the accreditation process.

APR 11
The organization does not publicly misrepresent its accreditation status or the scope of facilities and services to which the accreditation applies.*

Rationale for APR 11
Organizations accredited by the Joint Commission must be accurate when describing to the public the nature and meaning of their accreditation. On request, the Joint Commission's Department of Communications will provide accredited organizations with appropriate guidelines for characterizing the accreditation award. An organization may not engage in any false or misleading advertising with respect to the accreditation award. Any such advertising may be grounds for denying or revoking accreditation.

Elements of Performance for APR 11
1. The organization accurately represents its accreditation status as to the scope of facilities and services to which the accreditation applies.

2. The organization does not engage in any false or misleading advertising with respect to the accreditation award.

APR 12
Accredited organizations or organizations seeking accreditation are not permitted to use Joint Commission full-time, part-time, or intermittent surveyors to provide any accreditation-related consulting services.

MC

---

* *See also* pages APP-11–APP-12.

Rationale for APR 12

Consulting services include, but are not limited to, the following:

- Helping an organization to meet Joint Commission standards
- Conducting mock surveys for an organization
- Providing consultation to an organization to address Priority Focus Process (PFP) information

Element of Performance for APR 12

1. The organization does not use Joint Commission full-time, part-time, or intermittent surveyors to provide any accreditation-related consulting services.

Survey Observers

APR 13

An organization that applies for survey is obligated to accept Joint Commission surveyor management staff and/or a member of the Board of Commissioners to observe a survey under two specific circumstances:

- Observation and mentoring of surveyors as part of surveyor management and development
- Preceptorship of new surveyors

The observer will not participate in the on-site survey process in any fashion, including the scoring of standards compliance. The presence of an observer will not result in any additional charge to the organization nor will it be accepted as "de facto" grounds for score revisions or decision appeal.

Element of Performance for APR 13

1. The organization accepts Joint Commission surveyor management staff and/or a member of the Board of Commissioners to observe a survey under either of the two specific circumstances.

Long Term Care—Medicare Certified

MC

APR 15

The organization notifies the Joint Commission within 24 hours when, at any time during the accreditation cycle, any state agency SNF/NF survey has resulted in termination from the Medicare/Medicaid program.

Element of Performance for APR 15

1. The Joint Commission has been notified that the SNF/NF has been terminated from the Medicare/Medicaid program.

National Patient Safety Goals

This chapter addresses the National Patient Safety Goals and requirements. Organizations providing care relevant to each of the goals will be responsible for implementing the applicable requirements or, with Joint Commission approval, effective alternatives.

As with Joint Commission standards, accredited organizations are evaluated for continuous compliance with the specific requirements associated with the National Patient Safety Goals. Compliance with these requirements is assessed by the Joint Commission through on-site surveys and Evidence of Standards Compliance (ESC). In mid-cycle the organization also assesses its own compliance in the PPR.* Organizations are judged to be either compliant or not compliant with each goal. If an organization does not fully comply with all the requirements associated with a goal, the organization will be assigned a requirement for improvement for the goal in the same way that noncompliance with an EP for a standard generates a requirement for improvement for that standard. Failure to resolve a requirement for improvement for a goal can ultimately lead to loss of accreditation.

Note: *You might notice that some goals appear to be misnumbered or "missing" from the numerical sequence. This is not a typographical error. Some goals do not apply to long term care and therefore have not been included in this chapter.*

The purpose of the Joint Commission's National Patient Safety Goals is to promote specific improvements in resident safety. The goals highlight problematic areas in health care and describe evidence and expert-based solutions to these problems. Recognizing that sound system design is intrinsic to the delivery of safe, high-quality health care, the goals focus on systemwide solutions, wherever possible.

Although the requirements associated with the National Patient Safety Goals are generally more prescriptive than Joint Commission standards requirements, organizations may request Joint Commission approval of specific alternative approaches to meeting National Patient Safety Goal requirements. The Joint Commission also provides guidance on how to achieve effective compliance with each goal's requirements. This guidance includes detailed answers to Frequently Asked Questions (FAQs).

The National Patient Safety Goals are derived primarily from informal recommendations made in the Joint Commission's safety newsletter, *Sentinel Event Alert.* The Sentinel Event database, which contains de-identified aggregate information on sentinel events reported to the Joint Commission, is the primary, but not the sole, source of information from which the alerts, as well as the National Patient Safety Goals, are derived. A broadly representative Sentinel Event Advisory Group works with Joint Commission staff on a continuing basis to determine priorities for, and develop, goals and associated requirements. As part of this development process, candidate goals and requirements are sent to the field for review and comment. Selected existing and new goals and requirements are annually recommended by the Advisory

MC

---

* For those programs required to complete a PPR.

Group to the Joint Commission's Board of Commissioners for final review and approval. The Advisory Group also assists the Joint Commission in evaluating potential alternatives to goal requirements that have been suggested by individual organizations.

Goal 1

Improve the accuracy of resident identification.

Requirement 1A

Use at least two resident identifiers (neither to be the resident's room number) whenever administering medications or blood products; taking blood samples and other specimens for clinical testing, or providing any other treatments or procedures.

Note: *The preceding requirement is not scored here. It is scored at standard PC.5.10, EP 4.* See *page MC-26.*

Requirement 1B

Prior to the start of any invasive procedure, conduct a final verification process, such as a "time out," to confirm the correct resident, procedure, site, using active—not passive—communication techniques.

Goal 2

Improve the effectiveness of communication among caregivers.

Requirement 2A

For verbal or telephone orders or for telephonic reporting of critical test results, verify the complete order or test result by having the person receiving the order or test result read-back the complete order or test result.

Note: *The preceding requirement is not scored here. It is scored at standard IM.6.50, EP 4.* See *page MC-75.*

Requirement 2B

Standardize a list of abbreviations, acronyms, and symbols that are *not* to be used throughout the organization.

Note: *The preceding requirement is not scored here. It is scored at standard IM.3.10, EP 2.* See *page MC-72.*

MC

Goal 3

Improve the safety of using medications.

Requirement 3A

Remove concentrated electrolytes (including, but not limited to, potassium chloride, potassium phosphate, and sodium chloride > 0.9%) from resident care units.

Note: *The preceding requirement is not scored here. It is scored at standard MM.2.20, EP 9. See page MC-31.*

Requirement 3B

Standardize and limit the number of drug concentrations available in the organization.

Note: *The preceding requirement is not scored here. It is scored at standard MM.2.20, EP 8. See page MC-31.*

Requirement 3C

Identify and, at a minimum, annually review a list of look-alike/sound-alike drugs used in the organization, and take action to prevent errors involving the interchange of these drugs.

Goal 5

Improve the safety of using infusion pumps.

Requirement 5A

Ensure free-flow protection on all general-use and PCA (resident controlled analgesia) intravenous infusion pumps used in the organization.

Goal 7

Reduce the risk of health care–associated infections.

Requirement 7A

Comply with current Centers for Disease Control and Prevention (CDC) hand hygiene guidelines.*

Requirement 7B

Manage as sentinel events all identified cases of unanticipated death or major permanent loss of function associated with a health care–associated infection.

Goal 8

Accurately and completely reconcile medications across the continuum of care.

---

* Organizations are required to comply with all 1A, 1B, and 1C CDC recommendations or requirements.

Requirement 8A

During 2005, for full implementation by January 2006, develop a process for obtaining and documenting a complete list of the resident's current medications upon the resident's admission to the organization and with the involvement of the resident. This process includes a comparison of the medications the organization provides to those on the list.

Requirement 8B

A complete list of the resident's medications is communicated to the next provider of service when it refers or transfers a resident to another setting, service, practitioner, or level of care within or outside the organization.

Goal 9 ▬▬▬▬▬▬▬

Reduce the risk of resident harm resulting from falls.

Requirement 9A

Assess and periodically reassess each resident's risk for falling, including the potential risk associated with the resident's medication regimen, and take action to address any identified risks.

Requirement 9B

Implement a fall reduction program, including a transfer protocol, and evaluate the effectiveness of the program.

Goal 10 ▬▬▬▬▬▬▬

Reduce the risk of influenza and pneumococcal disease in institutionalized older adults.

Requirement 10A

Develop and implement a protocol for administration and documentation of the flu vaccine.

Requirement 10B

Develop and implement a protocol for administration and documentation of the pneumococcus vaccine.

Requirement 10C

Develop and implement a protocol to identify new cases of influenza and to manage an outbreak.

MC

Standards

The following is a list of all standards for Medicare/Medicaid Certification–Based Long Term Care Accreditation. They are presented here for your convenience without footnotes or other explanatory text. If you have a question about a term used here, please check the Glossary.

Note: *A revised standard numbering system is being used with the reformatted standards. The revised numbering system allows for more flexibility to add standards while maintaining the current label for each standard.*

Ethics, Rights, and Responsibilities

RI.1.10   The organization follows ethical behavior in its care, treatment, and services and business practices.

RI.2.90   Residents and, when appropriate, their families are informed about the outcomes of care, treatment, and services that have been provided, including unanticipated outcomes.

RI.2.160   Residents have the right to pain management.

Provision of Care, Treatment, and Services

PC.5.10   The organization provides care, treatment, and services for each resident according to the plan for care, treatment, and services.

PC.6.10   The resident receives education and training specific to the resident's needs and as appropriate to the care, treatment, and services provided.

PC.9.10   Blood and blood components are administered safely, as appropriate to the setting.

PC.16.10   The organization establishes policies and procedures that define the context in which waived test results are used in resident care, treatment, and services.

PC.16.20   The organization identifies the staff responsible for performing and supervising waived testing.

PC.16.30   Staff performing tests have adequate, specific training and orientation to perform the tests and demonstrate satisfactory levels of competence.

PC.16.40   Approved policies and procedures governing specific testing-related processes are current and readily available.

MC

PC.16.50 Quality control checks, as defined by the organization, are conducted on each procedure.

PC.16.60 Appropriate quality control and test records are maintained.

Medication Management

MM.2.20 Medications are properly and safely stored throughout the organization.

Improving Organization Performance

PI.1.10 The organization collects data to monitor its performance.

PI.2.10 Data are systematically aggregated and analyzed.

PI.2.20 Undesirable patterns or trends in performance are analyzed.

PI.2.30 Processes for identifying and managing sentinel events are defined and implemented.

PI.3.10 Information from data analysis is used to make changes that improve performance and resident safety and reduce the risk of sentinel events.

PI.3.20 An ongoing, proactive program for identifying and reducing unanticipated adverse events and safety risks to residents is defined and implemented.

Leadership

LD.1.20 Governance responsibilities are defined in writing, as applicable.

LD.1.30 The organization complies with applicable law and regulation.

LD.3.50 Services provided by consultation, contractual arrangements, or other agreements are provided safely and effectively.

LD.3.60 Communication is effective throughout the organization.

LD.3.70 The leaders define the required qualifications and competence of those staff who provide care, treatment, and services, and recommend a sufficient number of qualified and competent staff to provide care, treatment, and services.

LD.3.90 The leaders develop and implement policies and procedures for care, treatment, and services.

MC

LD.3.120   The leaders plan for and support the provision and coordination of resident education activities.

LD.4.10   The leaders set expectations, plan, and manage processes to measure, assess, and improve the organization's governance, management, clinical, and support activities.

LD.4.20   New or modified services or processes are designed well.

LD.4.40   The leaders ensure that an integrated resident safety program is implemented throughout the organization.

LD.4.50   The leaders set performance improvement priorities and identify how the organization adjusts priorities in response to unusual or urgent events.

LD.4.60   The leaders allocate adequate resources for measuring, assessing, and improving the organization's performance and improving resident safety.

LD.4.70   The leaders measure and assess the effectiveness of the performance improvement and safety improvement activities.

Management of the Environment of Care

EC.1.10   The organization manages safety risks.

EC.1.20   The organization maintains a safe environment.

EC.1.30   The organization develops and implements a policy to prohibit smoking except in specified circumstances.

EC.3.10   The organization manages its hazardous materials and waste risks.

EC.4.10   The organization addresses emergency management.

EC.6.10   The organization manages medical equipment risks.

EC.6.20   Medical equipment is maintained, tested, and inspected.

EC.7.10   The organization manages its utility risks.

EC.7.30   The organization maintains, tests, and inspects its utility systems.

EC.7.50   The organization maintains, tests, and inspects its medical gas and vacuum systems.

MC

EC.9.10   The organization monitors conditions in the environment.

EC.9.20   The organization analyzes identified environment issues and develops recommendations for resolving them.

EC.9.30   The organization improves the environment.

Management of Human Resources

HR.1.30   The organization uses data on clinical/service screening indicators in combination with human resource screening indicators to assess staffing effectiveness.

HR.2.10   Orientation provides initial job training and information.

HR.2.20   Staff members, licensed independent practitioners, students, and volunteers, as appropriate, can describe or demonstrate their roles and responsibilities, based on specific job duties or responsibilities, relative to safety.

HR.2.30   Ongoing education, including in-services, training, and other activities, maintains and improves competence.

HR.3.10   Competence to perform job responsibilities is assessed, demonstrated, and maintained.

HR.4.10   There is a process for ensuring the competence of all practitioners permitted by law and the organization to practice independently.

HR.4.20   Individuals permitted by law and the organization to practice independently are granted clinical privileges.

HR.4.30   The organization has a process for granting temporary clinical privileges, when appropriate.

HR.4.40   There are mechanisms, including a fair hearing and appeal process, for addressing adverse decisions regarding reappointment denial, reduction, suspension, or revocation of clinical privileges that may relate to quality of care, treatment, and service issues.

MC

HR.4.50   Clinical privileges and appointments/reappointments are reviewed and revised at least every two years.

Management of Information

IM.1.10   The organization plans and designs information management processes to meet internal and external information needs.

IM.2.10   Information privacy and confidentiality are maintained.

IM.3.10   The organization has processes in place to effectively manage information, including the capturing, reporting, processing, storing, retrieving, disseminating, and displaying of clinical/service and non-clinical data and information.

IM.4.10   The information management system provides information for use in decision making.

IM.5.10   Knowledge-based information resources are readily available, current, and authoritative.

IM.6.50   Designated qualified personnel accept and transcribe verbal orders from authorized individuals.

IM.6.130   Clinical record documentation includes the provision of education and its effectiveness.

MC

Understanding the Parts of This Section

To help you navigate this reformatted standards section, it may be helpful to think of its parts this way:

- The **standard** is the goal
- The **rationale** explains why it's important to achieve this goal
- The **elements of performance (EPs)** identify the step(s) needed to achieve this goal

These parts are defined as follows.

Standard A statement that defines the performance expectations and/or structures or processes that must be in place for an organization to provide safe, high-quality care, treatment, and services. An organization is either compliant or not compliant with a standard.

Accreditation decisions are based on simple counts of the standards that are determined to be not compliant.

Rationale A statement that provides background, justification, or additional information about a standard. A standard's rationale is not scored. In some instances, the rationale for a standard is self-evident. Therefore, not every standard has a written rationale.

Elements of performance (EPs) The specific performance expectations and/or structures or processes that must be in place for an organization to provide safe, high-quality care, treatment, and services. The scoring of EP compliance determines an organization's overall compliance with a standard. EPs are evaluated on the following scale:

0	Insufficient compliance
1	Partial compliance
2	Satisfactory compliance
NA	Not applicable

You will find a **measure of success (MOS)** icon—**Ⓜ**—next to some EPs. MOS need to be developed for certain EPs when a standard is judged to be not compliant. An MOS is defined as a quantifiable measure, usually related to an audit, that can be used to determine whether an action has been effective and is being sustained.*

Assessing Your Compliance

When you are familiar with the parts of this chapter, you can begin to assess your compliance with its requirements. The scoring category designations are provided next to each EP for your convenience. If you would like to assess your organization's performance, mark your scores for the EPs and standards by following the simple steps described in the following sections. **Note:** *You are **not** required to complete this scoring grid. It is provided simply to help you assess your own performance.*

MC

---

* For more information about MOS, *see* "The New Joint Commission Accreditation Process" chapter in this book.

Two components are scored for each EP: (1) compliance with the requirement itself **and** (2) compliance with the track record* for that requirement. Scoring has been simplified and track record achievements (which have always been part of the scoring) have been appropriately modified.

Note: *Some standards and EPs do not apply to a particular type of organization; these standards and EPs are marked "not applicable" and the related text is not included. Your organization is not expected to comply with standards and EPs marked "not applicable."*

In addition, some standards and EPs that do apply to organizations may not apply to the specific care, treatment, and services that your individual organization provides. Although these standards and EPs are included in the book, you are not expected to comply with them. If you are unsure about the standards or EPs that apply to your organization, please contact the Joint Commission's Standards Interpretation Group at 630/792-5900.

Step 1: Score Your Compliance with Each Element of Performance

Before you can determine your compliance with the standards, you must score your compliance with each EP. There are three scoring criterion categories: A, B, and C (described in the following sections). Please note that for each EP scoring criterion category, your organization must meet the performance requirement itself and the track record achievements (*see* "Track Record Achievements").

Category A

These EPs relate to the presence or absence of the requirement(s) and are scored either yes (2) or no (0); however, a score of 1 for partial compliance is also possible based on track record achievements.

If an A EP has multiple components designated by bullets, your organization must be compliant with all the bullets to receive a score of 2. If your organization does not meet one or more requirements in the bullets, you will receive a score of 0.

Category B

Category B EPs are scored in two steps:
1. As with category A EPs, category B EPs relate to the presence or absence of the requirement(s). If your organization *does not meet* the requirement(s), the EP is scored 0; there is no need to assess your compliance with the principles of good process design
2. If your organization *does meet* the requirement(s), but there is concern about the quality or comprehensiveness of the effort, then and only then should you assess the qualitative aspect of the EP. That is, review the applicable principles of good process design and ask how the principles were applied in the situation under discussion. Good process design has the following characteristics:

---

* **Track record** The amount of time that an organization has been in compliance with a standard, EP, or other requirement.

MC

- Is consistent with your organization's mission, values, and goals
- Meets the needs of residents
- Reflects the use of currently accepted practices (doing the right thing, using resources responsibly, using practice guidelines)
- Incorporates current safety information and knowledge such as sentinel event data and National Patient Safety Goals and Requirements
- Incorporates relevant performance improvement results

This two-part evaluation applies to both simple and bulleted B EPs. First, the EPs are assessed to determine whether the requirements are present. If the EP has multiple components designated by bullets, as with the category A EPs, an organization must meet the requirements in *all* the bulleted items to get a score of 2. If an organization meets *none* of the requirements in the bullets, it receives a score of 0. If an organization meets *at least one, but not all*, of the bulleted requirements, it receives a score of 1.

Use the following rules to determine your EP score:

- Your EP score is 0 if your organization does not meet the requirement(s); you *do not* need to assess your compliance with the preceding applicable principles of good process design
- Your EP score is 1 if your organization does meet the requirement(s) but considered only *some* of the preceding applicable principles of good process design
- Your EP score is 2 if your organization does meet the requirement(s) *and* considered *all* the preceding principles of good process design

Category C

C EPs are scored 0, 1, or 2 based on the number of times your organization does not meet the EP. These EPs are frequency based and require totaling the number of occurrences (that is, results of performance or nonperformance) related to a particular EP. Each situation discovered by a surveyor(s) will be counted as a separate occurrence.

Note: *Multiple events of the same type related to a single resident and single practitioner/staff member are counted as* one occurrence only.

Use the following rules to determine your EP score:

- Your EP score is 2 if you find one or fewer occurrences of noncompliance with the EP
- Your EP score is 1 if you find two occurrences of noncompliance with the EP
- Your EP score is 0 if you find three or more occurrences of noncompliance with the EP

MC

If an EP in the C category has multiple requirements designated by bullets, the following scoring guidelines apply:

- If there are fewer than two findings in all bullets, the EP is scored 2
- If there are three or more findings in all bullets, the EP is scored 0
- In all other combinations of findings, the EP is scored 1

Track Record Achievements

In addition to meeting the requirement(s) in each EP, regardless of category, your organization must also meet the following track record achievements:

Score	Initial Survey	Full Survey
2	4 months or more	12 months or more
1	2 to 3 months	6 to 11 months
0	Fewer than 2 months	Fewer than 6 months

Sample Sizes

If during an on-site survey, your organization has been found to be not compliant with one or more standards, you must demonstrate Evidence of Standards Compliance (ESC) for each standard that is not compliant. The ESC must address compliance at the EP level; when an EP within a not compliant standard requires an MOS, your organization must demonstrate achievement with the MOS when completing the ESC.

Note: *Not every EP requires an MOS. EPs that do require an MOS are clearly marked in this chapter. Organizations are required to demonstrate achievement with an MOS only for EPs within a not compliant standard that require an MOS. Organizations do not need to demonstrate achievement with an MOS for any EP within a compliant standard.*

When demonstrating achievement with an MOS during the ESC process, your organization is **required** to use the following sample sizes, which were established because of their statistical significance, their relative simplicity in application, and their sensitivity to an organization's population size:

- For a population size of fewer than 30 cases,* sample 100% of available cases
- For a population size of 30 to 100 cases, sample 30 cases
- For a population size of 101 to 500 cases, sample 50 cases
- For a population size greater than 500 cases, sample 70 cases

When demonstrating an ESC, use the following percentages to determine your EP score: 90% through 100% of your sample size is compliant = score 2; 80% through 89% of your sample size is compliant = score 1; less than 80% of your sample size is compliant = score 0.

In addition, the following information should govern your organization's selection of samples:

- The appropriate sample size should be determined by the specific population related to the survey findings
- The sampling approach should involve either systematic random sampling (for example, your organization selects every second or third case for review) or simple random sampling (for example, your organization uses a series of random numbers generated by a computer to identify the cases to be reviewed)

---

* *Case* refers to a single instance in which a situation related to a survey finding occurs. For example, if a survey finding was related to **pain assessment**, a case would be any resident record. If a survey finding was related to **pain management**, a case would be any resident record for residents receiving pain management.

MC

- When submitting a clarifying ESC, if your organization selects records as part of its sample, the records should be from a period of no more than three months before the last date of the survey
- Assessment of MOS compliance is conducted for a four-month period following the date of ESC approval. Your organization should select records as a part of your sample following the date of ESC approval and use the required sample sizes. MOS percentage compliance rates are derived from the average of all four months.

Step 2: Use Your EP Scores to Gauge Your Compliance with the Standards

Now that you have evaluated and scored each EP for a particular standard, use these simple rules to determine your compliance with the standard itself:

- Your organization is not in compliance (that is, not compliant) with the standard if any EP is scored 0
- Otherwise, your organization is compliant with a standard if 65% or more of its EPs are scored 2

MC

Standards, Rationales, Elements of Performance, and Scoring

Ethics, Rights, and Responsibilities

Standard RI.1.10

The organization follows ethical behavior in its care, treatment, and services and business practices.

Elements of Performance for RI.1.10

B   1.   The organization identifies ethical issues and issues prone to conflict.

B   2.   The organization develops and implements a process to handle these issues when they arise.

B   3.   The organization's policies and procedures reflect ethical practices for marketing, admission, transfer, discharge, and billing.

B   4.   Marketing materials accurately represent the organization and address the care, treatment, and services that the organization can provide, directly or by contractual arrangement.

C Ⓜ   5.   Residents receive information about charges for which they will be responsible.

B   6.   The effectiveness and safety of care, treatment, and services does not depend on the resident's ability to pay.

C Ⓜ   7.   The leaders ensure that care, treatment, and services are not negatively affected when the organization grants a staff member's request to be excused from participating in an aspect of the care, treatment, and services.

C Ⓜ   8.   Residents are informed whenever services, charges, or coverage change.

Standard RI.2.90

Residents and, when appropriate, their families are informed about the outcomes of care, treatment, and services that have been provided, including unanticipated outcomes.

Elements of Performance for RI.2.90

At a minimum, the resident and when appropriate, his or her family, is informed about the following (EPs 1–2):

C Ⓜ   1.   Outcomes of care, treatment, and services that have been provided that the resident (or family) must be knowledgeable about to participate in current and future decisions affecting the resident's care, treatment, and services.

C Ⓜ 2. Unanticipated outcomes of care, treatment, and services that relate to sentinel events considered reviewable* by the Joint Commission.

C Ⓜ 3. The responsible licensed independent practitioner or his or her designee informs the resident (and when appropriate, his or her family) about those unanticipated outcomes of care, treatment, and services (*see* EP 2 above).[†]

Standard RI.2.160 ━━━━━━━━━━━━━━━━━━━━━━━━━━━━━━━━━━

Residents have the right to pain management.

Rationale for RI.2.160

Residents may experience pain. Unrelieved pain has adverse physical and psychological effects. The organization respects and supports the right of residents to pain management. In accordance with the organization's mission, this may occur through referral.

Element of Performance for RI.2.160

B 1. The organization plans, supports, and coordinates activities and resources to ensure that pain is recognized and addressed appropriately and in accordance with the care, treatment, and services provided including the following:
- Assessing for pain
- Educating all relevant providers about assessing and managing pain
- Educating residents and families, when appropriate, about their roles in managing pain and the potential limitations and side effects of pain treatments

Provision of Care, Treatment, and Services[‡]

Standard PC.5.10 ━━━━━━━━━━━━━━━━━━━━━━━━━━━━━━━━━━

The organization provides care, treatment, and services for each resident according to the plan for care, treatment, and services.

MC

---

* *See* the "Sentinel Events" chapter of this book for a definition of reviewable sentinel events.

[†] In settings where there is no licensed independent practitioner, the staff member responsible for the care of the resident is responsible for sharing information about such outcomes.

[‡] This chapter is a compilation of the former "Assessment," "Care," "Education," and "Continuum of Care" chapters.

Elements of Performance for PC.5.10

C Ⓜ 1. The organization provides care, treatment, and services for each resident according to the plan for care, treatment, and services.

A 4. The organization uses at least two resident identifiers (neither to be the resident's room number) whenever taking blood samples or administering medications, or blood, or blood products.

Standard PC.6.10

The resident receives education and training specific to the resident's needs and as appropriate to the care, treatment, and services provided.

Rationale for PC.6.10

Residents must be given sufficient information to make decisions and to take responsibility for self-management activities related to their needs. Residents and, as appropriate, their families are educated to improve individual outcomes by promoting healthy behavior and appropriately involving residents in their care, treatment, and service decisions.

Elements of Performance for PC.6.10

B 1. Education provided is appropriate to the resident's needs.

C Ⓜ 2. The assessment of learning needs addresses cultural and religious beliefs, emotional barriers, desire and motivation to learn, physical or cognitive limitations, and barriers to communication as appropriate.

B 3. As appropriate to the resident's condition and assessed needs and the organization's scope of services, the resident is educated about the following:
- The plan for care, treatment, and services
- His or her condition or illness and preventive interventions
- Basic health practices and safety
- The safe and effective use of medications
- Nutrition interventions, modified diets, or oral health
- Safe and effective use of medical equipment or supplies when provided by the organization
- Understanding pain, the risk for pain, the importance of effective pain management, the pain assessment process, and methods for pain management
- Habilitation or rehabilitation techniques to help them reach the maximum independence possible
- Environmental and physical plant safety issues, such as fire safety, evacuation, storage of chemical agents, and so on
- Use of nonmedical equipment, including, but not limited to, operating call lights, beds, and personal appliances

MC

Standard PC.9.10 ▬▬▬▬▬▬▬▬▬▬▬▬▬▬▬▬▬▬▬▬▬▬▬▬

Blood and blood components are administered safely, as appropriate to the setting.

Element of Performance for PC.9.10

A   10. If the organization provides for the maintenance and transfusion of blood or blood components, it meets all applicable law and regulation.

Standard PC.16.10 ▬▬▬▬▬▬▬▬▬▬▬▬▬▬▬▬▬▬▬▬▬▬

The organization establishes policies and procedures that define the context in which waived test results are used in resident care, treatment, and services.

Elements of Performance for PC.16.10

B   1. Quantitative test result reports in the clinical record are accompanied by reference intervals specific to the test method used and are appropriate to the population served.

B   2. Criteria for confirmatory testing for each test, qualitative or quantitative, is specified in the written procedure as dictated by clinical usage and methodology limitations.

B   3. Actual usage is consistent with the organization's policies and the manufacturer's recommendations for each waived test.

Standard PC.16.20 ▬▬▬▬▬▬▬▬▬▬▬▬▬▬▬▬▬▬▬▬▬▬

The organization identifies the staff responsible for performing and supervising waived testing.

Elements of Performance for PC.16.20

B   1. Staff members who perform testing are identified.

B   2. Staff members who direct or supervise testing are identified.

> **Note:** *These individuals may be employees of the organization, contracted staff, or employees of a contracted service.*

Standard PC.16.30 ▬▬▬▬▬▬▬▬▬▬▬▬▬▬▬▬▬▬▬▬▬▬

Staff performing tests have adequate, specific training and orientation to perform the tests and demonstrate satisfactory levels of competence.

MC

Rationale for PC.16.30

For waived tests to be performed properly, the staff performing them must be qualified to do so. Staff members who perform waived testing have specific training in each test performed. This training may be acquired through organization or other training programs, such as those provided by other health care organizations or manufacturers.

Elements of Performance for PC.16.30

C Ⓜ 1. Current competence of testing staff is demonstrated.

C Ⓜ 2. Each staff member who performs testing has been trained specifically to each test he or she is authorized to perform.

C Ⓜ 3. Each staff member who performs testing has been oriented according to the organization's specific needs.

B 4. Testing that requires the use of an instrument is performed by staff with adequate and specific training on the use and care of that instrument.

C Ⓜ 5. Competence is assessed according to organization policy at defined intervals, but at least at the time of orientation and annually thereafter.

B 6. These assessments have considered the following:
- The frequency by which staff members perform tests
- The technical backgrounds of the staff
- The complexity of the test methodology and the consequences of an inaccurate result

B 7. Methods to assess current competency include at least two of the following:
- Performing a test on an unknown specimen
- Having the supervisor or qualified delegate periodically observe routine work
- Monitoring each user's quality control performance
- Having written testing that is specific to the method assessed

B 8. The organization evaluates and documents the information listed above.

> **Note:** *All staff who perform instrument-based testing, including (but not limited to) physicians, licensed independent practitioners, contracted staff, and RNs, must participate in training and competence demonstrations.*

Standard PC.16.40 ▬▬▬▬▬▬▬▬▬▬▬▬▬▬▬▬▬▬▬▬▬▬▬▬▬▬▬▬▬

Approved policies and procedures governing specific testing-related processes are current and readily available.

MC

Rationale for PC.16.40

Current and up-to-date policies and procedures are an important reference tool in managing laboratory testing activities, particularly when individual staff members perform them infrequently. Testing policies and procedures include requirements that are in compliance with the manufacturer's recommendations regarding all the following, as applicable:
- Specimen type (for example, a method for whole blood is not used for spinal fluid)

- Storage considerations for test components (for example, compliance with directions such as store away from direct light, temperature requirements, open container expiration dates, and so forth)
- Instrument maintenance and function checks such as calibration
- Quality control frequency and type
- Result follow-up recommendations (for example, out-of-range results' recommendation for retesting)
- Tests approved by the FDA for home use only are not used for professional purposes (for example, glucose meters cleared for home use only are not used in a hospital setting by nursing staff except as resident education)

Elements of Performance for PC.16.40

B   1.   Written policies and procedures address all the following items:
- Specimen collection, identification, and required labeling as appropriate
- Specimen preservation, as appropriate
- Instrument calibration
- Quality control and remedial action
- Equipment performance evaluation
- Test performance

B   2.   The policies and procedures for each item are applicable to the specific organization.

Note: *Reference to a manufacturer's manual is acceptable if appropriate modifications have been made to customize the manual's content for the organization.*

C Ⓜ   3.   Current and complete policies and procedures are readily available to the person performing the test.

A   4.   The director named on the waived testing certificate or a designee approves policies and procedures at defined intervals.

Standard PC.16.50 ▬▬▬▬▬▬▬▬▬▬▬▬▬▬▬▬▬▬▬▬▬▬▬▬

Quality control checks, as defined by the organization, are conducted on each procedure.

Elements of Performance for PC.16.50

B   1.   The organization has a written quality control plan that specifies how procedures will be controlled for quality, establishes timetables, and explains the rationale for choice of procedures and timetables.

B   2.   Quality control procedures are performed at least as frequently as recommended by the manufacturer, according to the organization's policies.

C Ⓜ   3.   For instrument-based waived testing, quality control requirements include two levels of control, if commercially available.

MC

C ⓜ 4. Quality control procedures are performed at least once each day on each instrument used for resident testing.

B 5. The documented quality control rationale is based on the following:
- How the test is used
- Reagent stability
- Manufacturers' recommendations
- The organization's experience with the test
- Currently accepted guidelines

B 6. At a minimum, manufacturers' instructions are followed.

Standard PC.16.60

Appropriate quality control and test records are maintained.

Elements of Performance for PC.16.60

C ⓜ 1. All quality control test results are documented, including internal, external, liquid, and electronic.

C ⓜ 2. Test results are documented.

> **Note:** *Test results may be located in the clinical record.*

B 3. Quality control records, instrument problems, and individual results are correlated.

B 4. A formal log is not required, but a functional audit trail is maintained that allows retrieval of results and associated quality control values for a minimum of two years.

Medication* Management

Standard MM.2.20

Medications are properly and safely stored throughout the organization.

Note: *The following EPs also apply to emergency medications.*

Elements of Performance for MM.2.20

1. Through 7. Not applicable

---

* For the purpose of these standards, *medication* includes prescription medications, sample medications, herbal remedies, vitamins, nutraceuticals, over-the-counter drugs, vaccines, diagnostic and contrast agents used on or administered to persons to diagnose, treat, or prevent disease or other abnormal conditions; radioactive medications; respiratory therapy treatments; parenteral nutrition; blood derivatives; intravenous solutions (plain, with electrolytes, and/or drugs); and any product designated by the Food and Drug Administration (FDA) as a drug. The definition of *medication* does not include enteral nutrition solutions (which are considered food products), oxygen, and other medical gases.

A   8. Drug concentrations available in the organization are standardized and limited in number.

A 🕦 9. Concentrated electrolytes are removed from care units or areas, unless resident safety is at risk if the concentrated electrolyte is not immediately available on a specific care unit or area and specific precautions are taken to prevent inadvertent administration.

Improving Organization Performance

Standard PI.1.10
The organization collects data to monitor its performance.

Rationale for PI.1.10
Data help determine performance improvement priorities. The data collected for high-priority and required areas are used to monitor the stability of existing processes, identify opportunities for improvement, identify changes that lead to improvement, or sustain improvement. Data collection helps identify specific areas that require further study. These areas are determined by considering the information provided by the data about process stability, risks, and sentinel events, and priorities set by the leaders. In addition, the organization identifies those areas needing improvement and identifies desired changes. Performance measures are used to determine whether the changes result in desired outcomes. The organization identifies the frequency and detail of data collection.

Note: *The organization also collects data on the following areas that will be scored in their respective chapters:*
- *Evaluation and improvement of conditions in the environment (see the "Management of the Environment of Care" chapter)*
- *Staffing effectiveness (see the "Management of Human Resources" chapter)*

Note: *For long term care organizations that serve residents with dementia, the organization may measure performance in the following areas: psychotropic drugs, incidents, acute behavioral events, family involvement, do-not-resuscitate orders, appropriate use of services, transfers, programs that meet resident needs, infection control, environmental adaptations, and safety.*

Elements of Performance for PI.1.10
B   1. The organization collects data for priorities identified by leaders (*see* standard LD.4.50).

A   2. The organization considers collecting data in the following areas:
- Staff opinions and needs
- Staff perceptions of risks to individuals and suggestions for improving resident safety

MC

   - Staff willingness to report unanticipated adverse events

B   3.   The organization collects data on the perceptions of care, treatment, and services* of residents including the following:
   - Their specific needs and expectations
   - How well the organization meets these needs and expectations
   - How the organization can improve resident safety
   - The effectiveness of pain management, when applicable

The organization collects data that measure the performance of each of the following potentially high-risk processes, when provided:

A   4.   Medication management

A   5.   Blood and blood product use

A   6.   Restraint use

A   8.   Behavior management and treatment

Relevant information developed from the following activities is integrated into performance improvement initiatives. This occurs in a way consistent with any organization policies or procedures intended to preserve any confidentiality or privilege of information established by applicable law.

B   13.   Risk management

B   14.   Utilization management

B   15.   Quality control

B   16.   Infection control surveillance and reporting

B   17.   Research, as applicable

Standard PI.2.10

Data are systematically aggregated and analyzed.

Rationale for PI.2.10

Aggregating and analyzing data means transforming data into information. Aggregating data at points in time enables the organization to judge a particular process's stability or a particular outcome's predictability in relation to performance expectations. Accumulated data are analyzed in such a way that current performance levels, patterns, or trends can be identified.

MC

---

* The Joint Commission is moving from the phrase *satisfaction with care, treatment, and services* toward the more inclusive phrase *perception of care, treatment, and services* to better measure the performance of organizations meeting the needs, expectations, and concerns of residents. By using this term, the organization will be prompted to assess not only residents' and/or families' satisfaction with care, treatment, and services, but also whether the organization meets their needs and expectations.

Elements of Performance for PI.2.10

B   1.   Collected data are aggregated and analyzed.

B   2.   Data are aggregated at the frequency appropriate to the activity or process being studied.

B   3.   Statistical tools and techniques are used to analyze and display data.

B   4.   Data are analyzed and compared internally over time and externally* with other sources of information when available.

B   5.   Comparative data are used to determine if there is excessive variability or unacceptable levels of performance, when available.

Standard PI.2.20 ▬▬▬▬▬▬▬▬▬▬▬▬▬▬▬▬

Undesirable patterns or trends in performance are analyzed.

Elements of Performance for PI.2.20

B   1.   Analysis is performed when data comparisons indicate that levels of performance, patterns, or trends vary substantially from those expected.

B   2.   Analysis occurs for those topics chosen by leaders as performance improvement priorities.

B   3.   Analysis is performed when undesirable variation occurs which changes priorities.

An analysis is performed for the following:

A   4.   All confirmed transfusion reactions, if applicable to the organization

A   5.   All serious adverse drug events, if applicable and as defined by the organization

A   6.   All significant medication errors, if applicable and as defined by the organization

A   9.   Hazardous conditions

A   10.   Staffing effectiveness issues

MC

Standard PI.2.30 ▬▬▬▬▬▬▬▬▬▬▬▬▬▬▬▬▬▬▬▬▬▬

Processes for identifying and managing sentinel events are defined and implemented.

---

* External sources of information include recent scientific, clinical, and management literature, including sentinel event alerts; well-formulated practice guidelines or parameters; performance measures; reference databases; other organizations with similar processes, and standards that are periodically reviewed and revised.

Rationale for PI.2.30

Identifying, reporting, analyzing, and managing sentinel events can help the organization prevent such incidents. Leaders define and implement such a program as part of the process to measure, assess, and improve the organization's performance.

Elements of Performance for PI.2.30

Processes for identifying and managing sentinel events include the following:

A 1. Defining *sentinel event* and communicating this definition throughout the organization (At a minimum, the organization's definition includes those events subject to review under the Joint Commission's Sentinel Event Policy as published in this manual and may include any process variation which does not affect the outcome or result in an adverse event, but for which a recurrence carries a significant chance of a serious adverse outcome or results in an adverse event, often referred to as a *near miss*.)

A 2. Reporting sentinel events through established channels in the organization and, as appropriate, to external agencies in accordance with law and regulation.

B 3. Conducting thorough and credible root cause analyses that focus on process and system factors.

B 4. Creating, documenting, and implementing a risk-reduction strategy and action plan that includes measuring the effectiveness of process and system improvements to reduce risk.

B 5. The processes are implemented.

Standard PI.3.10

Information from data analysis is used to make changes that improve performance and resident safety and reduce the risk of sentinel events.

Elements of Performance for PI.3.10

B 1. The organization uses the information from data analysis to identify and implement changes that will improve the quality of care, treatment, and services.

B 2. The organization identifies and implements changes that will reduce the risk of sentinel events.

B 3. The organization uses the information from data analysis to identify changes that will improve resident safety.

B 4. Changes made to improve processes or outcomes are evaluated to ensure that they achieve the expected results.

B 5. Appropriate actions are undertaken when planned improvements are not achieved or sustained.

Standard PI.3.20

An ongoing, proactive program for identifying and reducing unanticipated adverse events and safety risks to residents is defined and implemented.

Rationale for PI.3.20

Organizations should proactively seek to identify and reduce risks to the safety of residents. Such initiatives have the obvious advantage of *preventing* adverse events rather than simply *reacting* when they occur. This approach also avoids the barriers to understanding created by hindsight bias and the fear of disclosure, embarrassment, blame, and punishment that can happen after an event.

Elements of Performance for PI.3.20

The following proactive activities to reduce risks to residents are conducted:

A   1.   Selecting a high-risk process* to be analyzed (at least one high-risk process is chosen annually—the choice should be based in part on information published periodically by the Joint Commission about the most frequent sentinel events and risks)

B   2.   Describing the chosen process (for example, through the use of a flowchart)

B   3.   Identifying the ways in which the process could break down† or fail to perform its desired function

B   4.   Identifying the possible effects that a breakdown or failure of the process could have on residents and the seriousness of the possible effects

B   5.   Prioritizing the potential process breakdowns or failures

B   6.   Determining why the prioritized breakdowns or failures could occur, which may include performing a hypothetical root cause analysis

B   7.   Redesigning the process and/or underlying systems to minimize the risk of the effects on residents

B   8.   Testing and implementing the redesigned process

B   9.   Monitoring the effectiveness of the redesigned process

MC

---

* **High-risk process** A process that if not planned and/or implemented correctly, has a significant potential for impacting the safety of the resident.

† The ways in which processes could break down or fail to perform their desired function are many times referred to as *the failure modes.*

Leadership

Standard LD.1.20

Governance responsibilities are defined in writing, as applicable.

Elements of Performance for LD.1.20

A 1. Governance defines its responsibilities in writing, as applicable.

A 2. If the organization is part of a larger corporate structure, the scope and degree of leaders' involvement, authority, and responsibility in corporate policy decisions are described in writing.

B 3. Governance provides for organizational management and planning.

A 4. The organization's scope of services is defined in writing and approved by the governance.

A 5. Governance either selects the individual(s) responsible for operating the organization or approves one selected by corporate management or another group.

B 6. Governance provides for coordination and integration among the organization's leaders to establish policy, maintain quality care and resident safety, and provide for necessary resources.

A 7. Governance annually evaluates the organization's performance in relation to its vision, mission, and goals.

A 8. If the organization has an organized medical staff, the governance approves the medical staff's bylaws and rules and regulations.

Standard LD.1.30

The organization complies with applicable law and regulation.

Elements of Performance for LD.1.30

A 1. The organization provides all care, treatment, and services in accordance with applicable licensure requirements, law, rules, and regulation.*

A 2. The organization acts upon any reports and/or recommendations from authorized agencies, as appropriate.

A 3. The organization possesses a license, certificate, or permit, as required by applicable law and regulation, to provide the health care services for which the organization is seeking accreditation.

---

* Applicable law and regulation include, but are not limited to, individual and facility licensure, certification, Food and Drug Administration regulations, Drug Enforcement Agency regulations, Centers for Medicare & Medicaid Services regulations, Occupational Safety and Health Administration regulations, Department of Transportation regulations, Health Insurance Portability and Accountability Act of 1996, and other local, state, and federal law and regulation.

MC

Standard LD.3.50

Services provided by consultation, contractual arrangements, or other agreements are provided safely and effectively.

Elements of Performance for LD.3.50

A   1.   The leaders approve sources for the organization's services that are provided by consultation, contractual arrangements, or other agreements.

A   2.   The clinical leaders advise the organization's leaders on the sources of clinical services to be provided by consultation, contractual arrangements, or other agreements.

A   4.   The nature and scope of services provided by consultation, contractual arrangements, or other agreements are defined in writing.*

B   5.   Services provided by consultation, contractual arrangements, or other agreements meet applicable Joint Commission standards.

B   6.   The organization evaluates the contracted care, treatment, and services to determine whether they are being provided according to the contract and the level of safety and quality that the organization expects.

A   7.   The organization retains overall responsibility and authority for services furnished under a contract.

A   8.   All reference and contract lab services[†] meet the applicable federal regulations for clinical laboratories and maintain evidence of the same.

Standard LD.3.60

Communication is effective throughout the organization.

Elements of Performance for LD.3.60

B   1.   The leaders ensure processes are in place for communicating relevant information throughout the organization in a timely manner.

---

* When an organization contracts for resident care, treatment, and services rendered outside the organization *but* under the control of a Joint Commission–accredited organization, the primary organization can do the following:
- Specify in the contract that the contracting entity will ensure that all services provided by contracted individuals who are licensed independent practitioners will be within the scope of his or her privileges
  or
- Verify that all contracted individuals who are licensed independent practitioners and who will be providing resident care, treatment, and services have appropriate privileges, for example, by obtaining a copy of the list of privileges

When an organization contracts for resident care, treatment, and services rendered outside the organization and under the control of a non-Joint Commission–accredited organization, all licensed independent practitioners who will be providing services are privileged by the Joint Commission–accredited organization through the process described in the "Management of Human Resources" chapter in this book.

† A written agreement (such as a formal contract) is not required for reference laboratories; however, it is required for a contract service where a major portion of laboratory testing is provided by an outside laboratory.

MC

B   2.   Effective communication occurs in the organization, among the organization's programs, among related organizations, with outside organizations, and with residents and families, as appropriate.

B   3.   The leaders communicate the organization's mission and appropriate policies, plans, and goals to all staff.

Standard LD.3.70

The leaders define the required qualifications and competence of those staff who provide care, treatment, and services, and recommend a sufficient number of qualified and competent staff to provide care, treatment, and services.

Rationale for LD.3.70

The determination of competence and qualifications of staff is based on the following:
- The organization's mission
- The organization's care, treatment, and services
- The complexity of care, treatment, and services needed by residents
- The technology used
- The health status of staff, as required by law and regulation

Element of Performance for LD.3.70

B   1.   The leaders provide for the allocation of competent qualified staff.

Standard LD.3.90

The leaders develop and implement policies and procedures for care, treatment, and services.

Elements of Performance for LD.3.90

B   1.   The leaders develop policies and procedures that guide and support resident care, treatment, and services.

C Ⓜ   2.   Policies and procedures are consistently implemented.

Standard LD.3.120

The leaders plan for and support the provision and coordination of resident education activities.

Elements of Performance for LD.3.120

B   1.   The leaders plan and support resident education activities appropriate to the organization's mission and scope of services.

B   2.   The leaders identify and provide the resources necessary for achieving educational objectives.

Standard LD.4.10

The leaders set expectations, plan, and manage processes to measure, assess, and improve the organization's governance, management, clinical, and support activities.

Elements of Performance for LD.4.10

B   1.   The leaders set expectations for performance improvement.

B   2.   The leaders develop plans for performance improvement.

B   3.   The leaders manage processes to improve organization performance.

B   4.   The leaders participate in performance improvement activities.

B   5.   Appropriate individuals and professions from each relevant program, service, site, or department participate collaboratively in organization-wide performance improvement activities.

Standard LD.4.20

New or modified services or processes are designed well.

Elements of Performance for LD.4.20

The design of new or modified services or processes incorporates the following:

B   1.   The needs and expectations of residents, staff, and others.

B   2.   The results of performance improvement activities, when available.

B   3.   Information about potential risks to residents, when available.

B   4.   Current knowledge, when available and relevant (for example, practice guidelines, successful practices, information from relevant literature and clinical standards).

B   5.   Information about sentinel events, when available and relevant.

B   6.   Testing and analysis to determine whether the proposed design or redesign is an improvement.

B   7.   The leaders collaborate with staff and appropriate stakeholders to design services.

Standard LD.4.40

The leaders ensure that an integrated resident safety program is implemented throughout the organization.

Rationale for LD.4.40

The leaders should work to foster a safe environment throughout the organization by integrating safety priorities into all relevant organization processes, functions, and services. In pursuit of this effort, a resident safety program can work to improve safety by reducing the risk of system or process failures. As part of its

MC

responsibility to communicate objectives and coordinate efforts to integrate resident care and support services throughout the organization and with contracted services, leadership takes the lead in developing, implementing, and overseeing a resident safety program.

The standard does not require the creation of new structures or offices in the organization; rather, the standard emphasizes the need to integrate all resident-safety activities, both existing and newly created, with the organization's leadership identified as accountable for this integration.

Elements of Performance for LD.4.40

The resident safety program includes the following:

A 1. One or more qualified individuals or an interdisciplinary group assigned to manage the organizationwide safety program

B 2. Definition of the scope of the program's oversight, typically ranging from no-harm, frequently occurring "slips" to sentinel events with serious adverse outcomes

B 3. Integration into and participation of all components of the organization into the organizationwide program

B 4. Procedures for immediately responding to system or process failures, including care, treatment, or services for the affected individual(s), containing risk to others, and preserving factual information for subsequent analysis

B 5. Clear systems for internal and external reporting of information about system or process failures

B 6. Defined responses to various types of unanticipated adverse events and processes for conducting proactive risk-assessment/risk-reduction activities

B 7. Defined support systems* for staff members who have been involved in a sentinel event

A 8. Reports, at least annually, to the organization's governance or authority on system or process failures and actions taken to improve safety, both proactively and in response to actual occurrences

MC

Standard LD.4.50

The leaders set performance improvement priorities and identify how the organization adjusts priorities in response to unusual or urgent events.

---

* Support systems provide individuals with additional help and support as well as additional resources through the human resources function or an employee assistance program. Support systems recognize that conscientious health care workers who are involved in sentinel events are themselves victims of the event and require support. Support systems also focus on the process rather than blaming the involved individuals.

Elements of Performance for LD.4.50

B   1.   The leaders set priorities for performance improvement for organizationwide activities, staffing effectiveness, and resident health outcomes.

B   2.   The leaders give high priority to high-volume, high-risk, or problem-prone processes.

B   3.   Performance improvement activities are reprioritized in response to significant changes in the internal or external environment.

Standard LD.4.60

The leaders allocate adequate resources for measuring, assessing, and improving the organization's performance and improving resident safety.

Elements of Performance for LD.4.60

B   1.   Sufficient staff is assigned to conduct activities for performance improvement and safety improvement.

B   2.   Adequate time is provided for staff to participate in activities for performance improvement and safety improvement.

B   3.   Adequate information systems are provided to support activities for performance improvement and safety improvement.

B   4.   Staff is trained in performance improvement and safety improvement approaches and methods.

Standard LD.4.70

The leaders measure and assess the effectiveness of the performance improvement and safety improvement activities.

Elements of Performance for LD.4.70

B   1.   Leaders continually monitor the effectiveness of the performance improvement and safety improvement activities.

B   2.   The leaders develop and implement improvements for these activities.

B   3.   The leaders assess the adequacy of the human, information, physical, and financial resources allocated to support performance improvement and safety improvement activities.

MC

Management of the Environment of Care

Standard EC.1.10

The organization manages safety risks.

Rationale for EC.1.10

Each organization has inherent safety risks associated with providing services for residents, the performance of daily activities by staff, and the physical environment in which services occur. It is important that each organization identifies these risks and plans and implements processes to minimize the likelihood of those risks causing incidents.

Elements of Performance for EC.1.10

B 1. The organization develops and maintains a written management plan describing the processes it implements to effectively manage the environmental safety of residents, staff, and other people coming to the organization's facilities.

A 2. The organization identifies a person(s), as designated by leadership, to coordinate the development, implementation, and monitoring of the safety-management activities.

A 3. The organization identifies a person(s) to intervene whenever conditions immediately threaten life or health, or threaten damage to equipment or buildings.

B 4. The organization conducts comprehensive, proactive risk assessments that evaluate the potential adverse impact of buildings, grounds, equipment, occupants, and internal physical systems on the safety and health of residents, staff, and other people coming to the organization's facilities.

C Ⓜ 5. The organization uses the risks identified to select and implement procedures and controls to achieve the lowest potential for adverse impact on the safety and health of residents, staff, and other people coming to the organization's facilities.

C Ⓜ 6. The organization establishes safety policies and procedures that are practiced and reviewed as frequently as necessary, but at least every three years.

B 8. The organization ensures that a process exists for responding to product-safety recalls by appropriate organization staff.

B 9. The organization ensures that all grounds and equipment are maintained appropriately.

MC

Standard EC.1.20

The organization maintains a safe environment.

Rationale for EC.1.20

It is essential that the organization conduct periodic environmental tours to determine if its current processes for managing resident, public, and staff safety risks are being practiced correctly and are effective. These tours can also be used to assess staff knowledge and behaviors, identify new or altered risks in areas where construction or changes in services have occurred, and identify opportunities to improve the environment.

Elements of Performance for EC.1.20

B 1. The organization conducts environmental tours to identify environmental deficiencies, hazards, and unsafe practices.

C Ⓜ 2. The organization conducts environmental tours at least every six months in all areas where individuals are served.

C Ⓜ 3. The organization conducts environmental tours at least annually in areas where individuals are not served.

Standard EC.1.30

The organization develops and implements a policy to prohibit smoking except in specified circumstances.

Rationale for EC.1.30

This standard is intended to reduce the following risks:

● To people who smoke, including possible adverse effects on care, treatment, and services.
● Of passive smoking for others.
● Of fire.
● The standard prohibits smoking in all areas of all building(s) under the organization's control, except for residents in circumstances specified in the following EPs.

Elements of Performance for EC.1.30

B 1. The organization develops a policy regarding smoking in all areas of all building(s) under the organization's control.

B 2. The organization's policy prohibits smoking in all areas of all building(s) under the organization's control (no medical exceptions allowed) for all children or youth residents.

B 3. The organization's policy may permit residents to smoke in the organization's buildings when a resident meets criteria developed and approved by the organization's leaders.

MC

C Ⓜ 4. When residents are permitted to smoke in the organization's buildings, they smoke only under the following circumstance(s):
- In designated locations environmentally separate from care, treatment, and service areas*
- After the organization has taken measures to minimize fire risks

C Ⓜ 5. Residents who do smoke in the organization's buildings are provided education, including information about options for smoking cessation.

B 6. The organization identifies and implements a process(es) for monitoring compliance with the policy.

B 7. The organization develops strategies to eliminate the incidence of policy violations when identified.

Standard EC.3.10

The organization manages its hazardous materials (HAZMAT) and waste† risks.

Rationale for EC.3.10

Organizations must identify materials they use that need special handling and implement processes to minimize the risks of their unsafe use and improper disposal.

Elements of Performance for EC.3.10

B 1. The organization develops and maintains a written management plan describing the processes it implements to effectively manage hazardous materials and wastes.

B 2. The organization creates and maintains an inventory that identifies HAZMAT and waste used, stored, or generated using criteria consistent with applicable law and regulation (for example, the Environmental Protection Agency [EPA] and the Occupational Safety and Health Administration [OSHA]).

The organization establishes and implements processes for selecting, handling, storing, transporting, using, and disposing of hazardous materials and waste from receipt or generation through use and/or final disposal, including managing the following:

MC

---

* **Note:** *This does not require that a designated smoking area be a specific distance from care, treatment, and service areas. A physically separate, well-ventilated room (a designated area for authorized smoking by residents that is exhausted to the outside) is acceptable.*

† **HAZMAT and waste** Materials whose handling, use, and storage are guided or regulated by local, state, or federal regulation. Examples include OSHA's Regulations for Bloodborne Pathogens (regarding blood, other infectious materials, contaminated items that could release blood or other infectious materials, or contaminated sharps), the Nuclear Regulatory Commission's regulations for handling and disposal of radioactive waste, management of hazardous vapors (such as glutaraldehyde, ethylene oxide, and nitrous oxide), chemicals regulated by the EPA, Department of Transportation requirements, and hazardous energy sources (for example, ionizing or nonionizing radiation, lasers, microwaves, and ultrasound).

C Ⓜ 3. Chemicals

A 4. Chemotherapeutic materials

A 5. Radioactive materials

C Ⓜ 6. Infectious and regulated medical wastes, including sharps

B 7. The organization provides adequate and appropriate space and equipment for safely handling and storing HAZMAT and waste.

B 9. The organization identifies and implements emergency procedures that include the specific precautions, procedures, and protective equipment used during HAZMAT and waste spills or exposures.

A 10. The organization maintains documentation, including required permits, licenses, and adherence to other regulations.

C Ⓜ 11. The organization maintains required manifests for handling HAZMAT and waste.

C Ⓜ 12. The organization properly labels HAZMAT and waste.

B 13. The organization effectively separates HAZMAT and waste storage and processing areas from other areas of the facility.

Standard EC.4.10

The organization addresses emergency management.

Rationale for EC.4.10

An emergency* in the organization or its community could suddenly and significantly affect the need for the organization's services or its ability to provide those services. Therefore, an organization needs to have an emergency management plan that comprehensively describes its approach to emergencies in the organization or in its community.

Elements of Performance for EC.4.10

A 1. The organization conducts a hazard vulnerability analysis† to identify potential emergencies that could affect the need for its services or its ability to provide those services.

MC

---

* **Emergency** A natural or manmade event that significantly disrupts the environment of care (for example, damage to the organization's building[s] and grounds due to severe winds, storms, or earthquakes); that significantly disrupts care, treatment and services (for example, loss of utilities such as power, water, or telephones due to floods, civil disturbances, accidents, or emergencies within the organization or in its community); or that results in sudden, significantly changed, or increased demands for the organization's services (for example, bioterrorist attack, building collapse, plane crash in the organization's community). Some emergencies are called *disasters* or *potential injury creating events (PICEs)*.

† **Hazard vulnerability analysis** The identification of potential emergencies and the direct and indirect effects these emergencies may have on the organization's operations and the demand for its services.

A   2.   The organization establishes the following with the community:
- Priorities among the potential emergencies identified in the hazard vulnerability analysis
- The organization's role in relation to a communitywide emergency management program
- An all-hazards command structure within the organization that links with the community's command structure

B   3.   The organization develops and maintains a written emergency management plan describing the process for disaster readiness and emergency management, and implements it when appropriate.

A   4.   At a minimum, an emergency management plan is developed with the involvement of the organization's leaders including the administrator, the medical director, the nursing leader, and other clinical leaders.

B   5.   The plan identifies specific procedures that describe mitigation,* preparedness,† response, and recovery strategies, actions, and responsibilities for each priority emergency.

B   6.   The plan provides processes for initiating the response and recovery phases of the plan, including a description of how, when, and by whom the phases are to be activated.

B   7.   The plan provides processes for notifying staff when emergency response measures are initiated.

B   8.   The plan provides processes for notifying external authorities of emergencies, including possible community emergencies identified by the organization.

B   9.   The plan provides processes for identifying and assigning staff to cover all essential staff functions under emergency conditions.

B   10. The plan provides processes for managing the following under emergency conditions:
- Activities related to care, treatment, and services (for example, scheduling, modifying, or discontinuing services; controlling information about residents; referrals; transporting residents)
- Staff support activities (for example, housing, transportation, incident stress debriefing)
- Staff family support activities
- Logistics relating to critical supplies (for example, supplies, food, linen, water)
- Security (for example, access, crowd control, traffic control)
- Communication with the news media

MC

---

* **Mitigation activities** Those activities an organization undertakes in attempting to lessen the severity and impact of a potential emergency.

† **Preparedness activities** Those activities an organization undertakes to build capacity and identify resources that may be used if an emergency occurs.

B   12. The plan provides processes for evacuating the entire facility (both horizontally and, when applicable, vertically) when the environment cannot support adequate care, treatment, and services.

B   13. The plan provides processes for establishing an alternate care site(s) that has the capabilities to meet the needs of residents when the environment cannot support adequate care, treatment, and services, including processes for the following:
- Transporting residents, staff, and equipment to the alternative care site(s)
- Transferring to and from the alternative care site(s), the necessities of residents (for example, medications, medical records)
- Tracking of residents
- Interfacility communication between the organization and the alternative care site(s)

B   14. The plan provides processes for identifying care providers and other personnel during emergencies.

B   15. The plan provides processes for cooperative planning with health care organizations that together provide services to a contiguous geographic area (for example, among organizations serving a town or borough) to facilitate the timely sharing of information about the following:
- Essential elements of their command structures and control centers for emergency response
- Names and roles of individuals in their command structures and command center telephone numbers
- Resources and assets that could potentially be shared in an emergency response
- Names of residents and deceased individuals brought to their organizations to facilitate identifying and locating victims of the emergency

B   18. The plan identifies backup internal and external communication systems in the event of failure during emergencies.

B   19. The plan identifies alternate roles and responsibilities of staff during emergencies, including to whom they report in the organization's command structure and, when activated, in the community's command structure.

B   20. The plan identifies an alternative means of meeting essential building utility needs when the organization is designated by its emergency management plan to provide continuous service during an emergency (for example, electricity, water, ventilation, fuel sources, medical gas/vacuum systems).

B   21. The plan identifies means for radioactive, biological, and chemical isolation and decontamination.

MC

Standard EC.6.10 ▬▬▬▬▬▬▬▬▬▬▬▬▬▬▬▬▬▬▬▬▬▬

The organization manages medical equipment risks.

Rationale for EC.6.10

Medical equipment is a significant contributor to the quality of care. It is used in treatment, diagnostic activities, and monitoring of the residents. It is essential that the equipment is appropriate for the intended use; that staff, including licensed independent practitioners, be trained to use the equipment safely and effectively; and it is essential that equipment is maintained appropriately by qualified individuals.

Elements of Performance for EC.6.10

B   1.   The organization develops and maintains a written management plan describing the processes it implements to manage the effective, safe, and reliable operation of medical equipment.

B   2.   The organization identifies and implements a process(es) for selecting and acquiring medical equipment.*

B   3.   The organization establishes and uses risk criteria[†] for identifying, evaluating, and creating an inventory of equipment to be included in the medical equipment management plan before the equipment is used. These criteria address the following:
- Equipment function (diagnosis, care, treatment, life support, and monitoring)
- Physical risks associated with use
- Equipment incident history

B   4.   The organization identifies appropriate inspection and maintenance strategies for all equipment in the inventory for achieving effective, safe, and reliable operation of all equipment in the inventory.[‡]

B   5.   The organization defines intervals for inspecting, testing, and maintaining appropriate equipment in the inventory (that is, those pieces of equipment in the inventory benefiting from scheduled activities to minimize the clinical and physical risks) that are based upon criteria such as manufacturers' recommendations, risk levels, and current organization experience.

B   6.   The organization identifies and implements processes for monitoring and acting on equipment hazard notices and recalls.

MC

---

* **Note:** *The acquisition process includes initially evaluating the condition and function of the equipment when received and evaluating the training of users before use on residents.*

[†] **Note:** *The organization may choose not to use risk criteria to limit the types of equipment to be included in the medical equipment management plan, rather include all medical equipment.*

[‡] **Note:** *Organizations may use different strategies for different items as appropriate. For example, strategies such as predictive maintenance, interval-based inspections, corrective maintenance, or metered maintenance may be selected to ensure reliable performance.*

B   7.   The organization identifies and implements processes for monitoring and reporting incidents in which a medical device is suspected or attributed to the death, serious injury, or serious illness of any individual, as required by the Safe Medical Devices Act of 1990.

A   8.   The organization identifies and implements processes for emergency procedures that address the following:
- What to do in the event of equipment disruption or failure
- When and how to perform emergency clinical interventions when medical equipment fails
- Availability of backup equipment
- How to obtain repair services

Standard EC.6.20

Medical equipment is maintained, tested, and inspected.

Elements of Performance for EC.6.20

C 𝕄   1.   The organization documents a current, accurate, and separate inventory of all equipment identified in the medical equipment management plan, regardless of ownership.

A   2.   The organization documents performance and safety testing of all equipment identified in the medical equipment management program before initial use.

A   3.   The organization documents inspection and maintenance of equipment used for life support* that is consistent with maintenance strategies to minimize clinical and physical risks identified in the equipment management plan (*see* standard EC.6.10).

C 𝕄   4.   The organization documents inspection and maintenance of non–life support equipment in the inventory that is consistent with maintenance strategies to minimize clinical and physical risks identified in the equipment management plan (*see* standard EC.6.10).

      5.   Not applicable

A 𝕄   6.   The organization documents chemical and biological testing of water used in renal dialysis and other applicable tests based upon regulations, manufacturers' recommendations, and organization experience.

MC

Standard EC.7.10

The organization manages its utility risks.

---

* **Life support equipment** Those devices intended to sustain life and whose failure to perform their primary function, when used according to manufacturer's instructions and clinical protocol, is expected to result in imminent death in the absence of immediate intervention (examples include ventilators, anesthesia machines, and heart-lung bypass machines).

Rationale for EC.7.10

Utility systems* are essential to the proper operation of the environment of care and significantly contribute to effective, safe, and reliable provision of care to residents in health care organizations. It is important that health care organizations establish and maintain a utility systems management program to promote a safe, controlled, and comfortable environment that does the following:

- Ensures operational reliability of utility systems
- Reduces the potential for organization-acquired illness to be transmitted through the utility systems
- Assesses the reliability and minimizes potential risks of utility system failures

Elements of Performance for EC.7.10

1. Through 6. Not applicable

B   7. The organization develops and maintains a written management plan describing the processes it implements to manage the effective, safe, and reliable operation of utility systems.

B   8. The organization designs and installs utility systems that meet the resident care and operational needs of the services in the organization's buildings.

B   9. The organization establishes risk criteria† for identifying, evaluating, and creating an inventory of operating components of systems before the equipment is used.

These criteria address the following:
- Life support
- Infection control
- Support of the environment
- Equipment support
- Communication

B   10. The organization develops appropriate strategies for all utility systems equipment in the inventory for ensuring effective, safe, and reliable operation of all equipment in the inventory.‡

B   11. The organization defines intervals for inspecting, testing, and maintaining appropriate utility systems equipment in the inventory (that is, those pieces of equipment in the inventory benefiting from scheduled activities to minimize the clinical and physical risks) that are based upon cri-

MC

---

* **Utility systems** May include electrical distribution; emergency power; vertical and horizontal transport; heating, ventilating, and air conditioning; plumbing, boiler, and steam; piped gases; vacuum systems; or communication systems, including data-exchange systems.

† **Note:** *The organization may choose not to use risk criteria to limit the types of utility systems to be included in the utility management plan, but rather include all utility systems.*

‡ **Note:** *Organizations may use different strategies as appropriate. For example, strategies such as predictive maintenance, interval-based inspections, corrective maintenance, or metered maintenance may be selected to ensure reliable performance.*

teria such as manufacturers' recommendations, risk levels, and current organization experience.

A   12. The organization identifies and implements emergency procedures for responding to utility system disruptions or failures that address the following:
- What to do if utility systems malfunction
- Identification of an alternative source of organization-defined essential utilities
- Shutting off the malfunctioning systems and notifying staff in affected areas
- How and when to perform emergency clinical interventions when utility systems fail
- Obtaining repair services

B   13. The organization maps the distribution of utility systems.

C Ⓜ 14. The organization labels controls for a partial or complete emergency shutdown.

B   15. The organization identifies and implements processes to minimize pathogenic biological agents in cooling towers, domestic hot/cold water systems, and other aerosolizing water systems.

A   16. The organization designs, installs, and maintains ventilation equipment to provide appropriate pressure relationships, air-exchange rates, and filtration efficiencies for ventilation systems serving areas specially designed* to control airborne contaminants (such as biological agents, gases, fumes, and dust).

Standard EC.7.30

The organization maintains, tests, and inspects its utility systems.

Note: *Organizations that offer care, treatment, and services in leased facilities need to communicate maintenance expectations for building equipment not under their control to their landlord through contractual language, lease agreements, memos, and so forth. These organizations are not required to possess maintenance documentation, but must only have access to such documentation as needed and during survey. It is also important that the landlord communicate to the organization any building equipment problems identified that could negatively affect the safety or health of residents, staff, and other people coming to the organization, as well as the landlord's plan to resolve such issues.*

MC

---

* **Areas specially designed** Include spaces such as rooms for residents diagnosed or suspected of having airborne communicable diseases (for example, pulmonary or laryngeal tuberculosis), residents in protective-isolation rooms (for example, those receiving bone marrow transplants), laboratories, pharmacies, and sterile supply rooms.

Elements of Performance for EC.7.30

C ⓜ 1. The organization maintains documentation of a current, accurate, and separate inventory of utility components identified in the utility management plan.

A ⓜ 2. The organization maintains documentation of performance and safety testing of each critical component identified in the plan before initial use.

A ⓜ 3. The organization maintains documentation of maintenance of critical components of life support utility systems/equipment consistent with maintenance strategies identified in the utility management plan (*see* standard EC.7.10).

A ⓜ 4. The organization maintains documentation of maintenance of critical components of infection control utility systems/equipment for high-risk residents consistent with maintenance strategies identified in the utility management plan (*see* standard EC.7.10).

C ⓜ 5. The organization maintains documentation of maintenance of critical components of non–life support utility systems/equipment in the inventory consistent with maintenance strategies identified in the utility management plan (*see* standard EC.7.10).

A ⓜ 6. The practice ensures preventive maintenance and inspection performance and safety testing of each critical utility component that may pose a risk to resident safety or adversely impact the delivery of resident care.

Standard EC.7.50 ▬▬▬▬▬▬▬▬▬▬▬▬▬▬▬▬

The organization maintains, tests, and inspects its medical gas and vacuum systems.

Note: *This standard does not require organizations to have the medical gas and vacuum systems discussed in the following EPs. However, if an organization has these types of systems, then the following maintenance, testing, and inspection requirements apply.*

Elements of Performance for EC.7.50

A 1. The organization inspects, tests, and maintains critical components of piped medical gas systems including master signal panels, area alarms, automatic pressure switches, shutoff valves, flexible connectors, and outlets.

A 2. The organization tests piped medical gas and vacuum systems when the systems are installed, modified, or repaired including cross-connection testing, piping purity testing, and pressure testing.

A 3. The organization maintains the main supply valve and area shut-off valves of piped medical gas and vacuum systems to be accessible and clearly labeled.

MC

Standard EC.9.10

The organization monitors conditions in the environment.

Elements of Performance for EC.9.10

B 1. The organization establishes and implements process(es) for reporting and investigating the following:*
- Injuries to residents or others coming to the organization's facilities as well as incidents of property damage
- Occupational illnesses and injuries to staff
- Security incidents involving residents, staff, or others coming to the organization's facilities or property
- Hazardous materials and waste spills, exposures, and other related incidents
- Fire-safety management problems, deficiencies, and failures
- Equipment-management problems, failures, and user errors
- Utility systems management problems, failures, or user errors

B 2. The organization's leaders assign a person(s) (hereafter referred to as the "assigned person[s]") to monitor and respond to conditions in the organization's environment. The assigned individual performs the following tasks:
- Coordinates the ongoing, organizationwide collection of information about deficiencies and opportunities for improvement in the environment of care
- Coordinates the ongoing collection and dissemination of other sources of information, such as published hazard notices or recall reports
- Coordinates the preparation of summaries of deficiencies, problems, failures, and user errors related to managing the environment of care†
- Coordinates the preparation of summaries on findings, recommendations, actions taken, and results of performance improvement (PI) activities
- Participates in hazard surveillance and incident reporting
- Participates in developing safety policies and procedures

B 3. The organization establishes and implements a process(es) for ongoing monitoring of performance regarding actual or potential risk(s) in each of the environment of care management plans.‡

---

* Organizations have the flexibility to develop a single reporting method that addresses one or more of the items listed.

† **Note:** *Incidents involving residents may be reported to appropriate staff such as staff in quality assessment, improvement, or other functions. However, at least a summary of incidents is shared with the person designated to coordinate safety management activities (see standard EC.1.10). Review of incident reports often requires that various legal processes be followed to preserve confidentiality. Opportunities to improve care, treatment, and services or to prevent future similar incidents are not lost as a result of the legal process followed.*

‡ The environment of care plans are for managing safety, security, hazardous materials and waste, emergency management, fire safety, medical equipment, and utilities.

MC

A   4.   Each of the environment of care management plans are evaluated at least annually.

B   5.   The objectives, scope, performance, and effectiveness of each of the environment of care management plans are evaluated at least annually.

B   10.   Environmental safety monitoring and response activities are communicated to the resident safety program required in the "Leadership" chapter of this book.

Standard EC.9.20

The organization analyzes identified environment issues and develops recommendations for resolving them.

Elements of Performance for EC.9.20

B   1.   The organization establishes an ongoing process for resolving environment of care issues that involves representatives from clinical, administrative, and support services.

C Ⓜ   2.   A multidisciplinary improvement team meets at least bimonthly to address environment of care issues.*

B   3.   The organization analyzes environment of care issues in a timely manner.

B   4.   Recommendations are developed and approved as appropriate.

B   5.   Appropriate staff establishes measurement guidelines.

B   6.   Environment of care issues are communicated to the organization's leaders and person(s) responsible for PI activities.

A   8.   A recommendation for one or more PI activities is communicated at least annually to the organization's leaders based on the ongoing performance monitoring of the environment of care management plans.

B   9.   Recommendations for resolving environmental safety issues are communicated, when appropriate, to those responsible for managing the resident safety program required in the "Leadership" chapter of this book.

MC

Standard EC.9.30

The organization improves the environment.

Elements of Performance for EC.9.30

B   1.   Appropriate staff participates in implementing recommendations.

---

* **Note:** *Meetings held less frequently than bimonthly are acceptable when supported by current organization experience and the multidisciplinary improvement team's approval. Ongoing justification of meeting frequency depends on a satisfactory annual evaluation of performance as required by EC.9.10.*

B   2.   Appropriate staff monitors the effectiveness of the recommendation's implementation.

B   3.   Monitoring results are reported through appropriate channels, including the organization's leaders.

B   4.   Monitoring results are reported to the multidisciplinary improvement team responsible for resolving environment of care issues.

B   5.   Results of monitoring are reported (when appropriate) to those responsible for managing the resident safety program required in the "Leadership" chapter of this book.

Management of Human Resources

Standard HR.1.30

The organization uses data on clinical/service screening indicators* in combination with human resource screening indicators† to assess staffing effectiveness.‡

Rationale for HR.1.30

Multiple screening indicators that relate to resident outcomes, including clinical/service and human resources screening indicators, may be indicative of staffing effectiveness.

Elements of Performance for HR.1.30

A   1.   The organization selects a minimum of four screening indicators: two clinical/service and two human resources indicators. The focus is on the relationship between human resource and clinical/service screening indicators, with the clear understanding that no one indicator, in and of itself, can directly demonstrate staffing effectiveness.

A   2.   The organization selects at least one of the human resource and one of the clinical/service screening indicators from a list of Joint Commission–identified screening indicators. The organization chooses additional screening indicators based on its unique characteristics, specialties, and services.

B   3.   The organization determines the rationale for screening indicator selection.

MC

---

* An example of a clinical/service screening indicator is adverse drug events.

† Examples of human resource screening indicators are overtime and staff vacancy rate.

‡ **Staffing effectiveness** is defined as the number, competency, and skill mix of staff related to the provision of needed services.

B   4.   The organization defines the direct and indirect caregivers included in the human resource screening indicators based on the impact, if any, the absence of such caregivers is expected to have on resident outcomes.

B   5.   The organization uses the data collected and analyzed from the selected screening indicators to identify potential staffing effectiveness issues when performance varies from expected targets (for example, ranges of desired performance, external comparisons, or improvement goals).

B   6.   The organization analyzes data over time per screening indicator (for example, identification of trends or patterns using a line graph, run chart, or control chart) to determine the stability of a process.

B   7.   The organization analyzes all screening indicator data in combination (for example, a table or matrix report, multiple line graphs, spider or radar diagrams, or scatter diagrams).

A   8.   The organization analyzes screening indicator data at the level in which staffing needs are planned in the organization and in collaboration with other areas in the organization, as needed.

B   9.   The organization reports at least annually to the leaders on the aggregation and analysis of data related to staffing effectiveness (*see* standards PI.1.10 and PI.2.20) and any actions taken to improve staffing.

B   10.   The organization can provide evidence of actions taken, as appropriate, in response to analyzed data.

List of Joint Commission Screening Indicators for Long Term Care
1.   Prevalence of pressure ulcers (Clinical/Service)
2.   Resident satisfaction (Clinical/Service)
3.   Family satisfaction (Clinical/Service)
4.   Prevalence of falls (Clinical/Service)
5.   Resident complaints (Clinical/Service)
6.   Injuries to residents (Clinical/Service)
7.   Family complaints (Clinical/Service)
8.   Restraint use (Clinical/Service)
9.   Prevalence of weight loss (Clinical/Service)
10.   Elopements/wandering of residents (Clinical/Service)
11.   Adverse drug events (Clinical/Service)
12.   Prevalence of dehydration (Clinical/Service)
13.   Pain assessment and management (that is, wait time to receive medications) (Clinical/Service)
14.   Urinary tract infection rate (Clinical/Service)
15.   Change in resident functioning (Clinical/Service)
16.   Prevalence of malnutrition (Clinical/Service)
17.   Activities of daily living (ADLs) met or unmet (Clinical/Service)
18.   Prevalence of urinary catheter use (Clinical/Service)
19.   Average-time in activities (Clinical/Service)
20.   Antibiotic use (Clinical/Service)

MC

21. Unexpected hospital admissions or emergency department visits (Clinical/Service)
22. Prevalence of depression (Clinical/Service)
23. Prevalence of more than eight prescribed medications (Clinical/Service)
24. Pneumonia rate (Clinical/Service)
25. Antipsychotic medication usage (Clinical/Service)
26. Staff vacancy rate (Human Resource)
27. Staff turnover rate (Human Resource)
28. Staff satisfaction (Human Resource)
29. Use of overtime (Human Resource)
30. Staff injury rate (Human Resource)
31. Nursing hours per resident day (R.N., L.P.N., C.N.A.) compared to baseline such as actual versus planned or budgeted (Human Resource)
32. Staff training hours (Human Resource)
33. Agency usage/contract staff (Human Resource)
34. Understaffing as compared to organization's staffing plan (Human Resource)
35. Use of sick time (Human Resource)
36. Activity staff hours per resident day (Human Resource)
37. Number of dietary staff per resident (Human Resource)
38. Number of housekeeping staff per resident (Human Resource)
39. Average response time for consultation order (Human Resource)

Standard HR.2.10

Orientation provides initial job training and information.

Rationale for HR.2.10

Staff members, licensed independent practitioners (if applicable), students, and volunteers are oriented to their jobs as appropriate and the work environment before providing care, treatment, and services.

Elements of Performance for HR.2.10

As appropriate, each staff member, licensed independent practitioner, student, and volunteer is oriented to the following:

C Ⓜ 1. The organization's mission and goals.

C Ⓜ 2. Organizationwide policies and procedures (including safety and infection control) and relevant unit, setting, or program-specific policies and procedures.

C Ⓜ 3. Specific job duties and responsibilities and service, setting, or program-specific job duties and responsibilities related to safety and infection control.

C Ⓜ 4. Each activity he or she will be expected to perform, including each instrument and piece of equipment, each technique, and all related functions such as resident specimen identification and collection, qual-

MC

ity control and calibration, reporting of results, and notification of the supervisor when problems arise.

C Ⓜ 5. Cultural diversity and sensitivity.

C Ⓜ 6. Staff, students, and volunteers are educated about the rights of residents and ethical aspects of care, treatment, and services and the process used to address ethical issues.

C Ⓜ 7. Staff is oriented to the effects of psychotropic medications as appropriate.

Standard HR.2.20

Staff members, licensed independent practitioners, students, and volunteers, as appropriate, can describe or demonstrate their roles and responsibilities, based on specific job duties or responsibilities, relative to safety.

Rationale for HR.2.20

The human element is the most critical factor in any process, determining whether the right things are done correctly. The best policies and procedures for minimizing risks in the environment where care, treatment, and services are provided are meaningless if staff, licensed independent practitioners (if applicable), students, and volunteers do not know and understand them well enough to perform them properly.

It is important that everyday precautions identified by the health care organization for minimizing various risks, including those related to resident safety and environmental safety,* are properly implemented. It is also important that the appropriate emergency procedures be instituted should an incident or failure occur in the environment.

Elements of Performance for HR.2.20

Staff members, licensed independent practitioners, students, and volunteers, as appropriate, can describe or demonstrate the following:

C Ⓜ 1. Risks within the organization's environment

C Ⓜ 2. Actions to eliminate, minimize, or report risks

C Ⓜ 3. Procedures to follow in the event of an incident

C Ⓜ 4. Reporting processes for common problems, failures, and user errors

Standard HR.2.30

Ongoing education, including in-services, training, and other activities, maintains and improves competence.

---

* The "Management of the Environment of Care" chapter of this book identifies risks associated with the following categories: safety, security, hazardous materials and wastes, emergency management, medical equipment, and utility management.

MC

Elements of Performance for HR.2.30

The following occurs for staff, students, and volunteers who work in the same capacity as staff providing care, treatment, and services:

B   1. Training occurs when job responsibilities or duties change.

C Ⓜ 2. Participation in ongoing in-services, training, or other activities occurs to increase staff, student, or volunteer knowledge of work-related issues.

C Ⓜ 3. Ongoing in-services and other education and training are appropriate to the needs of the population(s) served and comply with law and regulation.

C Ⓜ 4. Ongoing in-services, training, or other activities emphasize specific job-related aspects of safety and infection prevention and control.

C Ⓜ 5. Ongoing in-services, training, or other education incorporate methods of team training, when appropriate.

C Ⓜ 6. Ongoing in-services, training, or other education reinforce the need and ways to report unanticipated adverse events.

C Ⓜ 7. Ongoing in-services or other education are offered in response to learning needs identified through performance improvement findings and other data analysis (that is, data from staff surveys, performance evaluations, or other needs assessments).

C Ⓜ 8. Ongoing education is documented.

B   10. Staff members are educated, as appropriate to their responsibilities, about psychotropic medications including the following:
- The need for a medication in relation to the resident's documented diagnosis and condition
- The potential for drug-drug and drug-food interactions
- Adverse reactions to psychotropic medications
- The use of a medication for an appropriate duration
- The optimal dose
- Frequent monitoring of the medication's effectiveness
- Nonmedication interventions and alternatives developed through interdisciplinary team assessment
- Reduction and discontinuation of a medication

MC

Standard HR.3.10

Competence to perform job responsibilities is assessed, demonstrated, and maintained.

Rationale for HR.3.10

Competence assessment is systematic and allows for a measurable assessment of the person's ability to perform required activities. Information used as part of competence assessment may include data from performance evaluations, performance improvement, and aggregate data on competence, as well as the assessment of learning needs.

Elements of Performance for HR.3.10

The competence assessment process for staff, students, and volunteers who work in the same capacity as staff providing care, treatment, and services is based on the following (EPs 1–7):

B   1. Populations served.

B   2. Defined competencies to be required.

B   3. Defined competencies to be assessed during orientation.

B   4. Defined competencies that need to be assessed and reassessed on an ongoing basis, based on techniques, procedures, technology, equipment, or skills needed to provide care, treatment, and services.

B   5. A defined time frame for how often competence assessments are performed for each person, minimally, once in the three-year accreditation cycle and in accordance with law and regulation.

B   6. Assessment methods (appropriate to determine the skill being assessed).

B   7. The use of qualified individuals to assess competence.

C Ⓜ 8. The organization assesses and documents each person's ability to carry out assigned responsibilities safely, competently, and in a timely manner upon completion of orientation.

C Ⓜ 9. The organization assesses each person according to its competence assessment process.

B   10. When improvement activities lead to a determination that a person with performance problems is unable or unwilling to improve, the organization modifies the person's job assignment or takes other appropriate action.

Standard HR.4.10

MC

There is a process for ensuring the competence of all practitioners permitted by law and the organization to practice independently.

Rationale for HR.4.10

Appropriate leaders of the organization formally approve the process for appointment and reappointment. The description of the process is sufficiently detailed to permit tracking of the steps involved when examining credential files.

Credentialing criteria specify requirements for practitioner membership in the organization. These criteria are designed to help establish an applicant's background and current competence. Moreover, they help assure the organization and its residents that the residents will receive quality care. The core criteria are the following:

- Current licensure
- Relevant education, training, or experience
- Current competence
- Ability to perform requested privileges

Each organization develops its own criteria for determining an applicant's ability to provide care, treatment, and services within the scope of clinical privileges requested. Criteria for renewing or revising clinical privileges include procedure outcomes and other results of performance improvement activities.

The organization may add other reasonable criteria, such as current evidence of adequate professional liability insurance or evidence of continuing medical education. The following principles summarize key concepts as they relate to privileging:

1. The organization administrator may substitute for the governing body.
2. An organized medical staff and bylaws are not required.
3. The medical director is comparable to the Medical Executive Committee (MEC) in settings where no organized medical staff exists.
4. In organizations without an organized medical staff, procedures for appointment, reappointment, and granting, renewal, or revision of clinical privileges are established by the medical director and approved by the governing body.
5. Privileges may be delineated by category and should address cognitive and technical skills.
6. Each organization defines its scope of care in such a way that practitioners can request privileges consistent with the scope of care.
7. In hospital-based long term care units, the long term care medical director reviews the credentials file and makes recommendations to the appropriate group or individual.
8. The organization's general credentialing process can be applied to determine credentials, but the privileges granted must be program and category specific.

Current licensure. Licensure is verified with the primary source at the time of appointment and initial granting of clinical privileges by a letter or secure electronic communication obtained from the appropriate state licensing board, if in a federal service. Verification of current licensure through the primary source through a secure electronic communication or by telephone is acceptable, if this verification is documented.

At the time of reappointment and renewal or revision of clinical privileges, current licensure is confirmed with the primary source or by viewing the applicant's current license or registration.

Relevant training and experience. At the time of appointment and initial granting of clinical privileges, the organization verifies relevant training or experience from the primary source(s), whenever feasible. Verification includes letters from professional schools, internships, residency, or postdoctoral programs. Relevant training and experience may be obtained by contacting the primary source via a secure electronic communication or by telephone, if this verification is docu-

MC

mented. For applicants who have just completed training in an approved residency or postdoctoral program, a letter from the program director is enough.

An external organization (for example, a credentials verification organization [CVO] or a Joint Commission–accredited health care organization functioning as a CVO) may be used to collect information from primary sources.

Note 1: *An organization may choose to use the credentialing information of a health care organization accredited by the Joint Commission (as long as it has determined that the organization meets the 10 CVO guidelines in Note 3 on page MC-63). The National Practitioner Data Bank (NPDB) must still be queried in this instance.*

The organization may choose to rely on a Joint Commission–accredited health care organization's credentialing information for some practitioners, while conducting the process itself for others.

Regardless of the source of credentialing information, leadership is responsible for reviewing the information on the licensed independent practitioner and making decisions regarding the assigning and renewal/revision of clinical responsibilities.

Note 2: *It may not always be feasible to obtain information from the primary source. In rare or occasional instances, a primary source such as an educational institution no longer exists, or the applicant's records have been lost or destroyed. Applicants may have received education, training, and experience partially or wholly in a foreign country, and for political or other reasons, information regarding their professional background is not accessible. When undue delay occurs in deriving information from a primary source, granting of clinical privileges is withheld pending receipt of this information. Under these circumstances, the applicant may be given temporary privileges for a limited time in accordance with rules and regulations or policies and procedures, as well as state and federal regulations. Designated equivalent sources or other reliable secondary sources may also be used if there has been a documented attempt to contact the primary source.*

Designated equivalent sources are selected agencies that have been determined to maintain a specific item(s) of credential information identical to information at the primary source. Their designated equivalent sources are the following:

- *The American Medical Association (AMA) Physician Masterfile for verification of a physician's medical school graduation and residency completion*
- *The American Board of Medical Specialties (ABMS) for verification of a physician's board certification*
- *The Education Commission for Foreign Medical Graduates (ECFMG) for verification of a physician's foreign medical school graduation*
- *The American Osteopathic Association (AOA) Physician Database for predoctoral education accredited by the AOA Bureau of Professional education; postdoctoral education approved by the AOA Council on Postdoctoral Training; and the Osteopathic Specialty Board Certification*
- *The Federation of State Medical Boards (FSMB) for all actions against a physician's medical license*

MC

These designated equivalent sources may be used by the organization or by a CVO used by the organization. There may be other designated equivalent sources for certain applicants, such as for licensure verification of an applicant in the federal service. The organization should communicate with the Joint Commission to determine whether a specific agency qualifies as a designated equivalent source under such special circumstances. The physician profiles from the AMA Physician Masterfile also include other primary source–reported information that is similar to primary source–verified information provided by a CVO. Use of this additional information is subject to the guidelines set forth in Note 3.

A primary source of verified information may designate to an agency the role of communicating credentials information. The delegated agency then becomes acceptable to be used as a primary source.

Note 3: *Any organization that bases its decisions in part on information obtained from a CVO should have confidence in the completeness, accuracy, and timeliness of that information. To achieve this level of confidence, the organization should evaluate the agency providing the information initially and then periodically as appropriate. The principles that guide such an evaluation include the following:*

- *The agency makes known to the user the data and information it can provide*
- *The agency provides documentation to the user describing how its data collection, information development, and verification process(es) are performed*
- *The user is given sufficient, clear information on database functions, including any limitations of information available from the agency (practitioners not included in the database), the time frame for agency responses to requests for information, and a summary overview of quality control processes related to data integrity, security, transmission accuracy, and technical specifications*
- *The user and agency agree on the format for transmitting credentials information about an individual from the CVO*
- *The user can easily discern what information transmitted by the CVO is from a primary source and what is not*
- *For information transmitted by the agency that can go out of date (licensure, board certification), the date the information was last updated from the primary source is provided by the CVO*
- *The CVO certifies that the information transmitted to the user accurately presents the information obtained by it*
- *The user can discern whether the information transmitted by the CVO from a primary source is all the primary source information in the CVO's possession pertinent to a given item or, if not, where additional information can be obtained*
- *The user can engage the CVO's quality control processes when necessary to resolve concerns about transmission errors, inconsistencies, or other data issues that may be identified from time to time*
- *The user has a formal arrangement with the CVO for communicating changes in credentialing information*

Current competence. Current competence at the time of appointment and initial granting of clinical privileges cannot be determined by board certification or admissibility alone. Instead, it is verified in writing by individuals personally acquainted

MC

with the applicant's professional and clinical performance, either in teaching facilities or in other organizations. Letters from authoritative sources provide the organization with information directly from the primary source(s). Such letters contain informed opinions about the applicant's scope and level of performance. The organization defines the number of reference letters required. Acceptable letters are those that describe the following:

- The applicant's actual clinical performance in general terms
- The applicant's satisfactory discharge of professional obligations as a licensed independent practitioner
- The applicant's acceptable ethical performance

Ideally, letters also address at least two aspects of current competence: the types and outcomes of medical conditions managed by the applicant as the responsible licensed independent practitioner and the applicant's clinical judgment and technical skills.

At the time of reappointment, current competence is determined by the results of performance improvement activities, peer recommendations, and/or the evaluation of the individual's professional performance, clinical judgment, and technical skills. Peer recommendations come from appropriate practitioners in the same professional specialty and preferably the same discipline as the applicant. If no peers on staff are knowledgeable about the applicant, a peer recommendation may be obtained from outside the organization. Peer recommendations refer, as appropriate, to relevant training or experience, current competence, and how well the applicant fulfilled organization-specific obligations. Sources for peer recommendations may include the following:

- A performance improvement committee, the majority of whose members are the applicant's peers
- A reference letter(s) or documented telephone conversation about the applicant from a peer(s) who is knowledgeable about the applicant's competence
- A department or major clinical service chair who is a peer

Ability to perform requested privileges. The applicant's ability to perform clinical privileges must be evaluated, and this evaluation is documented in the applicant's credentials file. Documentation may include the applicant's statement that no health problems exist that could affect his or her practice; this statement must be confirmed. Applicants applying for appointment or for initial clinical privileges need this statement confirmed by the director of a training program, staff at another organization at which the applicant holds privileges, or by an individual the organization designates.

MC

Applicants applying for reappointment or renewed or revised clinical privileges must have their health status confirmed by at least a countersignature on the applicant's statement by a licensed independent practitioner knowledgeable of the applicant's health status.

Elements of Performance for HR.4.10

B   10. The organization has a defined process approved by the leaders for appointing and reappointing licensed independent practitioners.

A   11. The following occur at the time of appointment and initial granting of clinical privileges:
- Current licensure, including all actions against the license, is verified with the primary source and documented
- Relevant training and experience are verified from the primary source
- Current competence is verified from a knowledgeable source
- The applicant's ability to perform the clinical privileges* requested is evaluated

A   12. In addition to the preceding criteria, the organization collects and evaluates information on restriction of privileges at other health care organizations.

B   13. The NPDB is queried in a timely manner and before finalizing appointments and granting initial privileges for information on adverse privilege actions taken by a health care organization.[†]

A   14. The leaders review all credentials information and decide whether to appoint the licensed independent practitioner to provide care, treatment, and services.

C ⓜ   15. The licensed independent practitioner is notified in writing of the governing body's decision.

B   16. Each credentials file demonstrates that the credentialing criteria are uniformly applied.

A   17. Individuals who do not possess a license, registration, or certification do not provide or have not provided health care services in the organization that would, under applicable law or regulation, require such a license, registration, or certification.

---

* The Americans with Disabilities Act (ADA) bars certain discrimination based on physical or mental impairment. To prevent such discrimination, the act prohibits or mandates various activities. Health care organizations need to determine the applicability of the ADA to their licensed independent practitioners. If applicable, the organization should examine its privileging or credentialing procedures as to how and when it ascertains and confirms an applicant's health status. For example, the act may prohibit inquiry as to an applicant's physical or mental health status before making an offer of membership and privileges, but may not prohibit such inquiry after an offer is extended (without specific reference to health matters) to perform the specific privileges requested. Thus, the inquiry may be made and confirmed as a component of the application process. The Joint Commission cannot provide legal advice to organizations. However, the Joint Commission has and will absolutely construe this standard in such a manner as to be consistent with organization efforts to comply with the ADA.

† Additional information received from the NPDB query that the organization may choose to use includes medical malpractice payments, licensure disciplinary actions, adverse actions affecting professional society membership, sanctions for Medicare and Medicaid, and adverse professional review actions taken by health care organizations against health care practitioners other than physicians and dentists.

MC

A   18. An individual who does not possess a license, registration, or certification does not provide or has not provided health care services in the organization that would, under applicable law or regulation, require such a license, registration, or certification and which could place the organization's residents at risk for a serious adverse outcome.

B   21. The governing body* does the following:
- Reviews recommendations made by the medical director
- Reviews documentation on which recommendations are based
- Reviews records of any hearings or appeals addressing adverse decisions
- Grants appropriate clinical privileges

Standard HR.4.20

Individuals permitted by law and the organization to practice independently are granted clinical privileges.

Elements of Performance for HR.4.20

B   1. Criteria for determining the licensed independent practitioner's clinical privileges are specified in writing and uniformly applied to all applicants.

C Ⓜ   2. Clinical privileges for licensed independent practitioners are delineated according to organization policy and based on the licensed independent practitioner's current credentials and competence, as well as the population(s) served and the types of care, treatment, and services provided in the organization.

A   3. Individuals with clinical privileges practice within the scope of their privileges.

Standard HR.4.30

The organization has a process for granting temporary clinical privileges, when appropriate.

Rationale for HR.4.30

Privileges for licensed independent practitioners can be issued to meet the important needs of residents for a limited period, as defined by policies and procedures or rules and regulations. Privileges can also be issued for new applicants for a period not to exceed 120 days.

---

* The organization administrator or a committee of two or more governing body members may substitute for a governing body.

Elements of Performance for HR.4.30

B   1.   Policies and procedures, rules, or regulations describe the process for granting temporary privileges for meeting the important needs of residents or for new applicants.

A   2.   To grant temporary privileges to meet the important needs of residents, there must be verification (which can be done by telephone) of current licensure and current competence.

A   3.   To grant temporary privileges for new applicants, there must be verification (which may be done by telephone) of the following:
   - Current licensure
   - Relevant education training or experience
   - Current competence
   - Ability to perform the clinical responsibilities privileges requested

A   4.   To grant temporary privileges for new applicants, the results of the NPDB query have been obtained and evaluated

A   5.   To grant temporary privileges for new applicants, the licensed independent practitioner applicant has the following:
   - A complete application
   - No current or previously successful challenge to licensure or registration
   - Not been subject to involuntary termination of professional or medical staff membership at another organization, when applicable to the discipline
   - Not been subject to involuntary limitation, reduction, denial, or loss of clinical responsibilities privileges, when applicable to the discipline

A   6.   The administrator or designee grants temporary clinical responsibilities privileges all for meeting important resident needs and for new applicants upon recommendation of clinical leadership or the medical director.

Standard HR.4.40

There are mechanisms, including a fair hearing and appeal process, for addressing adverse decisions regarding reappointment, denial, reduction, suspension, or revocation of clinical privileges that may relate to quality of care, treatment, and service issues.

MC

Rationale for HR.4.40

Mechanisms for fair hearing and appeals processes are designed to allow the affected individual a fair opportunity to defend herself or himself regarding the adverse decision to an unbiased hearing committee, and an opportunity to appeal the decision of the committee to the governance function. The purpose of a fair hearing and appeal is to assure full consideration and reconsideration of quality and safety issues and, under the current structure of reporting to the NPDB, to allow practitioners an opportunity to defend themselves.

Elements of Performance for HR.4.40

The organization has developed a fair hearing and appeals process that does the following:

B　　1.　Is designed to provide a uniform and fair process

B　　2.　Has a mechanism to schedule a hearing of such requests

B　　3.　Has identified the procedures for the hearings to follow

B　　4.　Identifies or defines the composition of the hearing committee

B　　5.　Provides for a mechanism to appeal an adverse decision through the governance function

Standard HR.4.50

Clinical privileges and appointments/reappointments are reviewed and revised at least every two years.

Elements of Performance for HR.4.50

A　　1.　Policies and procedures or rules and regulations specify a period of no more than two years between appointments and reappointments and between granting, renewing, and revising clinical privileges.

C ⓜ 2.　Credential files for licensed independent practitioners contain substantive information and indicate that clinical privileges are reviewed or revised at least every two years and are revised as needed; in addition, appointments and reappointments are made for a period of no more than two years.

A　　3.　A reappraisal is conducted at the time of reappointment or renewal or revision of clinical privileges.

A　　4.　The reappraisal addresses current competence and includes the following:
- Confirmation of adherence to organization policies and procedures, rules, or regulations
- Relevant information from organization performance improvement activities when evaluating professional performance, judgment, and clinical or technical skills
- Any results of review of the individual's clinical performance
- Clinical performance in the organization that is outside acceptable standards
- Relevant education, training, and experience, if changed since initial privileging and appointment, when available
- Verification of current licensure, including all actions against the license

MC

- A statement that the individual can perform the care, treatment, and services he or she has been providing
- Evaluation of restrictions on privileges at a hospital(s) or other health care organization(s)
- A query of the NPDB for information on adverse privilege actions taken by a health care entity, when appropriate to the discipline

B   5.   Credentials files contain clear evidence that the full range of privileges has been included in the reappraisal.

Management of Information

Standard IM.1.10

The organization plans and designs information management processes to meet internal and external information needs.

Rationale for IM.1.10

Organizations vary in size, complexity, governance, structure, decision-making processes, and resources. Information management systems and processes vary accordingly. Only by first identifying the information needs can one then evaluate the extent to which they are planned for, and at what performance level the needs are being met. Planning for the management of information does not require a formal written information plan, but does require evidence of a planned approach that identifies the organization's information needs and supports its goals and objectives.

Elements of Performance for IM.1.10

B   1.   The organization bases its information management processes on a thorough analysis of internal and external information needs.
- The analysis ascertains the flow of information in an organization, including information storage and feedback mechanisms.
- The analysis considers what data and information are needed within and among departments, services, or programs; within and among the staff, the administration, and governance structure; to support relationships with outside services and contractors; with licensing, accrediting, and regulatory bodies; with purchasers, payers, and employers; and to participate in national research and databases.

B   2.   To guide development of processes for managing information used internally and externally, the organization assesses its information management needs based on the following:
- Its mission
- Its goals
- Its services

MC

- Personnel
- Resident safety considerations
- Quality of care, treatment, and services
- Mode(s) of service delivery
- Resources
- Access to affordable technology
- Identification of barriers to effective communication among caregivers

B   3.   The organization bases management, staffing, and material resource allocations for information management on the scope and complexity of care, treatment, and services provided.

B   4.   Appropriate staff participates in assessment, selection, integration, and use of information management systems for clinical/service and organization information.

B   5.   The organization has an ongoing process to assess the needs of the organization, departments, and individuals for knowledge-based information and uses this assessment as a basis for planning.

Standard IM.2.10

Information privacy* and confidentiality† are maintained.

Rationale for IM.2.10

Confidentiality of data and information applies across all systems and automated, paper, and verbal communications, as well as to clinical/service, financial, and business records and employee-specific information. The capture, storage, and retrieval processes for data and information are designed to be performed on a timely‡ basis without compromising the data and information's confidentiality. Protecting privacy and confidentiality of information is the responsibility of the whole organization. In achieving this responsibility, the organization provides appropriate safeguards for resident privacy and the confidentiality of information. These safeguards are consistent with available technology and legitimate needs for accessibility of the information to authorized individuals for the delivery of care, treatment, and services and for effective functioning of the organization, research, and education.

Elements of Performance for IM.2.10

B   1.   The organization has developed a written process (in one or more policies) based on and consistent with applicable law that addresses the privacy and confidentiality of information.

---

* **Privacy** An individual's right to limit the disclosure of personal information.

† **Confidentiality** The safekeeping of data/information so as to restrict access to individuals who have need, reason, and permission for such access.

‡ Defined by organization policy and based on the intended use of the information.

B 2. The organization's policy, including significant changes to the policy, has been effectively communicated to applicable staff.

B 3. The organization has a process to monitor compliance with its policy.

B 4. The organization improves privacy and confidentiality by monitoring information and developments in technology.

C ⓜ 5. Individuals about whom personally identifiable health data and information may be maintained or collected are made aware of what uses and disclosures of the information will be made.

B 6. For uses and disclosures of health information, the removal of personal identifiers is encouraged to the extent possible, consistent with maintaining the usefulness of the information.

C ⓜ 7. Protected health information* is used for the purposes identified or as required by law and not further disclosed without resident authorization.

B 8. The organization preserves the confidentiality of data and information identified as sensitive and requires extraordinary means to preserve resident privacy.

Standard IM.3.10

The organization has processes in place to effectively manage information, including the capturing, reporting, processing, storing, retrieving, disseminating, and displaying of clinical/service and nonclinical data and information.

Rationale for IM.3.10

Records resulting from data capture and report generation† are used for communication and continuity of the resident's care or financial and business operations over time. Records are also used for other purposes, including litigation and risk management activities, reimbursement, and statistics. Improved data capture and report generation systems enhance the value of the records. Potential benefits include improved resident care quality and safety, improved efficiency effectiveness and reduced costs in resident care, and financial and business operations. To maximize the benefits of data capture and report generation, these processes

MC

---

* **Protected health information** Health information that contains information such that an individual person can be identified as the subject of that information.

† **Report generation** The process of analyzing, organizing, and presenting recorded information for authentication and inclusion in the resident's health care record or in financial or business records.

exhibit the following characteristics: unique ID, accuracy, completeness, timeliness,* interoperability,† retrievability,‡ authentication and accountability,§ auditability, confidentiality, and security.

The processing, storage, and retrieval functions are integral to electronic, computerized, and paper-based information systems in organizations. Important considerations for these functions include data elements, data accuracy, data confidentiality, data security, data integrity, permanence of storage (the time a medium can safely store information), ease of retrievability, aggregation of information, interoperability, clinical/service practice considerations, performance improvement, and decision support processing.

A goal for information storage is to be linked or centrally organized and accessible. This could include the organization having an index identifying where the information is stored and how to access it; or, as the organization moves to electronic systems, the organization creates all information systems to be interoperable within the enterprise. As more organizations automate various processes and activities, it is important to share critical data among systems. As challenges of interoperability have arisen, standards organizations have stepped in to develop industry standards. It is important that the organization is aware of the standards development organizations and their recommendations.

Internally and externally generated data and information are accurately disseminated to users. Access to accurate information is required to deliver, improve, analyze, and advance resident care and the systems that support health care delivery. Information may be accessed and disseminated through electronic information systems or paper-based records and reports. The use of information should be considered in developing forms, screen displays, and standard or ad hoc reports.

Elements of Performance for IM.3.10

B   1.   Uniform data definitions and data capture methods are used.
- Minimum data sets, terminology, definitions, classifications, vocabulary, and nomenclature are standardized as needed.
- Industry standards are used whenever possible.

A Ⓜ 2.   Abbreviations, acronyms, and symbols are standardized throughout the organization, and there is a list of abbreviations, acronyms, and symbols not to use.

MC

---

* **Timeliness** The time between the occurrence of an event and the availability of data about the event. Timeliness is related to the use of the data.

† **Interoperability** Enables authorized users to capture, share, and report information from any system, whether paper or electronic based.

‡ **Retrievability** The capability of efficiently finding relevant information.

§ **Accountability** All information is attributable to its source (person or device).

B   3.   Quality control systems are used to monitor data content and collection activities.
- The method used assures timely and economical data collection with the degree of accuracy, completeness, and discrimination necessary for their intended use.
- The method used minimizes bias in the data and regularly assesses the data's reliability, validity, and accuracy.
- Those responsible for collecting and reviewing the data are accountable for information accuracy and completeness.

B   4.   Storage and retrieval systems are designed to support organization needs for clinical/service and organization-specific information.
- Storage and retrieval systems are designed to balance the ability to retrieve data and information with the intended use for the data and information.
- Storage and retrieval systems are designed to balance security and confidentiality issues with accessibility.
- Systems for paper and electronic records are designed to reduce disruption or inaccessibility during such times as diminished staffing and scheduled and unscheduled downtimes of electronic information systems.

A   5.   Data and information are retained for sufficient time to comply with law and regulation.

B   6.   Data and information are retained for quality of care and other organization needs.

B   7.   The necessary expertise and tools are available for collecting, retrieving, and analyzing data and their transformation into information.

B   8.   Data are organized and transformed into information in formats useful to decision makers.

B   9.   Dissemination of data and information is timely and accurate.

B   10. Data and information are disseminated in standard formats and methods to meet user needs and provide for easy retrievability and interpretation.

B   11. Industry or organization standards are used whenever possible for data display and transmission.

MC

Information-Based Decision Making

Standard IM.4.10 ━━━━━━━━━━━━━━━━━━━━━━━━━━━━━━

The information management system provides information for use in decision making.

Rationale for IM.4.10

Information management supports timely and effective decision making at all organization levels. The information management processes support managerial and operational decisions, performance improvement activities, and resident care, treatment, and service decisions. Clinical and strategic decision making depends on information from multiple sources, including the resident record, knowledge-based information, comparative data/information, and aggregate data/information.

Elements of Performance for IM.4.10

To support clinical decision making, information found in the resident record must include the following:

C Ⓜ 1. Readily accessible throughout the system

C Ⓜ 2. Accurately recorded

C Ⓜ 3. Complete

C Ⓜ 4. Organized for efficient retrieval of needed data

C Ⓜ 5. Timely

B 6. Comparative performance data and information are available for decision making, if applicable.

B 7. The organization has the ability to collect and aggregate data and information to support care, treatment, and service delivery and operations, including the following:
- Individual care, treatment, and services and care, treatment, and service delivery
- Decision making
- Management and operations
- Analysis of trends over time
- Performance comparisons over time within the organization and with other organizations
- Performance improvement
- Infection control
- Resident safety

MC

Standard IM.5.10 ━━━━━━━━━━━━━━━━━━━━━━━━━━━━━

Knowledge-based information* resources are readily available, current, and authoritative.

---

* **Knowledge-based information** A collection of stored facts, models, and information that can be used for designing and redesigning processes and for problem solving. In the context of this manual, knowledge-based information is found in the clinical, scientific, and management literature.

Rationale for IM.5.10

Organization practitioners and staff have access to knowledge-based information to do the following:

- Help them acquire and maintain the knowledge and skills needed to maintain and improve competence
- Help with clinical/service and management decision making
- Provide appropriate information and education to residents and families
- Support performance improvement and resident safety activities
- Support the institution's educational and research needs

Elements of Performance for IM.5.10

B   2.   The organization provides access to information resources needed by staff in print, electronic, Internet, audio, and/or other appropriate form.*

B   3.   Knowledge-based resources are available at all times to clinical/service staff, through electronic means, after-hours access to an in-house collection, or other methods.

B   4.   The organization has a plan to provide for access to information during times when electronic systems are unavailable.

Standard IM.6.50

Designated qualified personnel accept and transcribe verbal orders from authorized individuals.

Rationale for IM.6.50

Processes for receiving, transcribing, and authenticating verbal orders are established to protect the quality of resident care, treatment, and services.

Elements of Performance for IM.6.50

A   1.   Qualified personnel are identified, as defined by organization policy and, as appropriate, in accordance with state and federal law, and authorized to receive and record verbal orders.

C Ⓜ   2.   Each verbal order is dated and identifies the names of the individuals who gave and received it, and the record indicates who implemented it.

A   3.   When required by state or federal law and regulation, verbal orders are authenticated within the specified time frame.

A   4.   Implement a process for taking verbal or telephone orders or receiving critical test results that require a verification read-back of the complete order or test result by the person receiving the order or test result.

MC

---

* Forms of information include current texts, periodicals, indexes, abstracts, reports, documents, databases, directories, discussion lists, successful practices, standards, protocols, practice guidelines, clinical trials and other resources.

Standard IM.6.130 ▬▬▬▬▬▬▬▬▬▬▬▬▬▬▬▬▬▬▬▬▬▬▬▬

Clinical record documentation includes the provision of education and its effectiveness.

Element of Performance for IM.6.130

C Ⓜ 1. The provision of and the resident's response to education are documented in the clinical record.

MC

Crosswalks of Standards*

Crosswalk of 2002–2003 Standards for Long Term Care to 2004 "Ethics, Rights, and Responsibilities" Standards for Long Term Care

This crosswalk is designed to show where the 2002–2003 standards requirements appeared in the reformatted "Ethics, Rights, and Responsibilities" (RI) standards for 2004. The left column, 2002–2003 Standards, lists consecutively each standard that was effective in 2002–2003. The middle column, 2004 Standards, indicates the RI standards, with revised numbers, which became effective January 1, 2004. The right column, Comments, identifies what changes occurred between the 2002–2003 standards and the 2004 standards.

2002–2003 Standards	2004 Standards	Comments
RI.1 The organization respects residents' rights and addresses ethical issues in providing care.	RI.2.10 The organization respects the rights of residents. RI.2.20 Residents receive information about their rights. RI.2.30 Residents are involved in decisions about care, treatment, and services provided. RI.2.80 The organization addresses the wishes of the resident relating to end-of-life decisions. RI.2.120 The organization addresses the resolution of complaints from residents and their families. RI.2.130 The organization respects the needs of residents for confidentiality, privacy, and security. RI.2.180 The organization protects research subjects and respects their rights during research, investigation, and clinical trials involving human subjects. HR.2.10 Orientation provides initial job training and information.	Requirement added to **RI.2.20** to address informing residents about policies and procedures regarding the handling of life-threatening emergencies.
RI.1.1 The resident is informed of his or her rights before or on admission.	RI.2.20 Residents receive information about their rights.	Reformatted and renumbered only.
RI.1.1.1 Residents are involved in resolving conflicts about care decisions.	RI.2.30 Residents are involved in decisions about care, treatment, and services provided.	Reformatted and renumbered only.
RI.1.2 Residents and, when appropriate, their families are informed about the outcomes of care, including unanticipated outcomes.	RI.2.90 Residents and, when appropriate, their families are informed about the outcomes of care, treatment, and services, including unanticipated outcomes.	Reformatted and renumbered only.
RI.2 The resident has a right to a quality of life that supports independent expression, choice, and decision making, consistent with applicable law and regulation.	RI.2.210 Residents have a right to a quality of life that supports independent expression, choice, and decision making, consistent with applicable law and regulation.	Reformatted and renumbered only.
RI.2.1 The resident has a right to considerate care that respects his or her personal values, beliefs, cultural and spiritual preferences, and life-long patterns of living.	RI.2.220 Residents receive care that respects their personal values, beliefs, cultural and spiritual preferences, and life-long patterns of living.	Reformatted and renumbered only.
RI.2.1.1 The resident has a right to personal freedom and dignity.	RI.2.10 The organization respects the rights of residents.	Reformatted and renumbered only.
RI.2.1.2 The resident has a right to impartial access to treatment or accommodations.	RI.2.20 Residents receive information about their rights.	Reformatted and renumbered only.

CW

---

* Crosswalks of 2002–2003 Standards to 2004 Standards are the same as published in the 2004 book. Some standards chapters have an additional crosswalk showing changes from 2004 to 2005–2006.

2002–2003 Standards	2004 Standards	Comments
RI.2.2 The resident has a right to confidentiality of information.	RI.2.130 The organization respects the needs of residents for confidentiality, privacy, and security. RI.2.20 Residents receive information about their rights.	Reformatted and renumbered only.
RI.2.3 The resident has a right to privacy, safety, and security.	RI.2.130 The organization respects the needs of residents for confidentiality, privacy, and security.	Reformatted and renumbered only.
RI.2.4 The resident has a right to exercise citizenship privileges.	RI.2.200 Residents have a right to exercise citizenship privileges.	Reformatted and renumbered only.
RI.2.5 The resident has a right to unlimited contact with visitors and others.	RI.2.110 Residents have a right to unlimited contact with visitors and others.	Reformatted and renumbered only.
RI.2.6 The resident has a right to appropriate assessment and management of pain.	RI.2.160 Residents have the right to pain management.	Reformatted and renumbered only.
RI.2.7 The resident has a right to freedom from chemical or physical restraint.	RI.2.230 Residents have a right to freedom from chemical or physical restraint.	Reformatted and renumbered only.
RI.2.8 The resident has a right to freedom from mental, physical, sexual, and verbal abuse, neglect, or exploitation.	RI.2.150 Residents have a right to be free from mental, physical, sexual, and verbal abuse, neglect, and exploitation. HR.1.20 The organization has a process to ensure that a person's qualifications are consistent with his or her job responsibilities.	Reformatted and renumbered only.
RI.2.9 The resident has the right to perform or refuse to perform tasks in or for the organization.	RI.2.190 In organizations that provide opportunities for work, a defined policy addresses situations in which residents work.	Reformatted and renumbered only.
RI.2.10 The resident has a right to participate or refuse to participate in social groups or community activities.	RI.2.240 Residents can participate or refuse to participate in social, spiritual, or community activities and groups.	Reformatted and renumbered only.
RI.2.11 The resident has a right to keep and use personal clothing and possessions.	RI.2.140 Residents have a right to an environment that preserves dignity and contributes to a positive self image.	Reformatted and renumbered only.
RI.2.12 The resident has a right to an environment that preserves dignity and contributes to a positive self-image.	RI.2.140 Residents have a right to an environment that preserves dignity and contributes to a positive self image.	Reformatted and renumbered only.
RI.2.13 The resident has a right to manage or delegate management of personal financial affairs.	RI.2.290 Residents have a right to manage or delegate management of personal financial affairs.	Reformatted and renumbered only.
RI.2.14 As appropriate to the care plan, the resident has a right to access transportation services.	RI.2.250 As appropriate to their care or service plan, residents can access transportation services.	Reformatted and renumbered only.
RI.2.15 The resident has a right to effective communication.	RI.2.100 The organization respects the resident's right to and need for effective communication.	Reformatted and renumbered only.
RI.2.16 The resident has a right to have complaints heard, reviewed, and, when possible, resolved.	RI.2.120 The organization addresses the resolution of complaints from residents and their families. RI.2.170 Residents have a right to access protective and advocacy services.	Reformatted and renumbered only.
RI.2.17 The resident has a right to a resident council.	RI.2.260 Residents have a right to a resident council.	Reformatted and renumbered only.
RI.2.18 The resident has a right to give informed consent.	RI.2.40 Informed consent is obtained.	Reformatted and renumbered only.
RI.2.19 Residents are involved in decisions to provide or withhold resuscitative services and provide, forgo, or withdraw life-sustaining treatment.	RI.2.80 The organization addresses the wishes of the resident relating to end-of-life decisions.	Reformatted and renumbered only.
RI.2.20 Residents are involved in decisions related to care at the end of their lives.	PC.8.70 Comfort and dignity are optimized during end-of-life care.	Reformatted and renumbered only.
RI.2.21 The resident has a right to select medical, dental, and other licensed independent practitioner care providers.	RI.2.270 Residents can select their medical, dental, and other licensed independent practitioner care providers.	Reformatted and renumbered only.

CW

2002–2003 Standards	2004 Standards	Comments
RI.2.22 The resident has a right to communicate with his or her medical, dental, and other licensed independent practitioner care providers.	**RI.2.280** Residents have a right to communicate with their medical, dental, and other licensed independent practitioner care providers.	Reformatted and renumbered only.
RI.2.23 The resident has a right to refuse care or treatment to the extent permitted by law.	**RI.2.70** Residents have the right to refuse care, treatment, or services in accordance with law and regulation.	Reformatted and renumbered only.
RI.2.24 The resident has a right to involve his or her family in making care or treatment decisions.	**RI.2.30** Residents are involved in decisions about care, treatment, and services provided.	Reformatted and renumbered only.
RI.2.25 The resident has a right to formulate advance directives.	**RI.2.80** The organization addresses the wishes of the resident relating to end-of-life decisions.	Reformatted and renumbered only.
RI.3 The organization respects and protects residents' rights during research, investigation, or clinical trials involving human subjects.	**RI.2.180** The organization protects research subjects and respects their rights during research, investigation, and clinical trials involving human subjects.	Requirements added to **RI.2.180** to address confidentiality and inclusion of research information in the clinical record, and handling of harmful consequences experienced as a result of the research.
RI.3.1 The resident has the right to participate in research, investigation, or clinical trials.	**RI.2.180** The organization protects research subjects and respects their rights during research, investigation, and clinical trials involving human subjects.	Reformatted and renumbered only.
RI.4 The organization practices ethical behavior regarding admissions, care, transfer, discharge, and billing.	**RI.1.10** The organization follows ethical behavior in its care, treatment, and services and business practices.	Part of the concept of **LD.2.4** (The leaders ensure comparable performance or resident care processes throughout the organization) was moved to **RI.1.10**. In addition, **HR.5** (The organization addresses staff requests to not participate in any aspect of resident care or treatment) and **HR.5.1** (The organization ensures that a resident's care or treatment is not negatively affected if the organization grants a staff request to not participate in an aspect of resident care or treatment) were moved to **RI.1.10**.
RI.4.1 The organization practices ethical behavior regarding marketing.	**RI.1.10** The organization follows ethical behavior in its care, treatment, and services and business practices.	Reformatted and renumbered only.
RI.4.2 The organization practices ethical behavior involving the relationship of the organization and its staff with other health care providers, educational institutions, and payers.	**RI.1.20** The organization addresses conflicts of interest.	Reformatted and renumbered only.
RI.4.3 The integrity of clinical decision making is not compromised regardless of how the organization compensates or shares financial risk with its leaders, managers, clinical staff, and licensed independent practitioners.	**RI.1.30** The integrity of decisions is based on identified care, treatment, and service needs of the residents.	Reformatted and renumbered only.
CC.6 An established procedure(s) is used to resolve denial-of-care conflicts. When care or services are subject to internal or external review that results in the denial of care, services, or payment, the organization makes decisions regarding the provision of ongoing care or discharge based on the assessed needs of the residents.	**RI.1.40** When care, treatment, and services are subject to internal or external review that results in the denial of care, treatment, services, or payment, the organization makes decisions regarding the provision of ongoing care, treatment, services, or discharge based on the assessed needs of the residents.	Reformatted and renumbered only.
PF.3.8 Education includes information about resident responsibilities in the resident's care.	**RI.3.10** Residents are given information about their responsibilities while receiving care, treatment, and services.	Reformatted and renumbered only.
	RI.2.50 Consent is obtained for recording or filming made for purposes other than the identification, diagnosis, or treatment of the residents.	New standard based on a Joint Commission standards clarification/FAQ.

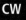

CW

Crosswalk of 2002–2003 Standards for Long Term Care to 2004 "Provision of Care, Treatment, and Services" Standards for Long Term Care

This crosswalk is designed to show where the 2002–2003 standards requirements appeared in the "Provision of Care, Treatment, and Services" (PC) standards for 2004. The left column, 2002–2003 Standards, lists consecutively each standard that was effective in 2002–2003. These standards are from the 2002–2003 "Continuum of Care," "Assessment of Residents," "Care and Treatment of Residents," and "Education of Residents" chapters. The middle column, 2004 Standards, indicates the new PC standards that became effective January 1, 2004. The right column, Comments, identifies what changes occurred between the 2002–2003 standards and the 2004 standards.

2002–2003 Standards	2004 Standards	Comments
CC.1 Within its capability, the organization has a process to provide access to the appropriate level of care and services based on the residents' assessed needs.	PC.1.10 The organization accepts for care, treatment, and services only those residents whose identified care, treatment, and services needs it can meet.	Reformatted and renumbered only.
CC.2 Individuals are accepted to appropriate care and services based on the organization's assessment procedures.	PC.1.10 The organization accepts for care, treatment, and services only those residents whose identified care, treatment, and services needs it can meet.	Reformatted and renumbered only.
CC.2.1 Criteria define the information necessary to determine the appropriate care, service, and setting.	PC.1.10 The organization accepts for care, treatment, and services only those residents whose identified care, treatment, and services needs it can meet.	Reformatted and renumbered only.
CC.3 The organization provides for continuity over time among the care and services provided to a resident.	PC.5.60 The organization coordinates the care, treatment, and services provided to a resident as part of the plan for care, treatment, and services and consistent with the scope of care, treatment, and services offered by the organization.	Reformatted and renumbered only.
CC.3.1 The organization provides for coordination of care and services among health professionals and settings.	PC.5.60 The organization coordinates the care, treatment, and services provided to a resident as part of the plan for care, treatment, and services and consistent with the organization's scope of care, treatment, and services.	Reformatted and renumbered only.
CC.4 Referral, transfer, discontinuation of services, or discharge of residents to other levels of care, health professionals, or settings are based on residents' assessed needs and each organization's capability to provide needed care and services.	PC.15.20 The transfer or discharge of a resident to another level of care, treatment, and services; different health professionals; or different settings is based on the resident's assessed needs and the organization's capabilities.	Reformatted and renumbered only.
CC.4.1 The follow-up process provides for continuing care based on the residents' needs.	PC.15.20 The transfer or discharge of a resident to another level of care, treatment, and services; different health professionals; or different settings is based on the resident's assessed needs and the organization's capabilities.	Reformatted and renumbered only.
CC.4.1.1 The residents are informed in a timely manner of the need for planning for discharge or transfer to another organization or level of care.	PC.15.20 The transfer or discharge of a resident to another level of care, treatment, and services; different health professionals; or different settings is based on the resident's assessed needs and the organization's capabilities.	Reformatted and renumbered only.
CC.4.1.2 Residents are transferred or discharged by order of their attending physician.	PC.15.10 A process addresses the needs for continuing care, treatment, and services after discharge or transfer.	Reformatted and renumbered only.
CC.4.1.3 The organization follows an established process for emergency discharge due to medical necessity.	PC.15.10 A process addresses the needs for continuing care, treatment, and services after discharge or transfer.	Reformatted and renumbered only.

CW

2002–2003 Standards	2004 Standards	Comments
CC.4.1.4 Residents are allowed to remain in a facility unless they meet specific criteria in accordance with law and regulation.	**PC.15.40** Residents are not transferred or discharged unless they meet specific criteria in accordance with law and regulation.	Reformatted and renumbered only.
CC.4.1.5 The organization informs residents and their families of its bed-hold policy.	**PC.15.50** The organization tells residents and their families of its bed-hold policy.	Reformatted and renumbered only.
CC.5 Appropriate information related to the care and services provided is exchanged when residents are accepted, referred, transferred, discontinued service, or discharged to receive further care or services.	**PC.15.30** When residents are transferred or discharged, appropriate information related to the care, treatment, and services provided is exchanged with other service providers.	Reformatted and renumbered only.
CC.6 An established procedure(s) is used to resolve denial-of-care conflicts. When care or services are subject to internal or external review that results in denial of care, services, or payment, the organization makes decisions regarding the provision of ongoing care or discharge based on the assessed needs of the residents.	No standard.	Covered in **RI.1.40.**
PE.1 Resident assessment process is defined by the organization.	**PC.2.20** The organization defines in writing the data and information gathered during assessment and reassessment.	Reformatted and renumbered only.
PE.1.1 A registered nurse coordinates the completion of each resident's assessment.	**PC.2.130** Initial assessments are performed as defined by the organization.	Reformatted and renumbered only.
PE.1.2 Each resident's initial assessment is completed within the time frame specified by organization policy, by law and regulation, not to exceed 14 days.	**PC.2.120** The organization defines in writing the time frame(s) for conducting the initial assessment(s).	Reformatted and renumbered only.
PE.1.2.1 The attending physician or authorized licensed independent practitioner performs each resident's medical assessment, including a medical history and physical examination, within required time frames.	**PC.2.120** The organization defines in writing the time frame(s) for conducting the initial assessment(s).	Reformatted and renumbered only.
PE.2 Each resident's physical, functional, psychosocial, and nutritional status is assessed.	**PC.2.130** Initial assessments are performed as defined by the organization.	Reformatted and renumbered only.
PE.2.1 Each resident's physical, functional, psychosocial, and nutritional status is initially assessed to determine the need for care, the type of care to be provided, and the need for further assessment. The initial assessment includes:	**PC.2.130** Initial assessments are performed as defined by the organization.	Reformatted and renumbered only.
PE.2.1.1 the resident's relevant past medical history and medical status, including current diagnosis, medications, allergies, treatments, results of diagnostic or laboratory studies, prognosis, limitations, and precautions;	**PC.2.20** The organization defines in writing the data and information gathered during assessment and reassessment.	Reformatted and renumbered only.
PE.2.1.2 the resident's neuropsychiatric status, including mental, affective, and cognitive status and needs, such as sleeping patterns or memory, recall ability, and decision-making ability, behavior patterns;	**PC.2.20** The organization defines in writing the data and information gathered during assessment and reassessment.	Reformatted and renumbered only.
PE.2.1.3 the resident's communication status, including hearing, speech, language, voice, and modes of expression;	**PC.2.20** The organization defines in writing the data and information gathered during assessment and reassessment.	Reformatted and renumbered only.
PE.2.1.4 the resident's rehabilitation status and needs, including previous and current functional status, ability to perform activities of daily living, mobility, balance, strength, bowel and bladder function, sensory capacity and impairments, ability to swallow, orientation, and rehabilitation potential;	**PC.2.20** The organization defines in writing the data and information gathered during assessment and reassessment.	Reformatted and renumbered only.

CW

2002–2003 Standards	2004 Standards	Comments
PE.2.1.5 the resident's psychosocial status, including level of functioning, cultural and ethnic factors, current emotional status, social skills, family circumstances, family relationships, current living situation, relevant past history, past roles, and response to current status;	**PC.2.20** The organization defines in writing the data and information gathered during assessment and reassessment.	Reformatted and renumbered only.
PE.2.1.5.1 the resident's spiritual status and needs, including spiritual orientation and the dying individual's concerns related to hope, despair, guilt, or forgiveness;	**PC.2.20** The organization defines in writing the data and information gathered during assessment and reassessment.	Reformatted and renumbered only.
PE.2.1.6 the resident's physical status, including musculoskeletal, cardiorespiratory, gastrointestinal, and integumentary status and foot care needs;	**PC.2.20** The organization defines in writing the data and information gathered during assessment and reassessment.	Reformatted and renumbered only.
PE.2.1.7 the resident's activities status, needs, and potential, including use of free time; personal preferences regarding schedules and grooming; preadmission hobbies, interests, and life-style; past and current recreational activities; and ability to participate in structured and group activities;	**PC.2.20** The organization defines in writing the data and information gathered during assessment and reassessment.	Reformatted and renumbered only.
PE.2.1.8 the resident's nutritional and hydration status and needs; potential nutritional risk and deficiencies; cultural, religious, or ethnic food preferences; special dietary requirements; and nutrient-intake patterns;	**PC.2.20** The organization defines in writing the data and information gathered during assessment and reassessment.	Reformatted and renumbered only.
PE.2.1.9 the resident's dental status and oral health, including the condition of the oral cavity, teeth, and tooth-supporting structures; the presence or absence of natural teeth or dentures; and the ability to function with or without natural teeth or dentures;	**PC.2.20** The organization defines in writing the data and information gathered during assessment and reassessment.	Reformatted and renumbered only.
PE.2.1.10 the resident's pain, including its origin, location, severity, alleviating and exacerbating factors, and current treatment and response to treatment;	**PC.8.10** When pain is identified, the resident is assessed and treated by the organization or referred for treatment.	Reformatted and renumbered only.
PE.2.1.11 the resident's response to stress caused by the illness and required treatment;	**PC.2.20** The organization defines in writing the data and information gathered during assessment and reassessment.	Reformatted and renumbered only.
PE.2.1.12 identifying ways to enhance the resident's activity and recreational skills, based on his or her cognitive abilities and the limitations of his or her illness or treatment; and	**PC.2.20** The organization defines in writing the data and information gathered during assessment and reassessment.	Reformatted and renumbered only.
PE.2.1.13 the resident's and family's educational needs, preferences, abilities, and readiness to learn.	**PC.2.20** The organization defines in writing the data and information gathered during assessment and reassessment.	Reformatted and renumbered only.
PE.2.2 The need for further assessment is identified.	**PC.2.20** The organization defines in writing the data and information gathered during assessment and reassessment.	Reformatted and renumbered only.
PE.2.2.1 The scope and intensity of any further assessments are determined by screening criteria, the resident's diagnosis, the treatment setting, the resident's desire for treatment, or the resident's response to previous treatment.	**PC.2.20** The organization defines in writing the data and information gathered during assessment and reassessment.	Reformatted and renumbered only.
PE.2.3 Each resident's discharge needs are assessed.	**PC.2.20** The organization defines in writing the data and information gathered during assessment and reassessment.	Reformatted and renumbered only.

CW

2002–2003 Standards	2004 Standards	Comments
PE.3 Each resident is reassessed at regularly specified intervals related to the course of treatment or when the resident's physical, psychosocial, functional, or nutritional status significantly changes, and at regular intervals required by law and regulation.	**PC.2.150** Residents are reassessed as needed.	Reformatted and renumbered only.
PC.4 Possible victims of abuse, neglect, and exploitation are identified using criteria developed by the organization.	**PC.3.10** Residents who may be victims of abuse, neglect, or exploitation are assessed (see standard **RI.2.150**).	Reformatted and renumbered only.
PE.4.1 Victims of alleged or suspected abuse, neglect, and exploitation are assessed.	**PC.3.10** Residents who may be victims of abuse, neglect, or exploitation are assessed (see standard **RI.2.150**).	Reformatted and renumbered only.
PE.4.1.1 Assessments are conducted with the resident's or legal guardian's consent, or as otherwise provided by law.	No standard.	Covered in **RI.2.40**.
PE.4.1.2 During such assessments, the organization collects, retains, and safeguards material pertinent to the investigation of the alleged abuse, neglect and exploitation.	No standard.	Covered in **IM.2.10**.
PE.4.1.3 During such assessments, the organization notifies and releases information to the proper authorities, as legally required.	**PC.3.10** Residents who may be victims of abuse, neglect, or exploitation are assessed (see standard **RI.2.150**).	Reformatted and renumbered only.
PE.5 Radiologic and other diagnostic services, including pathology and clinical laboratory services, are available 24 hours a day, seven days a week.	**PC.3.230** Diagnostic testing necessary for determining the resident's health care needs is performed.	Reformatted and renumbered only.
PE.5.1 Diagnostic testing relevant to the resident's health status is ordered, provided, and reported, as required.	**PC.3.230** Diagnostic testing necessary for determining the resident's health care needs is performed.	Reformatted and renumbered only.
PE.6 Waived testing, as classified under federal law and regulation, meets the following requirements:	No standard.	This was a nonscorable standard. The concept is addressed in the Introduction to the waived testing standards.
PE.6.1 The organization defines the extent that test results are used in a resident's care.	**PC.16.10** The organization defines the extent to which waived test results are used in resident care, treatment, and services (definitively or only as a screen).	Reformatted and renumbered only.
PE.6.2 Staff responsible for performing tests and those responsible for directing or supervising the testing are identified.	**PC.16.20** The organization identifies the staff responsible for performing and supervising waived testing.	Reformatted and renumbered only.
PE.6.3 Staff performing tests receive specific training and orientation and demonstrate satisfactory competence.	**PC.16.30** Staff performing tests has adequate, specific training and orientation to perform the tests and demonstrates satisfactory levels of competence.	Reformatted and renumbered only.
PE.6.4 Policies and procedures governing specific testing-related processes are current and readily available.	**PC.16.40** Approved policies and procedures for specific testing-related processes are current and readily available.	Reformatted and renumbered only.
PE.6.5 Quality control checks are conducted on each procedure as defined by the organization.	**PC.16.50** Quality control checks, as defined by the organization, are conducted on each procedure.	Reformatted and renumbered only.
PE.6.5.1 At a minimum, manufacturers' instructions are followed.	**PC.16.50** Quality control checks, as defined by the organization, are conducted on each procedure.	Reformatted and renumbered only.
PE.6.5.2 Appropriate quality-control and test records are maintained.	**PC.16.60** Appropriate quality-control and test records are maintained.	Reformatted and renumbered only.
PE.6.6 If the organization provides for the maintenance and transfusion of blood or blood components, it meets all applicable law and regulation.	**PC.9.10** Blood and blood components are administered safely.	Reformatted and renumbered only.
TX.1 A care-planning process is designed to ensure that the care and treatment planning is systematic and comprehensive.	**PC.4.10** Development of a plan for care, treatment, and services is individualized and appropriate to the resident's needs, strengths, limitations, and goals.	Reformatted and renumbered only.

CW

2002–2003 Standards	2004 Standards	Comments
TX.1.1 An interim care plan is developed.	**PC.4.10** Development of a plan for care, treatment, and services is individualized and appropriate to the resident's needs, strengths, limitations, and goals.	Reformatted and renumbered only.
TX.1.1.1 An individualized, interdisciplinary care plan is developed by an interdisciplinary team representing all appropriate health care professionals as soon as possible after admission, but no later than seven calendar days after comprehensive assessments are completed.	**PC.4.10** Development of a plan for care, treatment, and services is individualized and appropriate to the resident's needs, strengths, limitations, and goals.	Reformatted and renumbered only.
TX.1.2 Care planning is individualized to address the resident's problems, needs, and severity of condition, impairment, disability, or disease.	**PC.4.10** Development of a plan for care, treatment, and services is individualized and appropriate to the resident's needs, strengths, limitations, and goals.	Reformatted and renumbered only.
TX.1.2.1 Individualized care and treatment goals are reasonable and measurable.	**PC.4.10** Development of a plan for care, treatment, and services is individualized and appropriate to the resident's needs, strengths, limitations, and goals.	Reformatted and renumbered only.
TX.1.3 Care is planned through a coordinated and collaborative approach by the interdisciplinary team.	**PC.4.10** Development of a plan for care, treatment, and services is individualized and appropriate to the resident's needs, strengths, limitations, and goals.	Reformatted and renumbered only.
TX.1.3.1 Advance directives are incorporated into the care-planning process.	No standard.	Covered in **RI.2.30**.
TX.1.4 The attending physician prescribes the medical requirements of care for the residents he or she admits.	**PC.5.30** The attending physician prescribes the medical requirements of care for the residents he or she admits.	Reformatted and renumbered only.
TX.1.4.1 Residents and family participate in developing and reviewing the care plan.	No standard.	Covered in **RI.2.30**.
TX.1.4.2 Medical services are available to meet the resident's medical needs.	No standard.	Covered in **LD.3.10**.
TX.1.4.3 The attending physician visits the resident in accordance with the resident's needs, and at least once during the 30 days following admission.	**PC.5.40** The attending physician visits the resident in accordance with the resident's needs and at least once during the 30 days after admission.	Reformatted and renumbered only.
TX.1.4.4 Each attending physician designates an alternate physician whom the organization can contact to obtain regular or emergency care when the attending physician is not available.	**PC.5.30** The attending physician prescribes the medical requirements of care for the residents he or she admits.	Reformatted and renumbered only.
TX.1.4.5 Oral health services are available to meet residents' needs.	**PC.5.60** The organization coordinates the care, treatment, and services provided to a resident as part of the plan for care, treatment, and services and consistent with the organization's scope of care, treatment, and services.	Reformatted and renumbered only.
TX.1.5 Spiritual services are provided to meet residents' needs.	**PC.5.60** The organization coordinates the care, treatment, and services provided to a resident as part of the plan for care, treatment, and services and consistent with the organization's scope of care, treatment, and services.	Reformatted and renumbered only.
TX.1.5.1 Behavioral health services are provided to meet residents' psychosocial needs.	**PC.5.60** The organization coordinates the care, treatment, and services provided to a resident as part of the plan for care, treatment, and services and consistent with the organization's scope of care, treatment, and services.	Reformatted and renumbered only.
TX.1.5.2 Activity services are provided to meet residents' needs.	**PC.5.60** The organization coordinates the care, treatment, and services provided to a resident as part of the plan for care, treatment, and services and consistent with the organization's scope of care, treatment, and services.	Reformatted and renumbered only.

CW

2002–2003 Standards	2004 Standards	Comments
TX.1.5.3 Services are provided to assist with guardianship and conservatorship, when indicated.	**PC.5.60** The organization coordinates the care, treatment, and services provided to a resident as part of the plan for care, treatment, and services and consistent with the organization's scope of care, treatment, and services.	Reformatted and renumbered only.
TX.1.5.4 Services are provided to assist in the development of a family and visitor council.	**PC.5.60** The organization coordinates the care, treatment, and services provided to a resident as part of the plan for care, treatment, and services and consistent with the organization's scope of care, treatment, and services.	Reformatted and renumbered only.
TX.2 Planned care is provided in a collaborative and interdisciplinary manner.	**PC.5.50** Care, treatment, and services are provided in an interdisciplinary, collaborative manner.	Reformatted and renumbered only.
TX.2.1 Residents receive appropriate services and interventions in response to physical and functional problems and needs.	**PC.5.10** The organization provides care, treatment, and services for each resident according to the plan for care, treatment, and services.	Reformatted and renumbered only.
TX.2.2 Residents are clean and well-groomed.	**PC.8.20** When necessary, residents receive appropriate restorative services, including assistance with activities of daily living, such as eating, dressing, grooming, bathing, oral hygiene, ambulation, and toilet activities.	Reformatted and renumbered only.
TX.2.3 Residents are assisted with self-care, as appropriate.	**PC.8.20** When necessary, residents receive appropriate restorative services, including assistance with activities of daily living, such as eating, dressing, grooming, bathing, oral hygiene, ambulation, and toilet activities.	Reformatted and renumbered only.
TX.2.3.1 Residents are helped with dining activities.	**PC.8.20** When necessary, residents receive appropriate restorative services, including assistance with activities of daily living, such as eating, dressing, grooming, bathing, oral hygiene, ambulation, and toilet activities.	Reformatted and renumbered only.
TX.2.4 All reasonable steps are taken to keep residents safe from accident and injury.	**PC.8.20** When necessary, residents receive appropriate restorative services, including assistance with activities of daily living, such as eating, dressing, grooming, bathing, oral hygiene, ambulation, and toilet activities.	Reformatted and renumbered only.
TX.2.5 Residents receive care to prevent and treat health-related complications.	**PC.8.30** Residents at risk for health-related complications receive appropriate preventive care.	Reformatted and renumbered only.
TX.2.6 Residents are helped so they can participate in social and diversional activities according to their functional levels.	**PC. 8.40** Residents are helped so they can participate in social and diversional activities according to their functional levels.	Reformatted and renumbered only.
TX.3 The resident's response to care and services is evaluated.	**PC.2.150** Residents are reassessed as needed.	Reformatted and renumbered only.
TX.3.1 The care plan is evaluated and revised as necessary to reflect the resident's status and as required by law and regulation.	**PC.4.10** Development of a plan for care, treatment, and services is individualized and appropriate to the resident's needs, strengths, limitations, and goals.	Reformatted and renumbered only.
TX.4 Processes are designed and implemented to ensure that medications are safely and effectively used.	No standard.	Moved to "Medication Management" chapter.
TX.4.1 Only medications needed to treat the resident's conditions are prescribed.	No standard.	Moved to "Medication Management" chapter.
TX.4.2 The long term care organization has an inventory of medications available to meet residents' needs.	No standard.	Moved to "Medication Management" chapter.
TX.4.2.1 Medications are stored and distributed safely in accordance with defined policies and procedures.	No standard.	Moved to "Medication Management" chapter.

CW

2002–2003 Standards	2004 Standards	Comments
TX.4.2.2 Medications are stored under proper conditions of sanitation, temperature, light, moisture, ventilation, segregation, and security.	No standard.	Moved to "Medication Management" chapter.
TX.4.2.3 When medications are prepared in the pharmacy, proper conditions of sanitation, temperature, light, moisture, ventilation, segregation, safety, and security are maintained.	No standard.	Moved to "Medication Management" chapter.
TX.4.2.4 Medications are dispensed safely and accurately to residents for whom they are prescribed or ordered.	No standard.	Moved to "Medication Management" chapter.
TX.4.2.5 Records of dispensed medications are kept as required to maintain control and accountability.	No standard.	Moved to "Medication Management" chapter.
TX.4.3 Controlled drugs are reconciled.	No standard.	Moved to "Medication Management" chapter.
TX.4.4 Medications are appropriately labeled.	No standard.	Moved to "Medication Management" chapter.
TX.4.5 The medication-dose system(s) is effective.	No standard.	Moved to "Medication Management" chapter.
TX.4.6 Important resident medication information is used and communicated.	No standard.	Moved to "Medication Management" chapter.
TX.4.7 Pharmacy services are available at all times.	No standard.	Moved to "Medication Management" chapter.
TX.4.8 The emergency-medication system(s) is effective.	No standard.	Moved to "Medication Management" chapter.
TX.4.9 The organization designs and implements an effective medication-recall system.	No standard.	Moved to "Medication Management" chapter.
TX.4.10 Medications are safely and accurately administered.	No standard.	Moved to "Medication Management" chapter.
TX.4.11 Safe self-administration of medication is supported.	No standard.	Moved to "Medication Management" chapter.
TX.4.12 Investigational medications are safely controlled and administered.	No standard.	Moved to "Medication Management" chapter.
TX.4.13 The effect of medication on the resident is monitored on an ongoing basis.	No standard.	Moved to "Medication Management" chapter.
TX.4.13.1 Assessment of medication effects is based on staff observations, the resident's perceptions, and information from the medical record and medication profile.	No standard.	Moved to "Medication Management" chapter.
TX.4.13.2 Psychotropic medication use is monitored.	No standard.	Moved to "Medication Management" chapter.
TX.4.13.3 Findings of medication monitoring are used to improve or maintain the resident's clinical outcome.	No standard.	Moved to "Medication Management" chapter.
TX.4.14 Significant medication errors and significant adverse drug reactions are reported in a timely manner.	No standard.	Moved to "Medication Management" chapter.
TX.4.14.1 Nursing, pharmacy, and other appropriate staff collaboratively develop and maintain processes for defining, identifying, and reviewing, and responding to these significant medication errors.	No standard.	Moved to "Medication Management" chapter.
TX.4.14.2 Nursing, pharmacy, and other appropriate staff collaboratively develop and maintain processes for defining, identifying, and reviewing, and responding to these significant adverse drug reactions.	No standard.	Moved to "Medication Management" chapter.
TX.5 The interdisciplinary care plan includes a plan for nutrition care.	No standard.	This is covered by the broader care planning standard **PC.4.10**.

CW

2002–2003 Standards	2004 Standards	Comments
TX.5.1 When necessary, a therapeutic diet or nutrition product(s) is prescribed in a timely manner by authorized individuals and provided to support optimal nutritional status.	**PC.7.10** The organization has a process for preparing and/or distributing food and nutrition products.	Reformatted and renumbered only.
TX.5.2 Menus are planned and posted in areas accessible to residents.	**PC.7.10** The organization has a process for preparing and/or distributing food and nutrition products.	Reformatted and renumbered only.
TX.5.2.1 Cycled menus are rotated over a period of at least three weeks.	**PC.7.10** The organization has a process for preparing and/or distributing food and nutrition products.	Reformatted and renumbered only.
TX.5.3 Responsibilities for preparing and distributing food and nutrition products are fulfilled.	**PC.7.10** The organization has a process for preparing and/or distributing food and nutrition products.	Reformatted and renumbered only.
TX.5.4 Responsibilities for administering food and nutrition products are fulfilled.	**PC.7.10** The organization has a process for preparing and/or distributing food and nutrition products.	Reformatted and renumbered only.
TX.5.5 Food and nutrition products are stored and prepared under proper conditions of sanitation, temperature, light, moisture, ventilation, and security.	**PC.7.10** The organization has a process for preparing and/or distributing food and nutrition products.	Reformatted and renumbered only.
TX.5.6 Each resident's food and nutrition products are distributed and served or administered in a safe, accurate, timely, and acceptable manner.	**PC.7.10** The organization has a process for preparing and/or distributing food and nutrition products.	Reformatted and renumbered only.
TX.5.7 Each resident's nutrition and hydration status is monitored.	No standard.	This is covered by the broader care planning standard **PC.4.10**.
TX.5.8 The organization provides food or nutrition products when diets or diet schedules change.	**PC.7.10** The organization has a process for preparing and/or distributing food and nutrition products.	Reformatted and renumbered only.
TX.6 Qualified rehabilitation professionals develop an individualized rehabilitation plan with the resident and his or her family, social network, or support system.	No standard.	Covered by the broader assessment standards **PC.2.20, PC.2.120, PC.2.130, PC.2.150**.
TX.6.1 Qualified rehabilitation professionals provide rehabilitation services consistent with professional licensure laws, regulations, registration, and certification.	No standard.	Covered by the broader assessment standards **PC.2.20, PC.2.120, PC.2.130, PC.2.150**.
TX.6.2 Residents receive appropriate rehabilitation services and interventions in response to physical and functional problems and needs as described in the care plan.	No standard.	Covered by the broader provision of care standard **PC.5.10**.
TX.6.3 Reassessment of the resident receiving rehabilitation services is an ongoing process.	No standard.	Covered by the broader reassessment standard **PC.2.150**.
TX.6.4 Discharge planning from rehabilitation services is integrated into the functional rehabilitation assessment.	No standard.	Covered by the broader care planning standard **PC.4.10**.
TX.6.5 Rehabilitation outcomes are restoration, improvement, or the maintenance of the resident's optimal level of functioning, self-care, self-responsibility, independence, and quality of life.	No standard.	Covered by the broader provision of care standard **PC.5.10**.
TX.7 The care of the dying resident optimizes his or her comfort and dignity.	**PC.8.70** Comfort and dignity are optimized during end-of-life care.	Reformatted and renumbered only.
TX.8 The organization designs a system to achieve a restraint-free environment.	**PC.11.80** The organization designs a system to achieve a restraint-free environment.	Reformatted and renumbered only.
TX.8.1 When alternatives to the use of restraint are ineffective, restraint is safely and appropriately used.	**PC.11.90** When alternatives to restraint are ineffective, restraint is safely and appropriately used.	Reformatted and renumbered only.

CW

2002–2003 Standards	2004 Standards	Comments
TX.9 A presedation or preanesthesia assessment is performed for each patient before beginning moderate or deep sedation and before anesthesia induction.	**PC.13.20** Operative or other procedures and/or the administration of moderate or deep sedation or anesthesia are planned.	Reformatted and renumbered only.
TX.9.1 Moderate or deep sedation and anesthesia are provided by qualified individuals.	**PC.13.20** Operative or other procedures and/or the administration of moderate or deep sedation or anesthesia are planned.	Reformatted and renumbered only.
TX.9.1.1 Each patient's moderate or deep sedation and anesthesia care is planned.	**PC.13.20** Operative or other procedures and/or the administration of moderate or deep sedation or anesthesia are planned.	Reformatted and renumbered only.
TX.9.2 Sedation and anesthesia options and risks are discussed with the patient and family prior to administration.	No standard.	Covered by **RI.2.40**.
TX.9.3 Each patient's physiological status is monitored during sedation or anesthesia administration.	**PC.13.30** Residents are monitored during the procedure and/or administration of moderate or deep sedation or anesthesia.	Reformatted and renumbered only.
TX.9.4 The patient's postprocedure status is assessed on admission to and before discharge from the postsedation or postanesthesia recovery area.	**PC.13.40** Residents are monitored immediately after the procedure and/or administration of moderate or deep sedation or anesthesia.	Reformatted and renumbered only.
TX.9.4.1 Patients are discharged from the postsedation or postanesthesia recovery area and the organization by a qualified licensed independent practitioner or according to criteria approved by the licensed independent practitioner staff.	**PC.13.40** Residents are monitored immediately after the procedure and/or administration of moderate or deep sedation or anesthesia.	Reformatted and renumbered only.
TX.10 An assessment determines the appropriateness of procedures.	**PC.13.20** Operative or other procedures and/or the administration of moderate or deep sedation or anesthesia are planned.	Reformatted and renumbered only.
TX.10.1 Before obtaining informed consent, the risk, benefits, and potential complications associated with procedures are discussed with patients.	No standard.	Covered by **RI.2.40**.
PF.1 The organization plans for and supports the provision and coordination of resident education activities.	No standard.	Covered by **LD.3.120**.
PF.1.1 The organization identifies and provides the resources necessary for achieving educational objectives.	No standard.	Covered by **LD.3.120**.
PF.2 The resident education process is coordinated among appropriate staff or disciplines that are providing care or services.	**PC.6.30** The resident receives education and training specific to the resident's abilities as appropriate to the care, treatment, and services provided by the organization.	Reformatted and renumbered only.
PF.3 The resident receives education and training specific to the resident's assessed needs, abilities, learning preferences, and readiness to learn as appropriate to the care and services provided by the organization.	**PC.6.30** The resident receives education and training specific to the resident's abilities as appropriate to the care, treatment, and services provided by the organization.	Reformatted and renumbered only.
PF.3.1 Education includes self-care activities, as appropriate.	**PC.6.10** The resident receives education and training specific to the resident's needs and as appropriate to the care, treatment, and services provided.	Reformatted and renumbered only.
PF.3.2 Based on assessed needs, the resident is educated about how to safely and effectively use medications, according to law and regulation, and the organization's scope of services, as appropriate.	**PC.6.10** The resident receives education and training specific to the resident's needs and as appropriate to the care, treatment, and services provided.	Reformatted and renumbered only.
PF.3.3 The resident is educated about nutrition interventions, modified diets, or oral health, when applicable.	**PC.6.10** The resident receives education and training specific to the resident's needs and as appropriate to the care, treatment, and services provided.	Reformatted and renumbered only.

CW

2002–2003 Standards	2004 Standards	Comments
PF.3.4 The organization assures that the resident is educated about how to safely and effectively use medical equipment or supplies, as appropriate.	**PC.6.10** The resident receives education and training specific to the resident's needs and as appropriate to the care, treatment, and services provided.	Reformatted and renumbered only.
PF.3.5 Residents are educated about pain and managing pain as part of treatment, as appropriate.	**PC.6.10** The resident receives education and training specific to the resident's needs and as appropriate to the care, treatment, and services provided.	Reformatted and renumbered only.
PF.3.6 Residents are educated about habilitation or rehabilitation techniques to help them be more functionally independent, as appropriate.	**PC.6.10** The resident receives education and training specific to the resident's needs and as appropriate to the care, treatment, and services provided.	Reformatted and renumbered only.
PF.3.7 The resident is educated about other available resources, and when necessary, how to obtain further care, services, or treatment to meet his or her identified needs.	**PC.6.10** The resident receives education and training specific to the resident's needs and as appropriate to the care, treatment, and services provided.	Reformatted and renumbered only.
PF.3.8 Education includes information about resident responsibilities in the resident's care.	No standard.	Moved to **RI.3.10.**
PF.3.9 Residents are educated about basic health practices and safety.	**PC.6.10** The resident receives education and training specific to the resident's needs and as appropriate to the care, treatment, and services provided.	Reformatted and renumbered only.
PF.3.10 Discharge instructions are given to the resident and those responsible for providing continuing care.	**PC.15.20** The transfer or discharge of a resident to another level of care, treatment, and services; different health professionals; or different settings is based on the resident's assessed needs and the organization's capabilities.	Reformatted and renumbered only.
PF.3.11 Academic education is provided to children and adolescents either directly by the organization or through other arrangements, when appropriate.	**PC.6.50** The organization provides academic education to children and youth as needed.	Reformatted and renumbered only.
	PC.9.20 The organization responds to life-threatening emergencies according to organization policy and procedure.	Although this is a new standard, some of the concepts were contained in a 2003 standard addressing emergency medications (**TX.4.8**).

CW

Crosswalk of 2004 "Provision of Care, Treatment, and Services" Standards for Long Term Care to 2005–2006 "Provision of Care, Treatment, and Services" Standards for Long Term Care

This crosswalk is designed to show where the 2004 standards requirements appear in the reformatted "Provision of Care, Treatment, and Services" (PC) standards for 2005–2006. The left column, 2004 Standards, lists consecutively each standard that was effective in 2004. The middle column, 2005–2006 Standards, indicates the PC standards, with revised numbers. The right column, Comments, identifies what changes have occurred between the 2004 standards and the 2005–2006 standards.

2004 Standards	2005–2006 Standards	Comments
Standard PC.2.120 The organization defines in writing the time frame(s) for conducting the initial assessment(s).	**Standard PC.2.120** The organization defines in writing the time frame(s) for conducting the initial assessment(s).	Rewording of EP 9 for clarification.
Elements of Performance for PC.2.120 9. For subacute services, the organization initiates assessments within 24 hours before admission and completes them within 72 hours after admission for all disciplines pertinent to the reason for admission.	**Elements of Performance for PC.2.120** 9. For subacute services, the organization initiates assessments within 24 hours of admission and completes them within 48 hours after admission for all disciplines pertinent to the reason for admission.	

CW

2004 Standards	2005–2006 Standards	Comments

Sedation and Anesthesia Care for Subacute Services
 	
The standards for sedation and anesthesia care apply when residents in any setting, receive, for any purpose, by any route, the following:
• General, spinal, or other major regional sedation and anesthesia
or
• Sedation (with or without analgesia) that, in the manner used, may be reasonably expected to result in the loss of protective reflexes
 	
Because sedation is a continuum, it is not always possible to predict how an individual resident receiving sedation will respond. Therefore, each organization develops specific, appropriate protocols for the care of residents receiving sedation. These protocols are consistent with professional standards and address at least the following:
• Sufficient qualified individuals present to perform the procedure and to monitor the resident throughout administration and recovery
• Appropriate equipment for care and resuscitation
• Appropriate monitoring of vital signs— heart and respiratory rates and oxygenation
• Documentation of care
• Monitoring of outcomes
	Sedation and Anesthesia Care for Subacute Services
	
	The standards for sedation and anesthesia care apply when residents in any setting, receive, for any purpose, by any route, the following:
	• General, spinal, or other major regional anesthesia
	or
	• Moderate or deep sedation (with or without analgesia) that, in the manner used, may be reasonably expected to result in the loss of protective reflexes
	
	Because sedation is a continuum, it is not always possible to predict how an individual resident receiving sedation will respond. Therefore, each organization develops specific, appropriate protocols for the care of residents receiving sedation. These protocols are consistent with professional standards and address at least the following:
	• Sufficient qualified individuals present to perform the procedure and to monitor the resident throughout administration and recovery. The individuals providing moderate or deep sedation and anesthesia have at a minimum had competency-based education, training, and experience in the following:
	  ○ Evaluating residents before performing moderate or deep sedation and anesthesia
	  ○ Performing the moderate or deep sedation and anesthesia, including rescuing residents who slip into a deeper-than-desired level of sedation or analgesia These include the following:
	    – Moderate sedation - are qualified to rescue residents from deep sedation and are competent to manage a compromised airway and to provide adequate oxygenation and ventilation
	    – Deep sedation - are qualified to rescue residents from general anesthesia and are competent to manage an unstable cardiovascular system as well as a compromised airway and inadequate oxygenation and ventilation
	  ○ Appropriate equipment for care and resuscitation
	  ○ Appropriate monitoring of vital signs, including, but not limited to, heart rates and oxygenation using pulse oximetry equipment, respiratory frequency and adequacy of pulmonary ventilation, the monitoring of blood pressure at regular intervals, and cardiac monitoring (by EKG or use of continuous cardiac monitoring device) in patients with significant cardiovascular disease or when dysrhythmias are anticipated or detected
	  ○ Documentation of care
	  ○ Monitoring of outcomes
		Additions and changes to language in the introduction to the standards for sedation and anesthesia care (**PC.13s**).
		
		This information on qualifications was moved into the introduction from its former location as a footnote for EP 2 of **PC.13.20**.
		
		New language added for clarification.

CW

2004 Standards	2005–2006 Standards	Comments
Definitions of four levels of sedation and anesthesia include the following: **Minimal sedation (anxiolysis)** A drug-induced state during which residents respond normally to verbal commands. Although cognitive function and coordination may be impaired, ventilatory and coordination may be impaired, ventilatory and cardiovascular functions are unaffected.	Definitions of four levels of sedation and anesthesia include the following: **Minimal sedation (anxiolysis)** A drug-induced state during which residents respond normally to verbal commands. Although cognitive function and coordination may be impaired, ventilatory and coordination may be impaired, ventilatory and cardiovascular functions are unaffected.	This section is also from the introduction to the standards for sedation and anesthesia.
Moderate sedation/analgesia ("conscious sedation") A drug-induced depression of consciousness during which residents respond purposefully to verbal commands —either alone or accompanied by light tactile stimulation. No interventions are required to maintain a patent airway, and spontaneous ventilation is adequate. Cardiovascular function is usually maintained.	**Moderate sedation/analgesia ("conscious sedation")** A drug-induced depression of consciousness during which residents respond purposefully to verbal commands (note, reflex withdrawal from a painful stimulus is not considered a purposeful response) either alone or accompanied by light tactile stimulation. No interventions are required to maintain a patent airway, and spontaneous ventilation is adequate. Cardiovascular function is usually maintained.	New language added for clarification.
Standard PC.13.20 Operative or other procedures and/or the administration of moderate or deep sedation or anesthesia are planned. **Elements of Performance for PC.13.20** 2. Individuals administering moderate or deep sedation and anesthesia are qualified* and have the appropriate credentials to manage residents at whatever level of sedation or anesthesia is achieved, either intentionally or unintentionally.	**Standard PC.13.20** Operative or other procedures and/or the administration of moderate or deep sedation or anesthesia are planned. **Elements of Performance for PC.13.20** 2. Individuals administering moderate or deep sedation and anesthesia are qualified* and have the appropriate credentials to manage residents at whatever level of sedation or anesthesia is achieved, either intentionally or unintentionally.	The footnote in EP 2 (explaining our definition of who is qualified to administer sedation and anesthesia) was moved into the introduction to the standards for sedation and anesthesia.
Standard PC.13.40 Patients are monitored immediately after the procedure and/or administration of moderate or deep sedation or anesthesia. **Elements of Performance for PC.13.40** 5. Residents who have received anesthesia are discharged in the company of a responsible, designated adult.	**Standard PC.13.40** Patients are monitored immediately after the procedure and/or administration of moderate or deep sedation or anesthesia. **Elements of Performance for PC.13.40** 5. Residents who have received sedation or anesthesia are discharged in the company of a responsible, designated adult.	EP 5 was edited to clarify the requirement.

CW

* **qualified** The individuals providing moderate or deep sedation and anesthesia have at a minimum had competency-based education, training, and experience in the following:
1. Evaluating residents before moderate or deep sedation and anesthesia.
2. Performing moderate or deep sedation and anesthesia, including rescuing residents who slip into a deeper-than-desired level of sedation or analgesia. This includes the following:
   a. *Moderate* sedation - are qualified to rescue residents from deep sedation and are competent to manage a compromised airway and to provide adequate oxygenation and ventilation
   b. *Deep* sedation - are qualified to rescue residents from general anesthesia and are competent to manage an unstable cardiovascular system as well as a compromised airway and inadequate oxygenation and ventilation

2004 Standards	2005–2006 Standards	Comments
Medicare/Medicaid Certification–Based LTC Accreditation Standards		
Standard PC.2.20 The organization defines in writing the data and information gathered during assessment and reassessment.	**Standard PC.2.20** The organization defines in writing the data and information gathered during assessment and reassessment.	An explanatory footnote was added for EP 1.
Elements of Performance for PC.2.20 1. The organization's written definition of the data and information gathered during assessment and reassessment includes the following: • The scope of assessment and reassessment activities by each discipline • The content of the assessment and reassessment • The criteria for when an additional or more in-depth assessment is done	**Elements of Performance for PC.2.20** 1. The organization's written definition of the data and information gathered during assessment and reassessment includes the following: • The scope of assessment and reassessment activities by each discipline • The content of the assessment and reassessment • The criteria for when an additional or more in-depth assessment is done*	
Standard PC.13.20 Operative or other procedures and/or the administration of moderate or deep sedation or anesthesia are planned.	**Standard PC.13.20** Operative or other procedures and/or the administration of moderate or deep sedation or anesthesia are planned.	The wording of EP 7 was changed to more clearly reflect what the requirement is supposed to mean.
Elements of Performance for PC.13.20 Before the operative and other procedures or the administration of moderate or deep sedation or anesthesia: 7. Patient acuity is assessed to plan for the appropriate level of postprocedure care.	**Elements of Performance for PC.13.20** Before the operative and other procedures or the administration of moderate or deep sedation or anesthesia: 7. The anticipated needs of the resident are assessed to plan for the appropriate level of postprocedure care.	
Standard PC.5.10 The organization provides care, treatment, and services for each resident according to the plan for care, treatment, and services.	**Standard PC.5.10** The organization provides care, treatment, and services for each resident according to the plan for care, treatment, and services. **Elements of Performance for PC.5.10** 1. The organization provides care, treatment, and services for each resident according to the plan for care, treatment, and services. 2. Not applicable 3. Not applicable 4. The organization uses at least two resident identifiers (neither to be the resident's room number) whenever taking blood samples or administering medications, blood, or blood products.	The published *2004 CAMLTC* omitted reference to EP 2, 3 and 4 for standard **PC.5.10**. EP 2 and 3 are not applicable to long term care; however, EP 4 relates to resident safety and will be scored.

---

* For example, nutritional or functional risk assessments may be defined for at risk residents. In such cases, nutritional risk criteria should be developed by dieticians or other qualified individuals, and functional risk criteria should be developed by rehabilitation specialists or other qualified individuals.

Crosswalk of 2002–2003 Standards for Long Term Care to 2004 "Medication Management" Standards for Long Term Care

This crosswalk is designed to show where the 2002–2003 standards requirements appeared in the "Medication Management" (MM) standards for 2004. The left column, 2002–2003 Standards, lists consecutively each standard that was effective in 2002–2003. The middle column, 2004 Standards, indicates the MM standards that became effective January 1, 2004. The right column, Comments, identifies what changes occurred between the 2002–2003 standards and the 2004 standards.

2002–2003 Standards	2004 Standards	Comments
TX.4 Processes are designed and implemented to ensure that medications are safely and effectively used.	No standard.	Deleted here; this concept is covered by the specific standards composing the "Medication Management" chapter.
TX.4.1 Only medications needed to treat the resident's conditions are prescribed.	**MM.3.10** Only medications needed to treat the resident's condition are ordered.	Reformatted and renumbered only.
TX.4.2 The long term care organization has an inventory of medications available to meet residents' needs.	**MM.2.10** Medications available for dispensing or administration are selected, listed, and procured based on criteria.	Reformatted and renumbered only.
TX.4.2.1 Medications are stored and distributed safely in accordance with defined policies and procedures.	**MM.2.10** Medications available for dispensing or administration are selected, listed, and procured based on criteria. **MM.2.40** A process is established to safely manage medications brought into the organization by residents or their families. **MM.4.80** Medications returned to the pharmacy are appropriately managed. **MM.7.40** Investigational medications are safely controlled and administered.	Reformatted and renumbered only.
TX.4.2.2 Medications are stored under proper conditions of sanitation, temperature, light, moisture, ventilation, segregation, and security.	**MM.2.20** Medications are properly and safely stored throughout the organization. **MM.7.40** Investigational medications are safely controlled and administered.	Reformatted and renumbered only.
TX.4.2.3 When medications are prepared in the pharmacy, proper conditions of sanitation, temperature, light, moisture, ventilation, segregation, safety, and security are maintained.	**MM.4.20** Medications are prepared safely.	Reformatted and renumbered only.
TX.4.2.4 Medications are dispensed safely and accurately to residents for whom they are prescribed or ordered.	**MM.4.10** All prescriptions or medication orders are reviewed for appropriateness. **MM.4.40** Medications are dispensed safely.	Reformatted and renumbered only.
TX.4.2.5 Records of dispensed medications are kept as required to maintain control and accountability.	**MM.4.40** Medications are dispensed safely.	Concept is also covered by **IM.6.10**.
TX.4.3 Controlled drugs are reconciled.	**MM.2.20** Medications are properly and safely stored throughout the organization.	Reformatted and renumbered only.
TX.4.4 Medications are appropriately labeled.	**MM.4.30** Medications are appropriately labeled.	Reformatted and renumbered only.
TX.4.5 The medication-dose system(s) is effective.	**MM.4.40** Medications are dispensed safely.	Reformatted and renumbered only.
TX.4.6 Important resident medication information is used and communicated.	**MM.1.10** Resident-specific information is readily accessible to those involved in the medication management system.	Reformatted and renumbered only.

CW

2002–2003 Standards	2004 Standards	Comments
TX.4.7 Pharmacy services are available at all times.	**MM.4.50** The organization has a system for safely providing medications to meet resident needs when the pharmacy is closed. **MM.4.60** If the organization does not operate a pharmacy but routinely administers medications, the organization has a process for obtaining medications from a pharmacy.	Also see **LD.3.10**.
TX.4.8 The emergency-medication system(s) is effective.	**MM.2.30** Emergency medications and/or supplies (if any) are consistently available, controlled, and secure in the organization's resident care areas.	Reformatted and renumbered only.
TX.4.9 The organization designs and implements an effective medication-recall system.	**MM.4.70** Medications dispensed by the organization are retrieved when recalled or discontinued by the manufacturer or the Food and Drug Administration for safety reasons.	Reformatted and renumbered only.
TX.4.10 Medications are safely and accurately administered.	**MM.3.20** Medication orders are written clearly and transcribed accurately. **MM.5.10** Medications are safely and accurately administered.	Reformatted and renumbered only.
TX.4.11 Safe self-administration of medication is supported.	**MM.2.40** A process is established to safely manage medications brought into the organization by residents or their families. **MM.5.20** Self-administered medications are safely and accurately administered.	Reformatted and renumbered only.
TX.4.12 Investigational medications are safely controlled and administered.	**MM.7.10** The organization develops processes for managing high-risk or high-alert medications. **MM.7.40** Investigational medications are safely controlled and administered.	Reformatted and renumbered only.
TX.4.13 The effect of medication on the resident is monitored on an ongoing basis.	No standard.	This standard was not scorable. The issue is addressed at **TX.4.13.1** (*see* the following standard).
TX.4.13.1 Assessment of medication effects is based on staff observations, the resident's perceptions, and information from the medical record and medication profile.	**MM.6.10** The effects of medication(s) on residents are monitored.	Reformatted and renumbered only.
TX.4.13.2 Psychotropic medication use is monitored.	**MM.7.20** Psychotropic medication use is monitored.	Reformatted and renumbered only.
TX.4.13.3 Findings of medication monitoring are used to improve or maintain the resident's clinical outcome.	No standard.	Deleted here; the concept is covered in Overview, embodied in all the MM standards, and also addressed at **PC.4.10**.
TX.4.14 Significant medication errors and significant adverse drug reactions are reported in a timely manner.	No standard.	This standard was not scorable and has been deleted. *See* **TX.4.14.1**.
TX.4.14.1 Nursing, pharmacy, and other appropriate staff collaboratively develop and maintain processes for defining, identifying, and reviewing, and responding to these significant medication errors.	**MM.6.20** The organization responds appropriately to actual or potential adverse drug events and medication errors.	Reformatted and renumbered only.
TX.4.14.2 Nursing, pharmacy, and other appropriate staff collaboratively develop and maintain processes for defining, identifying, and reviewing, and responding to these significant adverse drug reactions.	**MM.6.20** The organization responds appropriately to actual or potential adverse drug events and medication errors.	Reformatted and renumbered only.
	MM.8.10 The organization evaluates its medication management system.	Moved to this chapter from **PI.3.1.1**.

CW

Crosswalk of 2004 "Medication Management" Standards for Long Term Care to 2005–2006 "Medication Management" Standards for Long Term Care

This crosswalk is designed to show where the 2004 standards requirements appear in the reformatted "Medication Management" (MM) standards for 2005–2006. The left column, 2004 Standards, lists consecutively each standard that was effective in 2004. The middle column, 2005–2006 Standards, indicates the MM standards, with revised numbers. The right column, Comments, identifies what changes have occurred between the 2004 standards and the 2005–2006 standards.

2004 Standards	2005–2006 Standards	Comments
Standard MM.2.10 Medications available for dispensing or administration are selected, listed, and procured based on criteria.	**Standard MM.2.10** Medications available for dispensing or administration are selected, listed, and procured based on criteria.	The change to EP 3 was to include a word that was inadvertently omitted from the previous version.
Elements of Performance for MM.2.10 3. A list of medications for dispensing or administration (including strength and dosage) is maintained and readily available. **Note:** *Sample medications are not required to be on this list.*	**Elements of Performance for MM.2.10** 3. A list of medications for dispensing or administration (including strength and dosage form) is maintained and readily available. **Note:** *Sample medications are not required to be on this list.*	
Standard MM.4.30 Medications are appropriately labeled.	**Standard MM.4.30** Medications are appropriately labeled.	EP 4 was edited to more accurately reflect what the requirement should be.
Elements of Performance for MM.4.30 4. When preparing medications for multiple residents or the person preparing the medications is not the person administering the medication, the label also includes the following: • Resident name • Resident location • Directions for use and any applicable cautionary statements either on the label or attached as an accessory label (for example, "requires refrigeration," "for IM use only")	**Elements of Performance for MM.4.30** 4. When preparing individualized medications for multiple specific residents or the person preparing the individualized medications is not the person administering the medication, the label also includes the following: • Resident name • Resident location • Directions for use and any applicable cautionary statements either on the label or attached as an accessory label (for example, "requires refrigeration," "for IM use only")	

CW

Crosswalk of 2002–2003 "Surveillance, Prevention, and Control of Infection" Standards for Long Term Care to 2004 "Surveillance, Prevention, and Control of Infection" Standards for Long Term Care

This crosswalk is designed to show where the 2002–2003 "Surveillance, Prevention, and Control of Infection" (IC) standards requirements appeared in the reformatted IC standards for 2004. The left column, 2002–2003 Standards, lists consecutively each IC standard that was effective in 2002–2003. The middle column, 2004 Standards, indicates the IC standards, with revised numbers, which became effective January 1, 2004. The right column, Comments, identifies what changes occurred between the 2002–2003 standards and the 2004 standards.

2002–2003 Standards	2004 Standards	Comments
IC.1 The organization designs an infection control program to reduce the risks of acquired or transmitted infections.	IC.1.10 The organization designs an infection control program to reduce the risks of acquired or transmitted infections.	Reformatted and renumbered only.
IC.1.2 The organization oversees the infection control program to reduce the risk of nosocomial infections in residents and health care workers.	IC.1.20 The organization oversees the infection control program to reduce the risk of endemic and epidemic nosocomial infections in residents and health care workers.	Reformatted and renumbered only.
IC.1.3 The organization's infection control program includes surveillance activities.	IC.1.30 The organization's infection control program includes surveillance activities.	Reformatted and renumbered only.
IC.1.4 The organization's infection control program includes identification activities.	IC.1.40 The organization's infection control program includes identification activities.	Reformatted and renumbered only.
IC.1.5 The organization's infection control program includes prevention activities.	IC.1.50 The organization's infection control program includes prevention activities.	Reformatted and renumbered only.
IC.1.6 The organization's infection control program includes activities to control transmission of an identified infection.	IC.1.60 The organization's infection control program includes activities to control transmission of an identified infection.	Reformatted and renumbered only.
IC.1.7 The organization's infection control program includes reporting activities.	IC.1.70 The organization's infection control program includes reporting activities.	Reformatted and renumbered only.
IC.2. The organization implements all components of its infection control program.	IC.2.10 The organization implements all components of its infection control program.	Reformatted and renumbered only.
IC.2.1 The organization implements its surveillance activities.	IC.2.10 The organization implements all components of its infection control program.	Reformatted and renumbered only.
IC.2.2 The organization implements its identification activities.	IC.2.10 The organization implements all components of its infection control program.	Reformatted and renumbered only.
IC.2.3 The organization implements its prevention activities.	IC.2.10 The organization implements all components of its infection control program.	Reformatted and renumbered only.
IC.2.4 The organization implements its control activities.	IC.2.10 The organization implements all components of its infection control program.	Reformatted and renumbered only.
IC.2.5 The organization implements its reporting activities.	IC.2.10 The organization implements all components of its infection control program.	Reformatted and renumbered only.

CW

Crosswalk of 2004 "Surveillance, Prevention, and Control of Infection" Standards for Long Term Care to 2005–2006 "Surveillance, Prevention, and Control of Infection" Standards for Long Term Care

This crosswalk is designed to show where the 2004 standards requirements appear in the reformatted "Surveillance, Prevention, and Control of Infection" (IC) standards for 2005–2006. The left column, 2004 Standards, lists consecutively each standard that was effective in 2004. The right column, 2005–2006 Standards, indicates the IC standards, with revised numbers.

2004 Standards	2005–2006 Standards
IC.1.10 The organization designs an infection control program to reduce the risks of acquired or transmitted infections.	
EP 1	
EP 2	IC.2.10, EP 1 IC.3.10, EP 1 IC.7.10, EP 1
EP 3	IC.1.10, EP 3 IC.1.10, EP 8
EP 4	IC.9.10, EP 1 IC.9.10, EP 2
EP 5	IC.2.10, EP 1
EP 6	IC.1.10, EP 4
IC.1.20 The organization oversees the infection control program to reduce the risk of endemic and epidemic nosocomial infections in residents and health care workers.	
EP1	IC.1.10, EP 3 IC.8.10, EP 1 IC.8.10, EP 2
EP2	IC.1.10, EP2 IC.7.10, EP 2 IC.7.10, EP 3 IC.7.10, EP 4
EP 3	IC.1.10, EP 7
IC.1.30 The organization's infection control program includes surveillance activities.	
EP 1	IC.1.10, EP 7
EP 2	
EP 3	
EP 4	IC.2.10, EP 3
IC.1.40 The organization's infection control program includes identification activities.	
EP 1	
EP 2	IC.2.10, EP 3
EP 3	IC.4.10, EP 4
EP 4	IC.1.10, EP 7

CW

2004 Standards	2005–2006 Standards
IC.1.50 The organization's infection control program includes prevention activities.	
EP 1	IC.3.10, EP 2 IC.4.10, EP 6
EP 2	IC.3.10, EP 2 IC.4.10, EP 1
EP 3	IC.3.10, EP 2 IC.3.10, EP 3
EP 4	IC.3.10, EP 2 IC.3.10, EP 5
EP 5	IC.3.10, EP 2
EP 6	IC.3.10, EP 2 IC.3.10, EP 5 IC.4.10, EP 3
EP 7	IC.3.10, EP 2 IC.3.10, EP 5 IC.4.10, EP 3
EP 8	IC.3.10, EP 2 IC.3.10, EP 5
EP 9	IC.3.10, EP 2
EP 10	IC.3.10, EP 2
EP 11	IC.3.10, EP 2 IC.4.10, EP 7
IC.1.60 The organization's infection control program includes activities to control the transmission of an identified infection.	
EP 1	IC.3.10, EP 2 IC.3.10, EP 5
EP 2	IC.1.10, EP 6 IC.3.10, EP 2 IC.4.10, EP 5
EP 3	IC.1.10, EP 6 IC.3.10, EP 2
EP 4	IC.1.10, EP 6 IC.3.10, EP 2 IC.4.10, EP 5
IC.1.70 The organization's infection control program includes reporting activities.	
EP 1	IC.1.10, EP 7
EP 2	
EP 3	IC 1.10, EP 5
IC.2.10 The organization implements all components of its infection control program.	
EP 1	IC.1.10, EP 1
EP 2	IC.1.10, EP 1
EP 3	IC.1.10, EP 1
EP 4	IC.1.10, EP 1

CW

CW – 23

Crosswalk of 2002–2003 Standards for Long Term Care to 2004 "Improving Organization Performance" Standards for Long Term Care

This crosswalk is designed to show where the 2002–2003 standards requirements appeared in the reformatted "Improving Organization Performance" (PI) standards for 2004. The left column, 2002–2003 Standards, lists consecutively each standard that was effective in 2002–2003. The middle column, 2004 Standards, indicates the PI standards, with revised numbers, which became effective January 1, 2004. The right column, Comments, identifies what changes occurred between the 2002–2003 standards and the 2004 standards.

2002–2003 Standards	2004 Standards	Comments
Overview.	No standard.	Substantially revised and streamlined. Dimensions of performance eliminated. Language added relative to safety standards.
PI.1 The leaders establish a planned, systematic, organizationwide approach to process design and performance measurement, analysis, and improvement.	No standard.	This standard is now located in the "Leadership" chapter.
PI.1.1 The activities are planned in a collaborative and interdisciplinary manner.	No standard.	This standard is now an element of performance (EP) in the "Leadership" chapter.
PI.2 New or modified processes are designed well.	No standard.	This standard is now located in the "Leadership" chapter.
PI.2.1 Performance expectations are established for new and modified processes.	No standard.	Requirement is deleted. Concept is inherent in remaining standards.
PI.2.2 The performance of new and modified processes is measured.	No standard.	Requirement is deleted. Concept is inherent in remaining standards.
PI.3 Data are collected to monitor the stability of existing processes, identify opportunities for improvement, identify changes that will lead to improvement, or sustain improvements.	**PI.1.10** The organization collects data to monitor its performance.	The former **PI.3–PI.3.1.3** standards are reflected as EPs under standard **PI.1.10**. Several standards addressing data collection were consolidated into one standard.
PI.3.1 The organization collects data to monitor its performance.	**PI.1.10** The organization collects data to monitor its performance.	See preceding comment.
PI.3.1.1 The organization collects data to monitor the performance of processes that involve risks or may result in sentinel events.	**PI.1.10** The organization collects data to monitor its performance.	See preceding comment.
PI.3.1.2 The organization collects data to monitor performance of areas targeted for further study.	**PI.1.10** The organization collects data to monitor its performance.	See preceding comment.
PI.3.1.3 The organization collects data to monitor improvements in performance.	**PI.1.10** The organization collects data to monitor its performance.	See preceding comment.
PI.4 Data are systematically aggregated and analyzed on an ongoing basis.	**PI.2.10** Data are systematically aggregated and analyzed.	Reformatted and renumbered only.
PI.4.1 Appropriate statistical techniques are used to analyze and display data.	**PI.2.10** Data are systematically aggregated and analyzed.	Reformatted and renumbered only.
PI.4.2 The organization compares its performance over time and with other sources of information.	**PI.2.10** Data are systematically aggregated and analyzed.	Reformatted and renumbered only.
PI.4.3 Undesirable patterns or trends in performance and sentinel events are intensively analyzed.	**PI.2.20** Undesirable patterns or trends in performance are analyzed. **PI.2.30** Processes for identifying and managing sentinel events are defined and implemented.	Reformatted and renumbered only.
PI.4.4 The organization identifies changes that will lead to improved performance and reduce the risk of sentinel events.	**PI.3.10** Information from data analysis is used to make changes that improve performance and resident safety and reduce the risk of sentinel events.	Reformatted and renumbered only.

CW

2002–2003 Standards	2004 Standards	Comments
PI.5 Improved performance is achieved and sustained.	**PI.3.10** Information from data analysis is used to make changes that improve performance and resident safety and reduce the risk of sentinel events.	Reformatted and renumbered only.
LD.5.3 Leaders ensure that the processes for identifying and managing sentinel events are defined and implemented.	**PI.2.30** Processes for identifying and managing sentinel events are defined and implemented.	The former Leadership standard was moved to the "Improving Organization Performance" chapter to better reflect the relationship to Improving Organization Performance activities.
LD.6.1 Leaders ensure that an ongoing, proactive program for identifying risks to resident safety and reducing medical/health care errors is defined and implemented.	**PI.3.20** An ongoing, proactive program for identifying and reducing unanticipated adverse events and safety risks to residents is defined and implemented.	The former Leadership standard was moved to the "Improving Organization Performance" chapter to better reflect the relationship to Improving Organization Performance activities.

CW

Crosswalk of 2004 "Improving Organization Performance" Standards for Long Term Care to 2005–2006 "Improving Organization Performance" Standards for Long Term Care

This crosswalk is designed to show where the 2004 standards requirements appear in the reformatted "Improving Organization Performance" (PI) standards for 2005–2006. The left column, 2004 Standards, lists consecutively each standard that was effective in 2004. The middle column, 2005–2006 Standards, indicates the PI standards, with revised numbers. The right column, Comments, identifies what changes have occurred between the 2004 standards and the 2005–2006 standards.

2004 Standards	2005–2006 Standards	Comments
Medicare/Medicaid Certification–Based LTC Accreditation Standards		
	Standard PI.3.20 An ongoing, proactive program for identifying and reducing unanticipated adverse events and safety risks to residents is defined and implemented.	This standard was inadvertently omitted from the list of requirements applicable for the Medicare/Medicaid Certification–based option.
	Rationale for PI.3.20 Organizations should proactively seek to identify and reduce risks to the safety of residents. Such initiatives have the obvious advantage of *preventing* adverse events rather than simply *reacting* when they occur. This approach also avoids the barriers to understanding created by hindsight bias and the fear of disclosure, embarrassment, blame, and punishment that can happen after an event.	
	Elements of Performance for PI.3.20 The following proactive activities to reduce risks to residents are conducted: 1. Selecting a high-risk process* to be analyzed (at least one high-risk process is chosen annually - the choice should be based in part on information published periodically by the Joint Commission about the most frequent sentinel events and risks) 2. Describing the chosen process (for example, through the use of a flowchart) 3. Identifying the ways in which the process could break down† or fail to perform its desired function 4. Identifying the possible effects that a breakdown or failure of the process could have on residents and the seriousness of the possible effects 5. Prioritizing the potential process breakdowns or failures 6. Determining why the prioritized breakdowns or failures could occur, which may include performing a hypothetical root cause analysis 7. Redesigning the process and/or underlying systems to minimize the risk of the effects on residents 8. Testing and implementing the redesigned process 9. Monitoring the effectiveness of the redesigned process	

CW

---

* **High-risk process** A process that, if not planned and/or implemented correctly, has a significant potential for impacting the safety of the resident.

† The ways in which processes could break down or fail to perform their desired function are many times referred to as *the failure modes*.

Crosswalk of 2002–2003 "Leadership" Standards for Long Term Care to 2004 "Leadership" Standards for Long Term Care

This crosswalk is designed to show where the 2002–2003 "Leadership" (LD) standards requirements appeared in the reformatted LD standards for 2004. The left column, 2002–2003 Standards, lists consecutively each LD standard that was effective in 2002–2003. The middle column, 2004 Standards, indicates the LD standards, with revised numbers, which became effective January 1, 2004. The right column, Comments, identifies what changes occurred between the 2002–2003 standards and the 2004 standards.

2002–2003 Standards	2004 Standards	Comments
Overview.	No standard.	Streamlined and restructured to match revisions to the order in which the standards appear.
LD.1 The governing body has ultimate responsibility and legal authority for the organization.	**LD.1.10** The organization identifies how it is governed.	Reformatted and renumbered only.
LD.1.1 The governing body fulfills its responsibilities as defined by the organization and law and regulation.	**LD.1.20** Governance responsibilities are defined in writing, as applicable.	Reformatted and renumbered only.
LD.2 The leaders are responsible for organizational planning.	**LD.3.10** The leaders engage in both short-term and long-term planning.	Reformatted and renumbered only.
LD.2.1 Planning includes developing a mission.	**LD.3.10** The leaders engage in both short-term and long-term planning.	Reformatted and renumbered only.
LD.2.1.1 Planning addresses the resident care and organization functions in this manual.	No standard.	Requirement deleted; concept is inherent in the remaining planning standards.
LD.2.1.2 When the organization is part of a multiorganization system, its leaders participate in policy decisions that affect their organization.	**LD.1.20** Governance responsibilities are defined in writing, as applicable.	Reformatted and renumbered only.
LD.2.2 The organization's leaders and appropriate staff collaborate to design services.	**LD.4.20** New or modified services or processes are designed well.	Reformatted and renumbered only.
LD.2.2.1 The design of resident care services is appropriate to the mission, scope, and level of care required by the residents.	**LD.3.10** The leaders engage in both short-term and long-term planning. **LD.4.20** New or modified services or processes are designed well.	Reformatted and renumbered only.
LD.2.2.2 The leaders are responsible for taking action on information about resident satisfaction.	No standard.	Addressed in the "Improving Organization Performance" chapter.
LD.2.2.3 Services are available in a timely manner to meet resident needs.	**LD.3.50** Services provided by consultation, contractual arrangements, or other agreements are provided safely and effectively.	Reformatted and renumbered only.
LD.2.3 The leaders and representatives from appropriate disciplines and services collaboratively develop an annual operating budget and, as required by law and regulation, a long-term capital expenditure plan and a strategy to monitor the plan's implementation.	**LD.2.50** The leaders develop and monitor an annual operating budget and, as appropriate, a long-term capital expenditure plan.	Reformatted and renumbered only.
LD.2.3.1 The governing body approves the annual operating budget and long-term capital expenditure plan.	**LD.2.50** The leaders develop and monitor an annual operating budget and, as appropriate, a long-term capital expenditure plan.	Reformatted and renumbered only.
LD.2.3.2 The budget-review process considers the care and services needed to meet resident needs.	**LD.2.50** The leaders develop and monitor an annual operating budget and, as appropriate, a long-term capital expenditure plan.	Reformatted and renumbered only.
LD.2.3.3 An independent public accountant conducts an annual review of the organization's financial statements, unless otherwise provided by law.	**LD.2.50** The leaders develop and monitor an annual operating budget and, as appropriate, a long-term capital expenditure plan.	Reformatted and renumbered only.
LD.2.4 The leaders ensure comparable performance of resident care processes throughout the organization.	**LD.3.20** Residents with comparable needs receive the same standard of care, treatment, and services throughout the organization.	Reformatted and renumbered only.

CW

2002–2003 Standards	2004 Standards	Comments
LD.2.5 Care and services provided are consistent with specific resident population needs, the goals of the organization, and the stated scope of services.	**LD.3.10** The leaders engage in both short-term and long-term planning.	Reformatted and renumbered only.
LD.2.5.1 The organization provides care and services according to professional standards of practice.	No standard.	Addressed in the "Provision of Care" chapter.
LD.2.6 The leaders develop programs for staff recruitment, retention, development, and continuing education.	**LD.3.70** The leaders define the required qualifications and competence of those staff who provide care, treatment, and services and recommend a sufficient number of qualified and competent staff to provide care, treatment, and services. **LD.3.20** Residents with comparable needs receive the same standard of care, treatment, and services throughout the organization.	Reformatted and renumbered only.
LD.2.7 A systematic process is designed for credentialing licensed independent practitioners.	No standard.	Addressed in the "Management of Human Resources" chapter.
LD.3 An individual who has administrative authority is appointed as required by law and regulation.	**LD.2.10** An individual(s) or designee(s) is responsible for operating the organization according to the authority conferred by governance.	Reformatted and renumbered only.
LD.3.1. A medical director ensures medical care provided to residents is adequate and appropriate.	**LD.2.40** The medical director's duties and responsibilities are defined.	Reformatted and renumbered only.
LD.3.1.1 The medical director's duties and responsibilities are delineated.	**LD.2.40** The medical director's duties and responsibilities are defined.	Reformatted and renumbered only.
LD.3.1.2 The organized medical staff, if one exists, is accountable to the governing body.	**LD.2.40** The medical director's duties and responsibilities are defined.	Reformatted and renumbered only.
LD.3.2 A full-time registered nurse directs nursing services.	**LD.2.30** A full-time registered nurse directs nursing services.	Reformatted and renumbered only.
LD.3.2.1 When the director of nursing is responsible for more than one organization or specialty program, an appropriately qualified registered nurse is identified and is responsible for the nursing staff activities in each setting.	**LD.2.30** A full-time registered nurse directs nursing services.	Reformatted and renumbered only.
LD.3.2.2 When the director of nursing is absent, responsibility for continuity and supervision of nursing care is delegated to a registered nurse.	**LD.2.30** A full-time registered nurse directs nursing services.	Reformatted and renumbered only.
LD.3.3 The leaders ensure that the organization complies with law and regulation.	**LD.1.30** The organization complies with applicable law and regulation.	Reformatted and renumbered only.
LD.3.3.1 The organization is licensed or certified by the appropriate agencies, when applicable.	**LD.1.30** The organization complies with applicable law and regulation.	Reformatted and renumbered only.
LD.3.4 Directors manage their departments or services, either personally or by delegation.	**LD.2.20** Each organizational program, service, site, or department has effective leadership.	Reformatted and renumbered only.
LD.4 Resident care is appropriately integrated throughout the organization.	**LD.2.20** Each organizational program, service, site, or department has effective leadership.	Reformatted and renumbered only.
LD.4.1 The leaders foster communication and coordination among individuals and services within the organization.	**LD.3.60** Communication is effective throughout the organization.	Reformatted and renumbered only.
LD.4.2 All service policies and procedures are developed in collaboration with associated services and approved by the leaders.	**LD.3.90** The leaders develop and implement policies and procedures for care, treatment, and services.	Reformatted and renumbered only.
LD.4.2.1 The leaders provide for mechanisms to measure, analyze, and manage variation in the performance of defined processes that affect resident safety.	**LD.4.40** The leaders ensure that an integrated resident safety program is implemented throughout the organization.	Reformatted and renumbered only.

CW

2002–2003 Standards	2004 Standards	Comments
LD.5 The leaders set expectations, develop plans, and manage processes to improve the organization's performance.	**LD.4.10** The leaders set expectations, plan, and manage processes to measure, assess, and improve the organization's governance, management, clinical, and support activities.	Reformatted and renumbered only.
LD.5.1 The leaders understand performance improvement principles and methods.	No standard.	Deleted as a specific requirement; concept is inherent in the standards in the **LD.4** section.
LD.5.2 The leaders adopt and implement a comprehensive approach to performance improvement.	No standard.	Deleted as a specific requirement; concept is inherent in the standards in the **LD.4** section.
LD.5.3 Leaders ensure that the processes for identifying and managing sentinel events are defined and implemented.	No standard.	Addressed in the "Improving Organization Performance" chapter.
LD.5.4 The leaders allocate adequate resources for assessing and improving the organization's performance and for improving resident safety.	**LD.4.60** The leaders allocate adequate resources for measuring, assessing, and improving the organization's performance and improving resident safety.	Reformatted and renumbered only.
LD.5.5 Relevant information is forwarded to leaders and individuals responsible for coordinating organizationwide performance improvement activities.	No standard.	Deleted as a specific requirement; concept is inherent in the standards in the **LD.4** section.
LD.5.5.1 The leaders assign responsibility for implementing performance improvement activities.	**LD.4.60** The leaders allocate adequate resources for measuring, assessing, and improving the organization's performance and improving resident safety.	Reformatted and renumbered only.
LD.5.6 The leaders analyze and assess the effectiveness of their contributions in improving performance and resident safety.	**LD.4.70** The leaders measure and assess the effectiveness of the performance improvement and safety improvement activities.	Reformatted and renumbered only.
LD.6 The leaders ensure implementation of an integrated resident safety program throughout the organization.	**LD.4.40** The leaders ensure that an integrated resident safety program is implemented throughout the organization.	Reformatted and renumbered only.
LD.6.1 Leaders ensure that an ongoing, proactive program for identifying risks to resident safety and reducing medical/health care errors is defined and implemented.	No standard.	Addressed in the "Improving Organization Performance" chapter
LD.6.2 Leaders ensure that resident safety issues are given a high priority and addressed when processes, functions, or services are designed or redesigned.	**LD.4.40** The leaders ensure that an integrated resident safety program is implemented throughout the organization.	Reformatted and renumbered only.
	LD.3.80 The leaders provide for adequate space, equipment, and other resources.	Moved from the "Management of the Environment of Care" chapter.
	LD.3.120 The leaders plan for and support the provision and coordination of resident education activities.	Moved from the former "Education of Residents" chapter.
	LD.3.130 Academic education is arranged for children and youth, when appropriate.	Moved from the former "Education of Residents" chapter.

CW

Crosswalk of 2004 "Leadership" Standards for Long Term Care to 2005–2006 "Leadership" Standards for Long Term Care

This crosswalk is designed to show where the 2004 standards requirements appear in the reformatted "Leadership" (LD) standards for 2005–2006. The left column, 2004 Standards, lists consecutively each standard that was effective in 2004. The middle column, 2005–2006 Standards, indicates the LD standards, with revised numbers. The right column, Comments, identifies what changes have occurred between the 2004 standards and the 2005–2006 standards.

2004 Standards	2005–2006 Standards	Comments
Standard LD.3.10 The leaders engage in both short-term and long-term planning.	**Standard LD.3.10** The leaders engage in both short-term and long-term planning. **Elements of Performance for LD.3.10** 26. Planning for care, treatment, and services addresses the following: • The needs and expectations of residents and, as appropriate, families and referral sources • Staff needs • The scope of care, treatment, and services needed by residents at all of the organization's locations • Resources (financial and human) for providing care and support services • Recruitment, retention, development, and continuing education needs of all staff • Data for measuring the performance of processes and outcomes of care	EP 26 was moved to **LD.3.10** from **LD.3.20**.
Standard LD.3.20 Residents with comparable needs receive the same standard of care, treatment, and services throughout the organization.	**Standard LD.3.20** Residents with comparable needs receive the same standard of care, treatment, and services throughout the organization.	EP 3 was moved from **LD.3.20** to **LD.3.10**.

CW

Crosswalk of 2002–2003 "Management of the Environment of Care" Standards for Long Term Care to 2004 "Management of the Environment of Care" Standards for Long Term Care

This crosswalk is designed to show where the 2002–2003 "Management of the Environment of Care" (EC) standards requirements appeared in the reformatted EC standards for 2004. The left column, 2002–2003 Standards, lists consecutively each EC standard that was effective in 2002–2003. The middle column, 2004 Standards, indicates the EC standards, with revised numbers, which became effective January 1, 2004. The right column, Comments, identifies what changes occurred between the 2002–2003 standards and the 2004 standards.

2002–2003 Standards	2004 Standards	Comments
EC.1 The organization plans for a safe, accessible, effective, and efficient environment consistent with its mission, services, law, and regulation.	No standard.	Concept is addressed in standards **EC.1.10** through **EC.7.50** and standard **LD.1.30**.
EC.1.1 The organization plans for a safe environment. **EC.1.1.1** The organization plans for worker safety. **EC.2.1** The organization implements its safety plan.	**EC.1.10** The organization manages safety risks.	a. Safety planning, safety implementation, and worker safety standards have been merged into one standard. b. EC education and staff knowledge requirements have been moved to new **HR.2.20** in the "Management of Human Resources" chapter. c. Requirements addressing reporting, monitoring, and annual evaluations have been moved to **EC.9.10**.
EC.1.1.2 The organization develops a policy regarding smoking.	**EC.1.30** The organization develops and implements a policy to prohibit smoking except in specified circumstances.	Standard has been revised from requiring a "no smoking" policy that must be absolutely enforced to requiring organizations to identify and implement monitoring processes and to take corrective actions when their "no smoking" policy is ineffective.
EC.1.2 The organization plans for a secure environment. **EC.2.2** The organization implements its security plan.	**EC.2.10** The organization identifies and manages its security risks.	a. Planning and implementation standards have been merged into one standard. b. EC education and staff knowledge requirements have been moved to new **HR.2.20** in the "Management of Human Resources" chapter. c. Requirements addressing reporting, monitoring, and annual evaluations have been moved to **EC.9.10**.
EC.1.3 The organization plans for managing hazardous materials and waste. **EC.2.3** The organization implements its plan for managing hazardous materials and waste.	**EC.3.10** The organization manages its hazardous materials and waste risks.	
EC.1.4 A plan addresses emergency management. **EC.2.4** The organization implements its emergency management plan.	**EC.4.10** The organization addresses emergency management.	
EC.1.5 The organization plans for fire prevention. **EC.2.5** The organization implements its fire prevention plan.	**EC.5.10** The organization manages fire-safety risks. **EC.5.50** The organization develops and implements activities to protect occupants during periods when a building does not meet the applicable provisions of the *Life Safety Code*®.*	a. Planning and implementation standards have been merged into one revised standard. b. EC education and staff knowledge requirements have been moved to new **HR.2.20** in the "Management of Human Resources" chapter. c. Requirements addressing reporting, monitoring, and annual evaluations have been moved to **EC.9.10**. d. Consolidated ILSM requirements into one new standard (**EC.5.50**).
EC.1.5.1 Newly constructed and existing environments of care are designed and maintained to comply with the *Life Safety Code*®.	**EC.5.20** Newly constructed and existing environments of care are designed and maintained to comply with the *Life Safety Code*®.	Reformatted and renumbered only.

---

* *Life Safety Code*® is a registered trademark of the National Fire Protection Association, Quincy, MA.

2002–2003 Standards	2004 Standards	Comments
EC.1.6 The organization plans for managing medical equipment. **EC.2.6** The organization implements its medical equipment management plan.	**EC.6.10** The organization manages medical equipment risks.	a. Planning and implementation standards have been merged into one revised standard. b. EC education and staff knowledge requirements have been moved to new **HR.2.20** in the "Management of Human Resources" chapter.
EC.1.7 The organization plans for managing utilities. **EC.2.7** The organization implements its plan for managing utility systems.	**EC.7.10** The organization manages its utility risks.	c. Requirements addressing reporting, monitoring, and annual evaluations have been moved to **EC.9.10**.
EC.1.7.1 The organization provides a reliable emergency power source as required by occupancy classification and services provided.	**EC.7.20** The organization provides a reliable emergency electrical power source.	Reformatted and renumbered only.
EC.2 The organization provides a safe, accessible, effective, and efficient environment consistent with its mission, services, law, and regulation.	No standard.	Concept is addressed in standards **EC.1.10** through **EC.7.50** and standard **LD.1.30**.
EC.2.8 Personnel have been oriented to and educated about the environment and possess the knowledge and skills to perform their responsibilities in the environment.	**HR.2.20** Staff members, licensed independent practitioners, students, and volunteers, as appropriate, can describe or demonstrate their roles and responsibilities, based on specific job duties or responsibilities, relative to safety.	Concept was moved to new **HR.2.20** in the "Management of Human Resources" chapter.
EC.2.9 The organization conducts emergency drills regularly.	No standard.	Concept is addressed in standards **EC.4.20** and **EC.5.30**.
EC.2.9.1 Drills are conducted regularly to test emergency preparedness.	**EC.4.20** The organization conducts drills regularly to test emergency management.	Reformatted and renumbered only.
EC.2.9.2 Fire drills are conducted regularly.	**EC.5.30** The organization conducts fire drills regularly.	Standard has been deleted because it is not scorable.
EC.2.10 Components and systems of the environment are maintained, tested, and inspected.	No standard.	Concept is addressed in standards **EC.1.20**, **EC.5.40**, **EC.6.20**, **EC.7.30**, **EC.7.40**, and **EC.7.50**.
EC.2.10.1 Safety elements of the environment of care are maintained, tested, and inspected.	**EC.1.20** The organization maintains a safe environment.	Reformatted and renumbered only.
EC.2.10.2 Fire safety elements in the environment of care are maintained, tested, and inspected.	**EC.5.40** The organization maintains fire-safety equipment and building features.	Reformatted and renumbered only.
EC.2.10.3 Medical equipment is maintained, tested, and inspected.	**EC.6.20** Medical equipment is maintained, tested, and inspected.	Reformatted and renumbered only.
EC.2.10.4 Utility systems are maintained, tested, and inspected.	**EC.7.30** The organization maintains, tests, and inspects its utility systems.	Reformatted and renumbered only.
	EC.7.50 The organization maintains, tests, and inspects its medical gas and vacuum systems.	Consolidated medical gas and vacuum requirements into one new standard (**EC.7.50**).
EC.2.10.4.1 Emergency power systems are maintained, tested, and inspected.	**EC.7.40** The organization maintains, tests, and inspects its emergency power systems.	Reformatted and renumbered only.
EC.3 The organization plans and provides for other environmental concerns.	No standard.	Concept is addressed in standards **EC.8.10** through **EC.8.30**.
EC.3.1 The organization establishes an environment that meets the needs of patients, encourages a positive self-image, and respects their human dignity.	**RI.2.140** Residents have a right to an environment that preserves dignity and contributes to a positive self-image. **EC.8.10** The organization establishes and maintains an appropriate environment.	Reformatted and renumbered only.
EC.3.2 The organization provides an environment with appropriate space and equipment.	**EC.8.10** The organization establishes and maintains an appropriate environment. **EC.8.20** The organization establishes and maintains an appropriate dining environment.	Consolidated dining environment requirements into one new standard (**EC.8.20**).
EC.3.2.1 The organization uses established design criteria when designing and building the environment.	**EC.8.30** The organization manages the design and building of the environment when it is renovated, altered, or newly created.	Reformatted and renumbered only.
EC.3.3 The built environment provides appropriate privacy to patients.	**RI.2.130** The organization respects the needs of residents for confidentiality, privacy, and security.	Concepts have been moved into the "Ethics, Rights, and Responsibilities" chapter.

CW

2002–2003 Standards	2004 Standards	Comments
EC.3.4 The built environment supports the development and maintenance of the patient's interests, skills, and opportunities for personal growth.	**EC.8.10** The organization establishes and maintains an appropriate environment.	Reformatted and renumbered only.
EC.4 The organization evaluates and improves conditions in the environment.	No standard.	Concept is addressed in standards **EC.9.10** through **EC.9.30**.
EC.4.1 The organization collects information about deficiencies and opportunities for improvement in the environment.	**EC.9.10** The organization monitors conditions in the environment.	Requirements from **EC.1** through **EC.1.7** addressing reporting, monitoring, and annual evaluations have been consolidated and moved to **EC.9.10**.
EC.4.2 The organization analyzes identified environment issues and develops recommendations for resolving them.	**EC.9.20** The organization analyzes identified environment issues and develops recommendations for resolving them.	Reformatted and renumbered only.
EC.4.3 The organization works to implement recommendations to improve the environment and monitor the effectiveness of the recommendation's implementation.	**EC.9.30** The organization improves the environment.	Reformatted and renumbered only.

CW

Crosswalk of 2002–2003 "Management of Human Resources" Standards for Long Term Care to 2004 "Management of Human Resources" Standards for Long Term Care

This crosswalk is designed to show where the 2002–2003 "Management of Human Resources" (HR) standards requirements appeared in the reformatted HR standards for 2004. The left column, 2002–2003 Standards, lists consecutively each HR standard that was effective in 2002–2003. The middle column, 2004 Standards, indicates the HR standards, with revised numbers, that became effective January 1, 2004. The right column, Comments, identifies what changes occurred between the 2002–2003 standards and the 2004 standards.

2004 Standards	2005–2006 Standards	Comments
Medicare/Medicaid Certification–Based LTC Accreditation Standards		
	Standard EC.5.20 Newly constructed and existing environments are designed and maintained to comply with the *Life Safety Code®*. **Elements of Performance for EC.5.20** 5. The organization is making sufficient progress toward the corrective actions described in a previously approved Statement of Conditions™.	A new EP was added (it corresponds to an existing decision rule) to correct for an anomaly in the scoring system that results in **EC.5.20** being inappropriately scored much more harshly than in the past.

Crosswalk of 2002–2003 "Management of Human Resources" Standards for Long Term Care to 2004 "Management of Human Resources" Standards for Long Term Care

This crosswalk is designed to show where the 2002–2003 "Management of Human Resources" (HR) standards requirements appeared in the reformatted HR standards for 2004. The left column, 2002–2003 Standards, lists consecutively each HR standard that was effective in 2002–2003. The middle column, 2004 Standards, indicates the HR standards, with revised numbers, that became effective January 1, 2004. The right column, Comments, identifies what changes occurred between the 2002–2003 standards and the 2004 standards.

2002–2003 Standards	2004 Standards	Comments
HR.1 The organization's leaders identify the qualifications and performance expectations for all staff positions to meet residents' needs.	**LD.3.70** The leaders define the required qualifications and competence of those staff who provide care, treatment, and services and recommend a sufficient number of qualified and competent staff to provide care, treatment, and services. **HR.1.20** The organization has a process to ensure that a person's qualifications are consistent with his or her job responsibilities.	Reformatted and renumbered only.
HR.2 The organization provides an adequate number of staff to successfully implement the resident-focused functions.	**HR.1.10** The organization provides an adequate number and mix of staff and licensed independent practitioners that are consistent with the organization's staffing plan.	Reformatted and renumbered only.
HR.2.1 The adequacy of staff is demonstrated by meeting residents'	**HR.1.10** The organization provides an adequate number and mix of staff and licensed independent practitioners that are consistent with the organization's staffing plan.	Reformatted and renumbered only.
HR.2.1.1 nursing care needs	**HR.1.10** The organization provides an adequate number and mix of staff and licensed independent practitioners that are consistent with the organization's staffing plan.	Reformatted and renumbered only.
HR.2.1.2 nutritional needs	**HR.1.10** The organization provides an adequate number and mix of staff and licensed independent practitioners that are consistent with the organization's staffing plan.	Reformatted and renumbered only.
HR.2.1.3 rehabilitation needs	**HR.1.10** The organization provides an adequate number and mix of staff and licensed independent practitioners that are consistent with the organization's staffing plan.	Reformatted and renumbered only.
HR.2.1.4 environmental needs	**HR.1.10** The organization provides an adequate number and mix of staff and licensed independent practitioners that are consistent with the organization's staffing plan.	Reformatted and renumbered only.
HR.2.1.5 social service needs	**HR.1.10** The organization provides an adequate number and mix of staff and licensed independent practitioners that are consistent with the organization's staffing plan.	Reformatted and renumbered only.
HR.2.1.6 activity needs	**HR.1.10** The organization provides an adequate number and mix of staff and licensed independent practitioners that are consistent with the organization's staffing plan.	Reformatted and renumbered only.

CW

2002–2003 Standards	2004 Standards	Comments
HR.2.1.7 oral health needs	**HR.1.10** The organization provides an adequate number and mix of staff and LIPs that are consistent with the organization's staffing plan.	Reformatted and renumbered only.
HR.2.1.8 other functional needs	**HR.1.10** The organization provides an adequate number and mix of staff and LIPs that are consistent with the organization's staffing plan.	Reformatted and renumbered only.
HR.2.2 The organization staff has qualifications that are commensurate with defined job responsibilities and applicable licensure, law and regulation, and certification to meet the residents'	**HR.1.20** The organization has a process to ensure that a person's qualifications are consistent with his or her job responsibilities.	EP 7 was added to clarify what is required by this standard. This EP was a requirement for other programs.
HR.2.2.1 nursing care needs	**HR.1.20** The organization has a process to ensure that a person's qualifications are consistent with his or her job responsibilities.	Reformatted and renumbered only.
HR.2.2.2 nutritional needs	**HR.1.20** The organization has a process to ensure that a person's qualifications are consistent with his or her job responsibilities.	Reformatted and renumbered only.
HR.2.2.3 rehabilitation needs		
HR.2.2.4 environmental needs		
HR.2.2.5 social service needs		
HR.2.2.6 activity needs		
HR.2.2.7 oral health needs		
HR.2.2.8 other functional needs		
HR.2.3 Nursing care is provided 24 hours a day, seven days a week.	**HR.1.10** The organization provides an adequate number and mix of staff and licensed independent practitioners that are consistent with the organization's staffing plan.	Reformatted and renumbered only.
HR.2.4 A registered nurse supervises at least eight consecutive hours a day, seven days a week.	**HR.1.10** The organization provides an adequate number and mix of staff and licensed independent practitioners that are consistent with the organization's staffing plan.	Reformatted and renumbered only.
HR.2.5 If any resident(s) requires a registered nurse's services, at least one registered nurse who is currently licensed by the state in which he or she practices is on duty on each shift seven days a week.	**HR.1.10** The organization provides an adequate number and mix of staff and licensed independent practitioners that are consistent with the organization's staffing plan.	Reformatted and renumbered only.
HR.3 The leaders ensure that the competence of all staff members is assessed, maintained, demonstrated, and improved continually.	**HR.3.10** Competence to perform job responsibilities is assessed, demonstrated, and maintained.	EPs (6 and 7) were added to clarify the requirements for this standard. These EPs were requirements for other programs.
HR.3.1 An orientation process provides initial job training and information.	**HR.2.10** Orientation provides initial job training and information. **HR.2.20** Staff members, licensed independent practitioners, students, and volunteers, as appropriate, can describe or demonstrate their roles and responsibilities based on specific job duties or responsibilities, relative to safety.	Reformatted and renumbered only.
HR.3.1.1 Volunteers are oriented to the organization.	**HR.2.10** Orientation provides initial job training and information.	Reformatted and renumbered only.
HR.3.2 Ongoing education, including in-service, training, and other activities, maintains and improves staff competence.	**HR.2.30** Ongoing education, including in-services, training, and other activities, maintains and improves competence.	Reformatted and renumbered only.
HR.3.3 The organization regularly collects aggregate data on competence patterns and trends to identify and respond to staff learning needs.	**HR.2.30** Ongoing education, including in-services, training, and other activities, maintains and improves competence.	Reformatted and renumbered only.
HR.4 The organization assesses each staff member's ability to meet the performance expectations stated in his or her job description.	**HR.3.20** The organization periodically conducts performance evaluations.	Reformatted and renumbered only.
HR.5 The organization addresses staff requests to not participate in any aspect of resident care or treatment.	**RI.1.10** The organization follows ethical behavior in its care, treatment, and services and business practices.	Reformatted and renumbered only.

CW

2002–2003 Standards	2004 Standards	Comments
HR.5.1 The organization ensures that a resident's care or treatment is not negatively affected if the organization grants a staff request to not participate in an aspect of resident care or treatment.	**RI.1.10** The organization follows ethical behavior in its care, treatment, and services, and business practices.	Reformatted and renumbered only.
HR.6 All individuals permitted by law and the organization to practice independently are appointed to do so through a defined process.	**HR.4.10** There is a process for ensuring the competence of all practitioners permitted by law and the organization to practice independently.	Reformatted and renumbered only.
HR.6.1 The credentialing criteria are designed to assure that care and treatment provided are adequate and appropriate.**HR.6.1.1** Credentials are verified.	**HR.4.10** There is a process for ensuring the competence of all practitioners permitted by law and the organization to practice independently.	Reformatted and renumbered only.
HR.6.1.2 The organization uniformly utilizes credentialing criteria for licensed independent practitioners applying to provide resident care or treatment under the organization's auspices.	**HR.4.10** There is a process for ensuring the competence of all practitioners permitted by law and the organization to practice independently.	Reformatted and renumbered only.
HR.6.1.3 All individuals who are permitted by law and the organization to provide resident care services independently in the organization are granted delineated privileges.	**HR.4.20** Practitioners permitted by law and the organization to practice independently are granted clinical privileges. **HR.4.30** The organization has a process for granting temporary clinical privileges, when appropriate.	Reformatted and renumbered only.
HR.6.1.4 Procedures for appointment, reappointment, and granting, renewal, or revision of privileges are explained to each applicant.	This requirement was deleted.	Reformatted and renumbered only.
HR.6.1.5 The organization uniformly applies professional criteria to all applicants as the basis for granting or continuing staff membership and for granting, renewing, or revising privileges.	**HR.4.20** Practitioners permitted by law and the organization to practice independently are granted clinical privileges.	Reformatted and renumbered only.
HR.6.1.6 Privileges and appointment or reappointment are granted for a period of no more than two years.	**HR.4.50** Clinical privileges and appointments/reappointments are reviewed and revised at least every two years.	Reformatted and renumbered only.
HR.6.1.7 All individuals with privileges provide services within the scope of privileges granted.	**HR.4.20** Practitioners permitted by law and the organization to practice independently are granted clinical privileges.	Reformatted and renumbered only.
HR.6.1.8 Reappointment and renewal or revision of privileges are based on a reappraisal of the individual at the time of reappointment or renewal or revision or privileges.	**HR.4.50** Clinical privileges and appointments/reappointments are reviewed and revised at least every two years.	Reformatted and renumbered only.
	HR.4.40 There are mechanisms, including a fair hearing and appeal process, for addressing adverse decisions regarding reappointment denial, reduction, suspension, or revocation of clinical privileges that may relate to quality of care, treatment, and service issues. This is a new requirement for long term care. This is currently required for all programs that require privileging.	Reformatted and renumbered only.

CW

Crosswalk of 2004 "Management of Human Resources" Standards for Long Term Care to 2005–2006 "Management of Human Resources" Standards for Long Term Care

This crosswalk is designed to show where the 2004 standards requirements appear in the reformatted "Management of Human Resources" (HR) standards for 2005–2006. The left column, 2004 Standards, lists consecutively each standard that was effective in 2004. The middle column, 2005–2006 Standards, indicates the HR standards, with revised numbers. The right column, Comments, identifies what changes have occurred between the 2004 standards and the 2005–2006 standards.

2004 Standards	2005–2006 Standards	Comments
HR.4.10 There is a process for ensuring the competence of all practitioners permitted by law and the organization to practice independently.	**HR.4.10** There is a process for ensuring the competence of all practitioners permitted by law and the organization to practice independently.	EP 7 was moved from **HR.4.20** to **HR.4.10** (where it became EP 21). EP 8 was deleted from **HR.4.20**, because it was very similar to **HR.4.10**, EP 15.
Elements of Performance for HR.4.10 12. In addition to the above criteria, the organization collects and verifies information on restriction of privileges at other health care organizations.	**Elements of Performance for HR.4.10** 12. In addition to the above criteria, the organization collects and evaluates information on restriction of privileges at other health care organizations.	
15. The LIP is notified in writing of the leaders' decision.	21. The governing body* does the following: • Reviews recommendations made by the medical director • Reviews documentation on which recommendations are based • Reviews records of any hearings or appeals addressing adverse decisions • Grants appropriate clinical privileges	
HR.4.20 Individuals permitted by law and the organization to practice independently are granted clinical privileges.	15. The licensed independent practitioner is notified in writing of the governing body's decision.	
Elements of Performance for HR.4.20 7. The governing body* does the following: • Reviews recommendations made by the medical director • Reviews documentation on which recommendations are based • Reviews records of any hearings or appeals addressing adverse decisions • Grants appropriate clinical privileges 8. The applicant is informed in writing of the governing body's decision.	**HR.4.20** Individuals permitted by law and the organization to practice independently are granted clinical privileges.	

CW

---

* The organization administrator or a committee of two or more governing body members may substitute for a governing body.

2004 Standards	2005–2006 Standards	Comments
HR.4.30 The organization has a process for granting temporary clinical privileges, when appropriate.	**HR.4.30** The organization has a process for granting temporary clinical privileges, when appropriate.	Clarifications were made to EPs 4, 5, and 6.
Elements of Performance for HR.4.30 4. The results of the NPDB query have been obtained and evaluated. 5. The applicant has the following: • A complete application • No current or previously successful challenge to licensure or registration • Not been subject to involuntary termination of professional or medical staff membership at another organization, when applicable to the discipline • Not been subject to involuntary limitation, reduction, denial, or loss of privileges, when applicable to the discipline 6. The administrator or designee grants temporary privileges upon recommendation of clinical leadership or the medical director.	**Elements of Performance for HR.4.30** 4. To grant temporary privileges for new applicants, the results of the NPDB query have been obtained and evaluated. 5. To grant temporary privileges for new applicants, the applicant has the following: • A complete application • No current or previously successful challenge to licensure or registration • Not been subject to involuntary termination of professional or medical staff membership at another organization, when applicable to the discipline • Not been subject to involuntary limitation, eduction, denial, or loss of privileges, when applicable to the discipline 6. The administrator or designee grants temporary privileges for meeting important resident needs and for new applicants, upon recommendation of clinical leadership or the medical director.	
HR.4.50 Clinical privileges and appointments/reappointments are reviewed and revised at least every two years.	**HR.4.50** Clinical privileges and appointments/reappointments are reviewed and revised at least every two years.	A clarification was made for EP 4.
Elements of Performance for HR.4.50 4. The reappraisal addresses current competency and includes the following: • Confirmation of adherence to organization policies and procedures, rules, or regulations • Relevant information from organization performance improvement activities when evaluating professional performance, judgment, and clinical or technical skills • Any results of peer review of the individual's clinical performance • Clinical performance in the organization that is outside acceptable standards • Relevant education, training, and experience, if changed since initial privileging and appointment • Verification of current licensure, including all actions against the license • A statement that the individual can perform the care, treatment, and services he or she has been providing • Restrictions on privileges at a hospital(s) or other health care organization(s) • A query of the NPDB for information on adverse privilege actions taken by a health care entity, when appropriate to the discipline	**Elements of Performance for HR.4.50** 4. The reappraisal addresses current competency and includes the following: • Confirmation of adherence to organization policies and procedures, rules, or regulations • Relevant information from organization performance improvement activities when evaluating professional performance, judgment, and clinical or technical skills • Any results of peer review of the individual's clinical performance • Clinical performance in the organization that is outside acceptable standards • Relevant education, training, and experience, if changed since initial privileging and appointment • Verification of current licensure, including all actions against the license • A statement that the individual can perform the care, treatment, and services he or she has been providing • Evaluation of restrictions on privileges at a hospital(s) or other health care organization(s) • A query of the NPDB for information on adverse privilege actions taken by a health care entity, when appropriate to the discipline	

CW

Crosswalk of 2002–2003 "Management of Information" Standards for Long Term Care to 2004 "Management of Information" Standards for Long Term Care

This crosswalk is designed to show where the 2002–2003 "Management of Information" (IM) standards requirements appeared in the reformatted IM standards for 2004. The left column, 2002–2003 Standards, lists consecutively each IM standard that was effective in 2002–2003. The middle column, 2004 Standards, indicates the IM standards, with revised numbers, which became effective January 1, 2004. The right column, Comments, identifies what changes occurred between the 2002–2003 standards and the 2004 standards.

2002–2003 Standards	2004 Standards	Comments
IM.1 The organization plans and designs information management processes to meet internal and external information needs.	**IM.1.10** The organization plans and designs information management processes to meet internal and external information needs.	Reformatted and renumbered only.
IM.2 Confidentiality, security, and integrity of data and information are maintained.	**IM.2.10** Information privacy and confidentiality are maintained.	New EPs were added to be consistent with HIPAA.
IM.2.1 Records and information are protected against loss, destruction, tampering, and unauthorized access or use.	**IM.2.20** Information security, including data integrity, is maintained. **IM.2.30** The organization has a process for maintaining continuity of information.	Some additional requirements were added to address electronic systems.
IM.3 Uniform data definitions and data capture methods are used whenever possible.	**IM.3.10** The organization has processes in place to effectively manage information, including the capturing, reporting, processing, storing, retrieving, disseminating, and displaying of clinical/service and nonclinical data and information.	Reformatted and renumbered only.
IM.4 The necessary expertise and tools are available for the analysis and transformation of data into information.	**IM.3.10** The organization has processes in place to effectively manage information, including the capturing, reporting, processing, storing, retrieving, disseminating, and displaying of clinical/service and nonclinical data and information. **IM.2.10** Information privacy and confidentiality are maintained.	Some additional requirements were added to address electronic systems.
IM.5 Transmission of data and information is timely and accurate.	**IM.3.10** The organization has processes in place to effectively manage information, including the capturing, reporting, processing, storing, retrieving, disseminating, and displaying of clinical/service and nonclinical data and information.	Reformatted and renumbered only.
IM.5.1 The format and methods for disseminating data and information are standardized, whenever possible.	**IM.3.10** The organization has processes in place to effectively manage information, including the capturing, reporting, processing, storing, retrieving, disseminating, and displaying of clinical/service and nonclinical data and information.	Reformatted and renumbered only.
IM.6 Adequate integration and interpretation capabilities are provided.	**IM.3.10** The organization has processes in place to effectively manage information, including the capturing, reporting, processing, storing, retrieving, disseminating, and displaying of clinical/service and nonclinical data and information. **IM.4.10** The information management system provides information for use in decision making.	Reformatted and renumbered only.
IM.7 The organization defines, captures, analyzes, transforms, transmits, and reports resident-specific data and information related to care processes and outcomes.	No standard.	Nonscorable standard. Concept is addressed in **IM.6.10** through **IM.6.170**.
IM.7.1 The organization initiates and maintains a medical record for every resident.	**IM.6.10** The organization has a complete and accurate clinical record for every individual assessed or treated.	Reformatted and renumbered only.

CW

2002–2003 Standards	2004 Standards	Comments
IM.7.1.1 The retention time of medical record information is determined by law and regulation and by its use for resident care, legal, research, or educational purpose.	**IM.6.10** The organization has a complete and accurate clinical record for every individual assessed or treated.	Reformatted and renumbered only.
IM.7.1.2 Only authorized individuals make entries in medical records.	**IM.6.10** The organization has a complete and accurate clinical record for every individual assessed or treated.	Reformatted and renumbered only.
IM.7.2 The medical record contains sufficient information to identify the resident, support the diagnosis, justify the treatment, document the course and results, and promote continuity of care among health care providers.	**IM.6.10** The organization has a complete and accurate clinical record for every individual assessed or treated. **IM.6.20** Records contain resident-specific information, as appropriate, to the care, treatment, and services provided.	Reformatted and renumbered only.
IM.7.3 Medical record documentation includes at least the following:	No standard.	Nonscorable standard. Only a lead-in phrase.
IM.7.3.1 The provision of and response to the activities program is documented at least quarterly;	**IM.6.70** Clinical record documentation includes the provision of and response to the activities program at least quarterly.	Reformatted and renumbered only.
IM.7.3.2 The provision of and response to nutrition care services is documented at least quarterly;	**IM.6.80** Clinical record documentation includes the provision of and response to nutrition care services at least quarterly.	Reformatted and renumbered only.
IM.7.3.3 The provision of and response to nursing care;	**IM.6.90** Clinical record documentation includes the provision of and response to nursing care.	Reformatted and renumbered only.
IM.7.3.4 The provision of and response to medical treatment and care;	**IM.6.100** Clinical record documentation includes the provision of and response to medical treatment and care.	Reformatted and renumbered only.
IM.7.3.5 The provision of and response to rehabilitation services;	**IM.6.110** Clinical record documentation includes the provision of and response to rehabilitation services.	Reformatted and renumbered only.
IM.7.3.6 The provision of and response to social service interventions;	**IM.6.120** Clinical record documentation includes the provision of and response to social service interventions.	Reformatted and renumbered only.
IM.7.3.7 The provision of education and its effectiveness;	**IM.6.130** Clinical record documentation includes the provision of education and its effectiveness.	Reformatted and renumbered only.
IM.7.3.8 Significant changes in the resident's condition, care, and treatment; and	**IM.6.140** Clinical record documentation includes significant changes in the resident's condition, care, and treatment.	Reformatted and renumbered only.
IM.7.3.9 Treatment provided to the resident by off-site source.	**IM.6.150** Treatment provided to the resident by off-site sources is documented in the clinical record.	Reformatted and renumbered only.
IM.7.4 The effects of medications on residents, and associated pharmacist's evaluation and physician consultation, are documented.	**IM.6.160** The effects of medications on residents, and associated pharmacist's evaluation and physician consultation, are documented	Reformatted and renumbered only.
IM.7.5 Discharge information provided to the resident or to the receiving organization is documented.	**IM.6.170** Discharge information provided to the resident or to the family, as appropriate and permissible, and/or to the receiving organization is documented.	Reformatted and renumbered only.
IM.7.6 Medical record data and information are managed in a timely manner.	**IM.6.10** The organization has a complete and accurate clinical record for every individual assessed or treated.	Reformatted and renumbered only.
IM.7.6.1 Medical records of discharged residents are completed within a time period specified in organization policy, not to exceed 30 days.	**IM.6.10** The organization has a complete and accurate clinical record for every individual assessed or treated.	Reformatted and renumbered only.
IM.7.7 Verbal orders of authorized individuals are accepted and transcribed by designated, qualified personnel.	**IM.6.50** Designated, qualified personnel accept and transcribe verbal orders from authorized individuals.	Reformatted and renumbered only.

CW

2002–2003 Standards	2004 Standards	Comments
IM.7.8 Every medical record entry is dated, its author identified and, when necessary, authenticated.	**IM.6.10** The organization has a complete and accurate clinical record for every individual assessed or treated.	Reformatted and renumbered only.
IM.7.9 The organization can quickly and routinely assemble all components of a resident's medical record as required, regardless of their location in the organization.	**IM.6.60** The organization can provide access to all relevant information from a resident's record when needed for use in resident care.	Reformatted and renumbered only.
IM.7.9.1 Medical records are periodically reviewed for completeness, accuracy, and timely completion of information, and action is taken as needed to resolve identified deficiencies.	**IM.6.10** The organization has a complete and accurate health or clinical record for every individual assessed or treated.	Reformatted and renumbered only.
IM.8 The organization collects and aggregates data and information to support care and service delivery and operations.	**IM.4.10** The information management system provides information for use in decision making.	Reformatted and renumbered only.
IM.9 Knowledge-based information systems, resources, and services meet the organization's needs.	**IM.5.10** Knowledge-based information resources are readily available, current, and authoritative.	Reformatted and renumbered only.
IM.9.1 Knowledge-based information resources are available, current, and authoritative.	**IM.5.10** Knowledge-based information resources are readily available, current, and authoritative.	Reformatted and renumbered only.
IM.10 Comparative performance data and information are defined, collected, analyzed, transmitted, reported, and used.	No standard.	Concepts addressed in the "Improving Organization Performance" and "Accreditation Participation Requirements" chapters.

CW

Glossary

abuse Intentional maltreatment of an individual which may cause injury, either physical or psychological. *See also* neglect.

> **mental abuse** Includes humiliation, harassment, and threats of punishment or deprivation.

> **physical abuse** Includes hitting, slapping, pinching, or kicking. Also includes controlling behavior through corporal punishment.

> **sexual abuse** Includes sexual harassment, sexual coercion, and sexual assault.

accountability *See* information management.

accreditation Determination by the Joint Commission's accrediting body that an eligible health care organization complies with applicable Joint Commission standards. *See also* accreditation decisions.

accreditation cycle A period of accreditation at the conclusion of which, accreditation expires unless a full survey is performed.

accreditation decisions Categories of accreditation that an organization can achieve based on a Joint Commission full survey. These decision categories are:

> **Accredited** The organization is in compliance with all standards at the time of the on-site survey or has successfully addressed all requirements for improvement in an ESC report within 90 days (45 days beginning July 1, 2005) following the survey.

> **Provisional Accreditation** The organization fails to successfully address all requirements for improvement in an ESC report within 90 days (45 days beginning July 1, 2005) following the survey.

> **Conditional Accreditation** The organization is not in substantial compliance with the standards, as usually evidenced by a count of the number of standards identified as not compliant at the time of survey, which is between two and three standard deviations above the mean number of not compliant standards for organizations in that accreditation program. The organization must remedy identified problem areas through preparation and submission of ESC and subsequently undergo an on-site, follow-up survey.

> **Preliminary Denial of Accreditation** There is justification to deny accreditation to the organization as usually evidenced by a count of the number of not compliant standards at the time of survey, which is at least three standard deviations above the mean number of standards identified as not compliant for organizations in that accreditation program. The decision is subject to appeal prior to the determination to deny accreditation; the appeal process may also result in a decision other than Denial of Accreditation.

> **Denial of Accreditation** The organization has been denied accreditation. All review and

GL

appeal opportunities have been exhausted.

Preliminary Accreditation The organization demonstrates compliance with selected standards in the first of two surveys conducted under the Early Survey Policy Option 1 (*see* definition).

accreditation process A continuous process whereby health care organizations are required to demonstrate to the Joint Commission that they are providing safe, high-quality care, as determined by compliance with Joint Commission standards, National Patient Safety Goals recommendations, and performance measurement requirements. Key components of this process are an on-site evaluation of an organization by Joint Commission surveyors, a Periodic Performance Review (PPR), and quarterly submission of performance measurement data to the Joint Commission, as applicable.

accreditation report A report of an organization's survey findings; the report includes organization strengths, requirements for improvement (*see* definition), and supplemental findings (*see* definition), as appropriate.

accreditation survey findings Findings from an on-site evaluation conducted by the Joint Commission's surveyors that results in an organization's accreditation decision.

activity services Structured activities designed to help an individual develop or maintain creative, physical, and social skills through participation in recreation, art, dance, drama, social, or other activities.

acuity The degree of psychosocial risk of health treatment or the degree of dependency or functional status of the resident.

administration **1.** The fiscal and general management of an organization, as distinct from the direct provision of services. **2.** *See* medication management, administration.

admitting privileges Authority issued to admit individuals to a health care organization. Individuals with admitting privileges may practice only within the scope of the clinical privileges granted by the organization's governing body.

advance directive A document or documentation allowing a person to give directions about future medical care or to designate another person(s) to make medical decisions if the individual loses decision-making capacity. Advance directives may include living wills, durable powers of attorney, do-not-resuscitate (DNR) orders, right to die, or similar documents listed in the Patient Self-Determination Act that express the resident's preferences.

advanced practice nurse A registered nurse who has gained additional knowledge and skills through successful completion of an organized program of nursing education that prepares nurses for advanced practice roles and has been certified by the Board of Nursing to engage in the practice of advanced practice nursing.

adverse drug event A resident injury resulting from a medication, either because of a pharmacological reaction to a normal dose, or because of a preventable adverse reaction to a drug resulting from an error.

GL

adverse drug reaction (ADR) Unintended, undesirable, or unexpected effects of prescribed medications or of medication errors that require discontinuing a medication or modifying the dose; require initial or prolonged hospitalization; result in disability; require treatment with a prescription medication; result in cognitive deterioration or impairment; are life threatening; result in death; or result in congenital anomalies.

advocate A person who represents the rights and interests of another individual as though they were the person's own, to realize the rights to which the individual is entitled, obtain needed services, and remove barriers to meeting the individual's needs. *See also* surrogate decision maker.

analyzing *See* information management.

anesthesia and sedation The administration to an individual, in any setting, for any purpose, by any route, medication to induce a partial or total loss of sensation for the purpose of conducting an operative or other procedure. Definitions of four levels of sedation and anesthesia include the following:

minimal sedation (anxiolysis) A drug-induced state during which residents respond normally to verbal commands. Although cognitive function and coordination may be impaired, ventilatory and cardiovascular functions are unaffected.

moderate sedation/analgesia (conscious sedation) A drug-induced depression of consciousness during which residents respond purposefully to verbal commands, either alone or accompanied by light tactile stimulation. Reflex withdrawal from a painful stimulus is not considered a purposeful response. No interventions are required to maintain a patent airway, and spontaneous ventilation is adequate. Cardiovascular function is usually maintained.

deep sedation/analgesia A drug-induced depression of consciousness during which residents cannot be easily aroused, but respond purposefully following repeated or painful stimulation. The ability to independently maintain ventilatory function may be impaired. Residents may require assistance in maintaining a patent airway and spontaneous ventilation may be inadequate. Cardiovascular function is usually maintained.

anesthesia Consists of general anesthesia and spinal or major regional anesthesia. It does *not* include local anesthesia. General anesthesia is a drug-induced loss of consciousness during which residents are not arousable, even by painful stimulation. The ability to independently maintain ventilatory function is often impaired. Residents often require assistance in maintaining a patent airway, and positive pressure ventilation may be required because of depressed spontaneous ventilation or drug-induced depression of neuromuscular function. Cardiovascular function may be impaired.

anesthetic gases Any gas delivered throught the respiratory system as a component of general anesthesia or sedation. This may include inhalation anesthetics distributed in liquid form that when vaporized produce an anesthetic gas (for example, isoflurane, sevoflurane) or nonliquid compresssed gases (for example, nitrous oxide). Oxygen is not included in this definition.

anesthetizing location   Any area used for the administration of anesthetic agents.

appeal process   The process afforded to an organization that receives a Preliminary Denial of Accreditation (*see* definition), which includes the organization having a right to make a presentation to a Review Hearing Panel (*see* definition) before the Accreditation Committee takes final action to deny accreditation.

assessment   1. For purposes of resident assessment, the process established by an organization for obtaining appropriate and necessary information about each individual seeking entry into a health care setting or service. The information is used to match an individual's need with the appropriate setting, care level, and intervention. **2.** For purposes of performance improvement, the systematic collection and review of resident-specific data.

auditability   *See* information management.

authenticate   To verify that an entry is complete, accurate, and final.

authentication   *See* information management.

best practices   Clinical, scientific, or professional practices that are recognized by a majority of professionals in a particular field.   These practices are typically evidence based and consensus driven.

biologicals   Medicines made from living organisms and their products,

including serums, vaccines, antigens, and antitoxins.

blood component   A fraction of separated whole blood, for example, red blood cells, plasma, platelets, and granulocytes.

blood derivative   A pooled blood product, such as albumin, gamma globulin, or Rh immune globulin whose use is considered significantly lower in risk than that of blood or blood components.

blood transfusion services   Services relating to transfusing and infusing individuals with blood, blood components, or blood derivatives.

blood usage measurement   An activity that entails measuring, assessing, and improving the ordering, distributing, handling, dispensing, administering, and monitoring of blood and blood components.

business occupancy   *See* occupancy.

bylaws   A governance framework that establishes the roles and responsibilities of a body and its members.

capture   *See* information management.

care plan   A written plan, based on data gathered during assessment, that identifies care needs, describes the strategy for providing services to meet those needs, documents treatment goals and objectives, outlines the criteria for terminating specified interventions, and documents the progress in meeting goals and objectives. The format of the plan in some organizations may be guided by resident-specific policies and procedures, protocols, practice guidelines, clinical paths, care maps, or a combination thereof. The care plan may

GL

include care, treatment, habilitation, and rehabilitation.

care planning (or planning of care) Individualized planning and provision of services that addresses the needs, safety, and well-being of the resident. The plan, which formulates strategies, goals, and objectives, may include narratives, policies and procedures, protocols, practice guidelines, clinical paths, care maps, or a combination of these.

chemical restraint *See* restraint.

CLIA '88 The Clinical Laboratory Improvement Amendments of 1988.

clinical or consultant pharmacist services The provision of professional care and services by a legally qualified pharmacist. This includes the assessment of the appropriateness of medication orders, the ongoing evaluation and review of the resident's medication regimen and pharmaceutical care plan, ongoing monitoring of medication effects in individual residents, provision of drug information, oversight of the medication management process to improve resident safety, and other cognitive medication- related services.

clinical privileges Authorization granted by the appropriate authority (for example, the governing body) to a practitioner to provide specific care, treatment, or services in an organization within well-defined limits, based on the following factors, as applicable: license, education, training, experience, competence, health status, and judgment.

clinical record *See* record.

clinical record services The activities designed to ensure the accuracy, completeness, timeliness, accessibil-

ity, and safe, secure, and confidential storage of individuals' medical records.

clinical service groups (CSGs) Groups of residents in distinct, clinical populations for which data are collected. Tracer residents are selected according to CSGs.

community The individuals, families, groups, agencies, facilities, or institutions within the geographic area served by a health care organization.

competence or competency A determination of an individual's skills, knowledge, and ability to meet defined expectations.

complex organization An organization that provides for more than one level of care (for example, acute, subacute, chronic) and type (for example, pediatric, dental, behavioral health) of health care service, usually in more than one type of setting (for example, hospital, behavioral, home). An example is an organization that provides acute care, long term care, and home care services.

complex organization survey A Joint Commission survey in which standards from more than one accreditation manual are used in assessing compliance. This type of survey may include using specialist surveyors appropriate to the standards selected for survey.

compliance with a standard (*see* definition) Meeting the requirements of a standard through compliance with its element(s) of performance (EPs).

component A health care delivery entity (for example, service, program, related entity) that meets survey eligibility criteria under one of the Joint Commission accreditation programs.

GL

Multiple components comprise a complex organization.

confidentiality   An individual's right, within the law, to personal and informational privacy, including his or her health care records. *See also* information management.

consultation   **1.** Provision of professional advice or services. **2.** For purposes of Joint Commission accreditation, advice that is given to staff members of surveyed organizations relating to compliance with standards that are the subject of the survey.

consultation report   **1.** A written opinion by a consultant that reflects, when appropriate, an examination of the individual and the individual's medical record(s). **2.** Information given verbally by a consultant to a care provider that reflects, when appropriate, an examination of the individual. The individual's care provider usually documents those opinions in the clinical/case record.

continuing care   Care provided over time; in various settings, programs, or services; spanning the illness-to-wellness continuum.

continuing education   Education beyond initial professional preparation that is relevant to the type of care delivered in an organization, that provides current knowledge relevant to an individual's field of practice or service responsibilities, and that may be related to findings from performance-improvement activities.

continuity   The degree to which the care of individuals is coordinated among practitioners, among organizations, and over time.

continuum of care   Matching the individual's ongoing needs with the appropriate level and type of care, treatment, or service within an organization or across multiple organizations.

contract   A formal agreement for care, treatment, or services with any organization, agency, or individual that specifies the services, personnel, products, or space provided by, to, or on behalf of the organization and specifies the consideration to be expended in exchange. The agreement is approved by the governing body or comparable entity.

contracted services   Services provided through a written agreement with another organization, agency, or individual. The agreement specifies the services or personnel to be provided on behalf of the applicant organization and the fees to provide these services or personnel.

control chart   A graphic display of data in the order they occur with statistically determined upper and lower limits of expected common-cause variation. A control chart is used to identify special causes of variation, to monitor a process for maintenance, and to determine if process changes have had the desired effect.

control limit   In statistics, an expected limit of common-cause variation, sometimes referred to as either an upper or a lower limit. Variation beyond a control limit is evidence that special causes are affecting a process. Control limits are calculated from process data and are not to be confused with engineering specifications or tolerance limits. Control limits are typically plotted on a control chart.

coordination of care   The process of coordinating care, treatment, or services provided by a health care organization, including referral to appropriate community resources and liaison with others (such as the individual's physician, other health care organizations, or community services involved in care, treatment, or services) to meet the ongoing identified needs of individuals, to ensure implementation of the plan of care, and to avoid unnecessary duplication of services.

credentialing The process of obtaining, verifying, and assessing the qualifications of a health care practitioner to provide resident care services in or for a health care organization.

credentials Documented evidence of licensure, education, training, experience, or other qualifications.

criteria 1. Expected level(s) of achievement, or specifications against which performance or quality may be compared. 2. For purposes of eligibility for a Joint Commission survey, the conditions necessary for health care organizations and networks to be surveyed for accreditation by the Joint Commission.

data *See* information management.

decentralized laboratory testing *See* point-of-care testing.

delineation of clinical privileges The listing of the specific clinical privileges an organization's staff member is permitted to perform in the organization.

dementia A deterioration of intellectual function associated with pathological changes in the brain that causes changes in behavior and personality. Dementia does not include loss of intellectual functioning caused by clouding conscious-

ness, as in delirium, nor that caused by depression or other functional mental disorders.

dental services Services provided by a dentist, or a qualified individual under the supervision of a dentist, to improve or maintain the health of an individual's teeth, oral cavity, and associated structures.

dentist An individual who has received the degree of either doctor of dental surgery or doctor of dental medicine and who is licensed to practice dentistry.

dietetic services The delivery of care pertaining to the provision of nutrition and food service to individuals.

director of nursing A registered professional nurse who is responsible for the full-time, direct supervision of nursing services and who is currently licensed by the state in which he or she practices. Attributes of this position may be further defined in regulatory statutes.

disaster *See* emergency.

disaster plan *See* emergency management plan.

discharge The point at which an individual's active involvement with an organization or program is terminated and the organization or program no longer maintains active responsibility for the care of the individual.

discharge planning A formalized process in a health care organization through which the need for a program of continuing and follow-up care is ascertained and, if warranted, initiated for each resident.

disinfection The use of a chemical procedure that eliminates virtually all recognized pathogenic microorganisms but not necessarily all microbial

GL

forms (e.g., bacterial endospores) on inanimate objects.

dispensing *See* medication management; pharmacy services.

drug *See* medication.

drug administration *See* medication management.

drug allergies A state of hypersensitivity induced by exposure to a particular drug antigen resulting in harmful immunologic reactions on subsequent drug exposures, such as a penicillin drug allergy. *See* medication.

drug dispensing *See* medication management.

e-App The electronic version of an organization's application for accreditation.

Early Survey Policy A policy that provides two options to organizations undergoing their first Joint Commission survey. Under both options, the organization undergoes two surveys. Under the first option, the first survey is limited in scope and successful completion results in Preliminary Accreditation (*see* accreditation decisions, Preliminary Accreditation). Under the second option, the first survey is a full survey, and successful completion can lead to the organization being Accredited (*see* accreditation decisions, Accredited). The second survey in both options is required and addresses all standards and a four-month track record of compliance with the standards.

effectiveness The degree to which care is provided in the correct manner, given the current state of knowledge, to achieve the desired or projected outcome(s) for the individual.

efficacy The degree to which the care of the individual has been shown

to accomplish the desired or projected outcome(s).

efficiency The relationship between the outcomes (results of care) and the resources used to deliver care.

elements of performance (EPs) The specific performance expectations and/or structures or processes that must be in place for an organization to provide safe, high-quality care, treatment, and services.

emergency **1.** An unexpected or sudden occasion, as in emergency surgery needed to prevent death or serious disability. **2.** A natural or man-made event that significantly disrupts the environment of care (for example, damage to the organization's building[s] and grounds due to severe winds, storms, or earthquakes); that significantly disrupts care, treatment, or services (for example, loss of utilities such as power, water, or telephones due to floods, civil disturbances, accidents, or emergencies in the organization or its community); or that results in sudden, significantly changed or increased demands for the organization's services (for example, a bioterrorist attack, building collapse, or plane crash in the organization's community). Some emergencies are called *disasters* or *potential injury creating events (PICEs)*.

emergency, life-threatening A situation (e.g., major trauma, neck injury) in which an individual requires resuscitation or other support to sustain life.

emergency management plan The organization's written document describing the process it would implement for managing the consequences of natural disasters or other emergencies that could disrupt the organization's ability to provide care, treatment, and services. The plan identifies specific procedures that describe mitigation, preparedness, response and recovery strategies, actions, and responsibilities. *See also* emergency, mitigation activities, preparedness activities.

encryption *See* information management.

endemic infection *See* infection, endemic infection.

enteral nutrition *See* nutrition, enteral nutrition.

entry The process by which an individual comes into a setting, including screening and/or assessment by the organization or the practitioner to determine the capacity of the organization or practitioner to provide the care, treatment, or services required to meet the individual's needs.

environmental tours Activities routinely used by the organization to determine the presence of unsafe conditions and whether the organization's current processes for managing environmental safety risks are being practiced correctly and effectively.

epidemic infection *See* infection, epidemic infection.

equipment management Activities selected and implemented by the organization to assess and control the clinical and physical risks of fixed and portable equipment used for diagnosis, treatment, monitoring, and care.

Evidence of Standards Compliance (ESC) report A report submitted by a surveyed organization within 45 days (90 days between January 1, 2004 and June 30, 2005) of its survey,

which details the action(s) that it took to bring itself into compliance with a standard or clarifies why the organization believes that it was in compliance with the standard for which it received a requirement for improvement. An ESC report must address compliance at the element of performance (EP) level and include a measure of success (MOS) (*see* definition) for all appropriate EP corrections.

exploitation Taking unjust advantage of another for one's own advantage or benefit.

failure modes and effect analysis *See* risk assessment, proactive.

family The person(s) who plays a significant role in an individual's life. This may include a person(s) not legally related to the individual. This person(s) is often referred to as a surrogate decision maker if authorized to make care decisions for the individual should he or she lose decision-making capacity. *See also* guardian; surrogate decision maker.

fire safety management Activities selected and implemented by the organization to assess and control the risks of fire, smoke, and other byproducts of combustion that could occur during the organization's provision of care, treatment, or services.

formulary A list of medications and associated information related to medication use.

free text *See* information management.

governance The individual(s), group, or agency that has ultimate authority and responsibility for establishing policy, maintaining quality of care, and providing for organization management and planning. Other names for this group include the board, board of

GL

trustees, board of governors, and board of commissioners.

guardian   A parent, trustee, conservator, committee, or other individual or agency empowered by law to act on behalf of or be responsible for an individual. *See also* family; surrogate decision maker.

hazard vulnerability analysis   The identification of potential emergencies and the direct and indirect effects these emergencies may have on the health care organization's operations and the demand for its services.

hazardous condition   Any set of circumstances (exclusive of the disease, disorder, or condition for which the resident is undergoing care, treatment, or services) defined by the organization that significantly increases the likelihood of a serious adverse outcome.

hazardous materials and waste   Materials whose handling, use, and storage are guided or defined by local, state, or federal regulation (for example, the Occupational Safety and Health Administration's Regulations for Bloodborne Pathogens regarding the disposal of blood and blood-soaked items; the Nuclear Regulatory Commission's regulations for the handling and disposal of radioactive waste), hazardous vapors (for example, gluteraldehyde, ethylene oxide, nitrous oxide), and hazardous energy sources (for example, ionizing or non-ionizing radiation, lasers, microwave, ultrasound). Although the Joint Commission considers infectious waste as falling into this category of materials, federal regulations do not define infectious or medical waste as hazardous waste.

hazardous materials and waste management   Activities selected and implemented by the organization to assess and control occupational and environmental hazards of materials and waste that require special handling. *See* hazardous materials and waste.

health care occupancy   *See* occupancy.

hospice   An organized program that consists of services provided and coordinated by an interdisciplinary team to meet the needs of residents who are diagnosed with a terminal illness and have a limited life span. The program specializes in palliative management of pain and other physical symptoms, meeting the psychosocial and spiritual needs of the resident and the resident family or other primary care person(s), utilization of volunteers, and provision of bereavement care to survivors. This includes, but is not limited to, all programs licensed as hospices, and Medicare-certified hospice programs. All services provided by the hospice (e.g., pharmacy and home medical equipment services) and care provided in all settings (inpatient, nursing home, etc.) are included.

human subject research   The use of individuals in the systematic study, observation, or evaluation of factors on preventing, assessing, treating, and understanding an illness. The term applies to all behavioral and medical experimental research that involves human beings as experimental subjects.

indicator   A measure used to determine, over time, an organization's performance of functions, processes, and outcomes.

GL

infection   The transmission of a pathogenic microorganism to a host, with subsequent invasion and multiplication, with or without resulting symptoms of disease.

>   **endemic infection**   The usual level or presence of an agent or disease in a defined population during a defined period.

>   **epidemic infection**   A higher-than-expected level of infection by a common agent in a defined population during a defined period.

>   **health care–associated infection**   An infection acquired while receiving care or services in the health care organization.

infection control program   An organized system of services designed to meet the needs of the organization or individual in relation to the surveillance, prevention, and control of infection.

information management   Terms applicable to information management functions:

*   **accountability**   All information is attributable to its source (person or device).

*   **analyzing**   The process that interprets data and transforms it into information.

*   **auditability**   The ability to do a methodical examination and verification of all information activities such as entering and accessing.

*   **authentication**   The validation of correctness for both the information itself and the person who is the author or user of the information.

*   **capture**   The process of recording representations of human thought, perceptions, or actions, as well as device- generated data or information that is gathered and/or computed about a resident as part of a health care encounter or about other matters in a health care organization.

*   **confidentiality**   The safekeeping of data/information so as to restrict access to individuals who have need, reason, and permission for such access.

*   **data**   Uninterpreted observations or facts.

*   **electronic health information**   A computerized format of the health care information in paper records that is used for the same range of purposes as paper records, namely to familiarize readers with the resident's status; to document care, treatment, and services; to plan for discharge; to document the need for care, treatment, and services; to assess the quality of care, treatment, and services; to determine reimbursement rates; to justify reimbursement claims; to pursue clinical or epidemiological research; and to measure outcomes of the care, treatment, and service process.

*   **encryption**   The process of transforming plain text (readable) into cipher text that is unreadable without a special software key.

*   **free text**   Free-flowing, nonstructured type of speaking, writing, or inputting information.

*   **integrity**   In the context of data security, data integrity means the protection of data from accidental or unauthorized intentional change.

*   **interactive text**   A more complex version of structured text, as it interactively prompts and provides

GL

feedback to the person using it. Typically, it uses a higher level of computer intelligence that inter-acts with the person who records information.

- **interoperability** Enables autho-rized users to capture, share, and report information from any sys-tem, whether paper based or elec-tronic based.

- **knowledge-based information** A collection of stored facts, mod-els, and information that can be used for designing and redesign-ing processes and for problem solving. In the context of the man-ual, knowledge-based information is found in the clinical, scientific, and management literature.

- **nonrepudiation** The inability to dispute a document's content or authorship.

- **privacy** An individual's right to limit the disclosure of personal information.

- **processing** The manipulation of data and information by editing and updating.

- **protected health information** Health information that contains information such that an individ-ual person can be identified as the subject of that information.

- **report generation** The process of analyzing, organizing, and pre-senting recorded information for authentication and inclusion in the resident's health care record or in financial or business records.

- **retrievability** The capability of efficiently finding relevant information.

- **security** The protection of data from intentional or unintentional destruction, modification, or disclosure.

- **structured text** A process that requires authors to put specific information into specific fields with passive guidance by the information system. In paper-based systems, a form encour-ages a practitioner to fill in fields or boxes. Electronic systems use the same principle for templates or macros, which are guides used to create standardized informa-tion documentation. The purpose is to produce data of more con-sistent quality, make information more usable for decision support, make information more complete and more easily retrievable, and save documentation time.

- **timeliness** The time between the occurrence of an event and the availability of data about the event. Timeliness is related to the use of data.

- **transmission** The sending of data and information from one location to another.

informed consent Agreement or permission accompanied by full notice about what is being consented to. A resident must be apprised of the nature, risks, and alternatives of a medical procedure or treatment before the physician or other health care professional begins any such course. After receiving this informa-tion, the resident then either consents to or refuses such a procedure or treatment.

initial survey An accreditation sur-vey of a health care organization not previously accredited by the Joint Commission, or an accreditation sur-vey of an organization performed

GL

without reference to any prior survey findings.

integrity *See* information management.

interactive text *See* information management.

interdisciplinary Communication; discussion; planning; evaluation; and care, treatment, and service activities that occur formally and informally between and among team members who are representatives of multiple disciplines.

interim life safety measures A series of 11 administrative actions intended to temporarily compensate for significant hazards posed by existing National Fire Protection Association 101® 2000 *Life Safety Code®* (*LSC*) deficiencies or construction activities. *See also Life Safety Code®*; fire safety management.

interoperability *See* information management.

intravenous (IV) admixture The preparation of a pharmaceutical product which requires the measured addition of a medication to a 50ml, or greater, bag or bottle of IV fluid (e.g., IV, IM, IT, SC, etc.). It does not include the drawing-up of medications into a syringe for immediate use (i.e., reconstitution), or the assembly and activation of an IV system that does not involve the measurement of the additive.

investigational medication A medication or placebo used as part of a research protocol or clinical trial.

involuntary seclusion An individual's separation from other individuals or from the individual's room against his or her will or the will of his or her legal representative.

Joint Commission on Accreditation of Healthcare Organizations An independent, not-for-profit organization dedicated to improving the quality of care in organized health care settings. Founded in 1951, its members represent the American College of Physicians–American Society of Internal Medicine, the American College of Surgeons, the American Dental Association, the American Hospital Association, the American Medical Association, the public, and the nursing profession. The Joint Commission engages in issues and activities concerning the advancement of health care safety and quality, including public policy initiatives, standards development, and accreditation and certification programs.

knowledge-based information *See* information management.

laboratory *See* pathology and clinical laboratory services.

leader An individual who sets expectations, develops plans, and implements procedures to assess and improve the quality of the organization's governance, management, clinical, and support functions, and processes. Leaders include (when applicable to the organization's structure) the owners, members of the governing body, the chief executive officer, director of nursing, medical director, and other senior managers, and the leaders of the licensed independent practitioners.

licensed independent practitioner Any individual permitted by law and by the organization to provide care, treatment, and services, without direction or supervision, within the scope of the individual's license and consistent with individually granted clinical privileges.

GL

licensure   A legal right that is granted by a government agency in compliance with a statute governing an occupation (such as medicine, nursing, psychiatry, or clinical social work) or the operation of an activity (such as in a long term care or residential treatment center).

Life Safety Code® (*LSC*)   A set of standards for the construction and operation of buildings, intended to provide a reasonable degree of safety to life during fires—prepared, published, and periodically revised by the National Fire Protection Association and adopted by the Joint Commission to evaluate health care organizations under its life-safety management program. *See also* fire safety management; interim life safety measures; occupancy.

life support equipment   Any device used for the purpose of sustaining life and whose failure to perform its primary function, when used according to manufacturer's instructions and clinical protocol, leads to resident death in the absence of immediate intervention (examples include ventilators, anesthesia machines, and heart-lung bypass machines).

long term care   The health and personal care services provided to chronically ill, aged, physically disabled, or developmentally disabled persons in an institution or in the place of residence. These persons are not in an acute phase of illness, but require convalescent, physical, supportive, and/or restorative services on a long-term basis.

long term care facility   An organization that provides nursing care and related services for individuals who require medical, nursing, rehabilita-tion, or subacute care services. Such a facility may be certified for participation in the Medicare and/or Medicaid program as a skilled nursing facility or a nursing facility.

long term care pharmacy services   Services that include the procurement, preparation, dispensing, and distribution of pharmaceutical products to residents of a nursing home or other long term care facility.

loss of protective reflexes   An inability to handle secretions without aspiration or to maintain a patent airway independently.

measure of success (MOS)   A numerical or quantifiable measure usually related to an audit that determines whether an action was effective and sustained due four months after Evidence of Standards Compliance report (*see* definition) approval.

measurement   The systematic process of data collection, repeated over time or at a single point in time.

medical equipment   Fixed and portable equipment used for the diagnosis, treatment, monitoring, and direct care of individuals. *See also* equipment management.

medical history   A component of the medical record consisting of an account of an individual's history, obtained whenever possible from the individual, and including at least the following information: chief complaint, details of the present illness or care needs, relevant past history, and relevant inventory by body systems.

medical record   *See* record.

medication   Any prescription medications; sample medications; herbal remedies; vitamins; nutriceuticals; over-the-counter drugs; vaccines;

GL

diagnostic and contrast agents used on or administered to persons to diagnose, treat, or prevent disease or other abnormal conditions; radioactive medications; respiratory therapy treatments; parenteral nutrition; blood derivatives; intravenous solutions (plain, with electrolytes and/or drugs); and any product designated by the Food and Drug Administration (FDA) as a drug. This definition of medication does not include enteral nutrition solutions (which are considered food products), oxygen, and other medical gases.

medication error   Any preventable event that may cause inappropriate medication use or jeopardize resident safety. *See also* adverse drug reaction; sentinel event.

medication history   A delineation of the drugs used by an individual (both past and present), including prescribed and unprescribed drugs and alcohol, along with any unusual reactions to those drugs. *See* medication.

medication management   The process an organization uses to provide medication therapy to individuals served by the organization. The steps in the medication management process include:

- **Selection**   Safe and appropriate selection of medications available for prescribing, storage, and/or use in the organization.

- **Procurement**   The task of obtaining selected medications from a source outside the organization. It does not include obtaining a medication from the organization's own pharmacy, which is considered part of the ordering and dispensing processes.

- **Storage**   The task of appropriately maintaining a supply of medications on the organization's premises.

- **Prescribing or Ordering**   Synonymous terms for when a licensed independent practitioner transmits a legal order or prescription to the organization directing the preparing, dispensing, and administering of a specific medication to a specific resident. It does not include requisitions for medication supplies.

- **Transcribing**   The process by which an order from a licensed independent practitioner is documented either in writing or electronically.

- **Preparing**   The compounding, manipulation, or other activity needed to get a medication ready for administration exactly as ordered by the licensed independent practitioner.

- **Dispensing**   Providing, furnishing, or otherwise making available a supply of medications to the individual for whom it was ordered or their representative by a licensed pharmacy according to a specific prescription or medication order, or by a licensed independent practitioner authorized by law to dispense. Dispensing does not involve providing an individual with a dose of medication previously dispensed by the pharmacy.

- **Administration**   The provision of a prescribed and prepared dose of an identified medication to the individual for whom it was ordered to achieve its pharmacological effect. This includes directly introducing the medication into or onto the individual's body.

GL

- **Self-administration** Independent use by a resident of a medication, including medications that may be held by the organization for independent use by the resident.
- **Monitoring** The ongoing evaluation of an individual to whom a medication was administered, to ascertain the effectiveness and efficacy of the medication therapy and prevent the occurrence of any serious adverse outcomes.

medication-management measurement The measurement, assessment, and improvement of the prescribing or ordering, preparing and dispensing, administering, and monitoring of medications.

mental abuse *See* abuse, mental abuse.

minimum data set An agreed-on and accepted set of terms and definitions constituting a core of data; a collection of related data items.

mission statement A written expression that sets forth the purpose of an organization or one of its components. The generation of a mission statement usually precedes the formation of goals and objectives.

mitigation activities Those activities an organization undertakes in attempting to lessen the severity and impact of a potential emergency. *See* emergency.

multidisciplinary team A group of clinical staff members composed of representatives from a range of professions, disciplines, or service areas.

near miss Used to describe any process variation that did not affect an outcome, but for which a recurrence carries a significant chance of a serious adverse outcome. Such a near miss falls within the scope of the definition of a sentinel event, but outside the scope of those sentinel events that are subject to review by the Joint Commission under its Sentinel Event Policy.

neglect The absence of minimal services or resources to meet basic needs. Neglect includes withholding or inadequately providing food and hydration (without physician, resident, or surrogate approval), clothing, medical care, and good hygiene. It may also include placing the individual in unsafe or unsupervised conditions. *See also* abuse.

network An entity offering comprehensive or specialty services that provides, or provides for, integrated health care services to a defined population of individuals. Networks are characterized by a centralized structure that coordinates and integrates services provided by components and practitioners participating in the network.

nonrepudiation *See* information management.

nursing The health profession dealing with nursing care and services as (1) defined by the Code of Ethics for Nurses with Interpretive Statements, Nursing's Social Policy Statement, Nurses' Bill of Rights, Scope and Standards of Nursing Practice of the American Nurses Association, and specialty nursing organizations; and (2) defined by relevant state, commonwealth, or territory nurse practice acts and other applicable laws and regulations.

nursing care Professional processes of assessment, diagnosis, planning, implementation, and evaluation based on the art and science of nursing to promote health, its recovery, or a peaceful and dignified death. This includes, but is not limited to, assisting individuals, families, communities, and/or populations in understanding health needs and carrying out therapeutic plans and activities.

nursing home   A nonhospital health care organization with inpatient beds and an organized professional staff that provides continuous nursing and other health-related, psychosocial, and personal services to residents who are not in an acute phase of illness, but who require continued care on an inpatient basis.

nursing services   One or more defined units or departments within a health care organization with accountability for the delivery of quality nursing care to individuals, families, communities, and/or populations. Personnel, fiscal, capital, and intellectual resources focus on resident safety via interdisciplinary collaboration, integrated data and information management, and communication within all planning, implementation, and evaluation activities.

nursing staff   Personnel within a health care organization who are accountable for providing and assisting in the provision of nursing care. Such personnel must include registered nurses (RNs), and may include others such as advanced practice registered nurses (APRNs), licensed practical or vocational nurses (LPNs/LVNs), and nursing assistants or other designated unlicensed assistive personnel.

nutriceuticals   Nutritional supplements formulated in a pharmaceutical dosage form and used with the intention of deriving medical or health benefits, including preventing and treating disease. Such products range from isolated nutrients, dietary supplements, and diets to genetically engineered "designer" foods, herbal products, and processed foods such as cereals, soups, and beverages.

nutrition   The sum of the processes by which one takes in and uses nutrients.

> **enteral nutrition**   Nutrition provided via the gastrointestinal tract. Enteral nutrition encompasses both oral (delivered through the mouth) and tube (provided through a tube or catheter that delivers nutrients distal to the mouth) routes.

> **parenteral nutrition**   Nutrients that are provided intravenously, bypassing the digestive tract, which may contain protein, sugar, fat, and added vitamins and minerals as needed by the resident. Other terms used are total parenteral nutrition (TPN), partial parenteral nutrition (PPN), and hyperalimentation (HA).

nutrition assessment   A comprehensive process for defining an individual's nutrition and hydration status using medical, nutrition and medication intake histories, physical examination, anthropomorphic measurements, and laboratory data.

nutrition care   Interventions and counseling to promote appropriate nutrition and fluid intake, based on nutrition and hydration assessment and information about food, other sources of nutrients, and meal preparation consistent with the individual's cultural background and socioeconomic status. Nutrition therapy, a component of medical treatment,

GL

includes enteral and parenteral nutrition. *See also* nutrition.

nutrition screening   A process used to indicate the need for a nutritional assessment to determine whether a resident is malnourished or at risk for malnourishment.

occupancy

ambulatory health care occupancy   An occupancy used to provide services or treatment to four or more residents at the same time that either (1) renders them incapable of providing their own means of self-preservation in an emergency or (2) provides outpatient surgical treatment requiring general anesthesia.

business occupancy   An occupancy used to provide outpatient care, treatment, or services that do not meet the criteria in the ambulatory health care occupancy definition (for example, three or fewer residents at the same time who are either rendered incapable of self-preservation in an emergency or are undergoing general anesthesia).

health care occupancy   An occupancy used for purposes such as medical or other care, treatment, or services provided to persons suffering from physical or mental illness, disease or infirmity; and for the care of infants, convalescents, or infirm aged persons. Health care occupancies provide sleeping facilities for four or more occupants and are occupied by persons who are mostly incapable of self-preservation because of age, physical or mental disability, or because of security measures not under the occupant's control. Health care occupancies include hospitals, nursing homes, and limited care facilities.

residential occupancy   An occupancy in which sleeping accommodations are provided for normal residential purposes and include all buildings designed to provide sleeping accommodations.

operative and other high-risk procedures   Surgical or other procedures that put the resident at risk of death or disability. This does not include use of medications that place residents at risk.

organization's strengths   Areas in which an organization's performance is exemplary, as evidenced by the implementation of innovative approaches to meeting Joint Commission standards. An organization will not be cited for having a strength if the organization has a related not compliant standard and/or partially compliant element of performance (EP).

organized medical staff   The governance structure of the medical staff, including the medical staff bylaws and rules and regulations to which the medical staff is subject. This structure is approved by the governing body of the organization. Long term care organizations do not necessarily have organized medical staffs.

parenteral nutrition   *See* nutrition, parenteral nutrition.

parenteral product   A sterile pharmaceutical preparation introduced into the body through a route other than the digestive tract, as by subcutaneous, intramuscular, or intravenous injection or infusion.

pathology and clinical laboratory services   The services that provide information on diagnosis, prevention, or treatment of disease or the assessment of health, through the examination of the structural and functional changes in tissues and organs of the body that cause or are caused by disease. It also includes the biological, microbiological, serological, chemical, immunohematological, hematological, or other examination of materials derived from the human body.

patient   An individual who receives care, treatment, or services. For hospice providers, the patient and family are considered a single unit of care. Synonyms used by various health care fields include client, resident, customer, patient and family unit, consumer, and health care consumer. *See also* resident.

patient tracer   The process of evaluating a patient's, client's, or resident's total care experience within a health care organization.

performance improvement   The continuous study and adaptation of a health care organization's functions and processes to increase the probability of achieving desired outcomes and to better meet the needs of individuals and other users of services.

Periodic Performance Review (PPR) An additional requirement of the accreditation process whereby an organization reviews its compliance with all applicable Joint Commission standards, completes and submits to the Joint Commission a plan of action (*see* definition) for any standard not in full compliance, including the identification of a measure of success (MOS) (*see* definition), and engages in a telephone discussion with a member of the Standards Interpretation Group staff to determine the acceptability of the plan of action. The PPR encourages organizations to be in continuous compliance with Joint Commission standards. At the time of the next full survey, surveyors validate that the MOS were implemented and effective.

pharmaceutical care and services Services provided directly or through written contract with another organization that include procuring, preparing, dispensing, and/or distributing pharmaceutical products and the ongoing monitoring of the recipient to identify, prevent, and resolve medication-related problems.

pharmacist   An individual who has a degree in pharmacy and is licensed and registered to prepare, preserve, compound, and dispense drugs and chemicals.

pharmacist, consultant   An individual who has a degree in pharmacy and is licensed and registered in accordance with pharmacy law and regulation. This individual provides services to a long term care facility, including conducting retrospective drug-regimen reviews (DRRs) of all residents' medications on at least a monthly basis; providing written recommendations (interventions) for medication order changes, as appropriate, based on the DRR; assessing medication use; consulting with the long term care facility on various drug-utilization management techniques such as formulary management, therapeutic interchange, generic substitution, drug-use evaluation, and disease management; and participating in a long term care facility's continuous quality improvement programs and on other resident care–oriented committees (for example, infection control).

GL

pharmacy A licensed location where drugs are stored and dispensed.

pharmacy services The provision of pharmaceutical care and services involving the preparation and dispensing of medications, and medication-related devices and supplies by a licensed pharmacy, with or without the provision of clinical or consultant pharmacist services.

physical abuse *See* abuse.

physical rehabilitation services The professional and technical care provided by rehabilitation professionals that assists physically disabled persons to attain, increase, or maintain functional capacity.

physical restraint *See* restraint.

physician A doctor of medicine or doctor of osteopathy who, by virtue of education, training, and demonstrated competence, is granted clinical privileges by the organization to perform a specific diagnostic or therapeutic procedure(s) and who is fully licensed to practice medicine.

physician assistant An individual who practices medicine with supervision by licensed physicians, providing residents with services ranging from primary medicine to specialized surgical care. The scope of practice is determined by state law, the supervising physician's delegation of responsibilities, the individual's education and experience, and the specialty and setting in which the individual works.

physician licensure The process by which a legal jurisdiction, such as a state, grants permission to a physician to practice medicine after finding that he or she has met acceptable qualification standards. Licensure also involves ongoing regulation of physicians by the legal jurisdiction, including the authority to revoke or otherwise restrict a physician's license to practice.

plan A detailed method, formulated beforehand, that identifies needs, lists strategies to meet those needs, and sets goals and objectives. The format of the plan may include narratives, policies and procedures, protocols, practice guidelines, clinical paths, care maps, or a combination of these.

plan for improvement For purposes of Joint Commission accreditation, an organization's written statement that details the procedures to be taken and timeframes to correct existing *Life Safety Code®* (*LSC*) deficiencies. *See also* Statement of Conditions™ (SOC); interim life safety measures; *Life Safety Code®*.

plan of action A plan detailing the action(s) that an organization will take to come into compliance with a Joint Commission standard. A plan of action must be completed for each element of performance (EP) (*see* definition) associated with a not compliant standard. A measure of success (MOS) (*see* definition) must also be included in the plan of action as indicated in the accreditation manual.

podiatrist An individual who has received the degree of doctor of podiatry medicine and who is licensed to practice podiatry.

point-of-care testing Analytical testing performed at sites outside the traditional laboratory environment, usually at or near where care is delivered to individuals. Testing may range from simple waived procedures, such as fecal occult blood, to more sophis-

GL

ticated chemical analyzers. The testing may be under the control of the main laboratory, the direction of another specialized laboratory (such as for arterial blood gas), or the nursing service. Testing may be categorized as waived, moderate, or high complexity under CLIA '88. Also called alternate site testing, decentralized laboratory testing, and distributed site testing.

policies and procedures The formal, approved description of how a governance, management, or clinical care process is defined, organized, and carried out.

practice guidelines Tools that describe processes found by clinical trials or by consensus opinion of experts to be the most effective in evaluating and/or treating a resident who has a specific symptom, condition, or diagnosis, or describe a specific procedure. Synonyms include practice parameter, protocol, preferred practice pattern, and guideline.

preadmission procedures An organization's process for obtaining appropriate and necessary information for each individual seeking admission into a health care setting or service. The information is used to match the individual need with the level of care required and to the appropriate setting.

Preliminary Denial of Accreditation *See* accreditation decisions.

preparedness activities Those activities an organization undertakes to build capacity and identify resources that may be used if an emergency occurs. *See* emergency.

prescribing or ordering *See* medication management.

primary source The original source of a specific credential that can verify the accuracy of a qualification reported by an individual health care practitioner. Examples include medical school, graduate medical education program, and state medical board.

priority focus areas (PFAs) Processes, systems, or structures in a health care organization that significantly impact the quality and safety of care. The PFAs are:

- Assessment and Care/Services
- Communication
- Credentialed Practitioners
- Equipment Use
- Infection Control
- Information Management
- Medication Management
- Organizational Structure
- Orientation and Training
- Patient Safety
- Physical Environment
- Quality Improvement Expertise and Activity
- Rights and Ethics
- Staffing

  primary PFA Every standard is linked to one or more PFAs. When a surveyor has findings under a standard, he or she determines which of the linked PFAs is most related to the specific finding—this becomes the *primary* PFA. For example, a finding under standard HR.1.10 may be assigned a primary PFA of Staffing. The organization's accreditation report is organized by PFA.

  secondary PFAs The additional PFAs that are also related to a spe-

GL

cific finding, in addition to the primary PFA. For example, a finding under standard HR.1.10 may be assigned a secondary PFA of Orientation and Training. The organization's accreditation report also lists the secondary PFAs.

Priority Focus Process (PFP) The process for standardizing the priorities for sampling during an organization's survey based on information collected about the organization prior to survey. The process also helps to focus the survey on areas that are critical to that organization's resident safety and quality-of-care processes. Examples of such information may include, but are not limited to, data from the organization's e-App (*see* definition); the organization's plan of action prepared as part of the Periodic Performance Review (PPR) (*see* definition) process; complaint and sentinel event information; data collected from external sources, such as MedPar data; performance measurement data; and previous survey results.

Priority Focus Tool (PFT) An automated tool that supports the Priority Focus Process (PFP) through the use of algorithms, or sets of rules, to transform a health care organization's data into information that guides the survey process.

privacy *See* information management.

privileging The process whereby a specific scope and content of resident care services (that is, clinical privileges) are authorized for a health care practitioner by a health care organization, based on evaluation of the individual's credentials and performance. *See* licensed independent practitioner.

processing *See* information management.

program An organized system of services designed to address the needs of an organization or individual.

protected health information *See* information management.

Provisional Accreditation *See* accreditation decisions.

psychoactive *See* psychotropic/psychopharmacologic medication.

psychotropic/psychopharmacologic medication Any medication whose intended purpose is to alter perception, mental status, or behavior. These include, but are not limited to, those drugs that produce drug dependence. Some examples of drug classes that are considered psychotropic/ psychopharmacologic medications include, but are not limited to, hypnotics, antipsychotics, long- and short-acting benzodiazepines, sedatives/anxiolytics, and antidepressants.

Public Information Policy A Joint Commission policy governing the disclosure of specific information about the performance of a health care organization or network, as well as accreditation-related information that remains confidential. This policy covers the Joint Commission's Quality Reports, information publicly disclosed on request, complaint information, aggregate performance data, data released to government agencies, and the Joint Commission's right to clarify information that an accredited organization releases about its accreditation status.

qualified individual An individual or staff member who is qualified to provide care, treatment, or services by virtue of the following: education,

GL

training, experience, competence, registration, certification or applicable licensure, or law or regulation. Examples of qualified individuals include: activities coordinator, administrator, audiologist, child psychiatrist, clinical chaplain, creative arts therapist, dietetic services supervisor, dietitian, registered dietitian, health information administrator, health information technician, licensed practical nurse (LPN), medical radiation physician, medical technologist, music therapist, occupational therapist, occupational therapy assistant, physiatrist, physical therapist assistant, physical therapist, psychiatric nurse, psychologist, radiologic technologist, recreational therapist, recreational therapist assistant or technician, respiratory care technician, respiratory therapist, respiratory therapy technician, social work assistant, social worker, and speech-language pathologist.

quality control　A process that consists of measuring performance, comparing performance against goals, and acting on the differences when performance falls short of defined goals.

quality of care　The degree to which health services for individuals and populations increase the likelihood of desired health outcomes and are consistent with current professional knowledge. Dimensions of performance include the following: resident perspective issues; safety of the care environment; and accessibility, appropriateness, continuity, effectiveness, efficacy, efficiency, and timeliness of care.

Quality Report　A report that is available to the public that provides information about an organization's accreditation decision and the effec-

tive date for the decision, any special quality awards the organization received, the accreditation services included in the organization's accreditation award, any disease-specific care certification(s) and the effective date of each certification received by the organization, the implementation of National Patient Safety Goals by the organization, the organization's performance against National Quality Improvement Goals and the organization's performance in relation to Patient Experience of Care measures.

range orders　Orders in which the dose or dosing interval varies over a prescribed range, depending on the situation or individual's status.

rationale for a standard　Background, justification, or additional information about a standard. A rationale is *not* scored. Not every standard has a rationale.

reassessment　Ongoing data collection, which begins on initial assessment, comparing the most recent data with the data collected at earlier assessments.

record　**1.** The account compiled by physicians and other health care professionals of a variety of resident health information, such as assessment findings, treatment details, and progress notes. **2.** (data source) Data obtained from the records or documentation maintained on a resident in any health care setting (for example, hospital, home care, long term care, practitioner office). Includes automated and paper medical record systems.

referral　The sending of an individual (1) from one clinician to another clinician or specialist, (2) from one setting or service to another, or (3) by one

GL

physician (the referring physician) to another physician(s) or other resource, either for consultation or care.

registered nurse (RN)   An individual who is qualified by an approved post-secondary program or baccalaureate or higher degree in nursing and licensed by the state, commonwealth, or territory to practice professional nursing.

report generation   *See* information management.

reprocessing   All operations performed to render a contaminated reusable or single-use device resident ready. The steps may include cleaning and disinfection/sterilization. The manufacturer of reusable devices and single- use devices that are marketed as nonsterile should provide validated reprocessing instructions in the labeling.

requirement for improvement   A survey finding cited in an organization's Accreditation Report that must be addressed in the organization's Evidence of Standards Compliance (ESC) report.

resident   The recipient of care from a long term care provider or assisted living community.

residential occupancy   *See* occupancy.

respiratory care services   Delivery of care to provide ventilatory support and associated services for individuals.

restorative services   Goal-directed interventions that assist or promote a resident's ability to attain his or her maximum functional potential.

restraint   Any method (chemical or physical) of restricting a resident's freedom of movement, including seclusion, physical activity, or normal access to his or her body that (1) is not a usual and customary part of a medical diagnostic or treatment procedure to which the resident or his or her legal representative has consented; (2) is not indicated to treat the resident's medical condition or symptoms; or (3) does not promote the resident's independent functioning.

> **chemical restraint**   The inappropriate use of a sedating psychotropic drug to manage or control behavior.

> **physical restraint**   Any method of physically restricting a person's freedom of movement, physical activity, or normal access to his or her body.

retrievability   *See* information management.

Review Hearing Panel   A panel of three individuals, including one member of the Joint Commission Accreditation Committee, which hears a presentation on the facts of the case by an organization in Preliminary Denial of Accreditation, should the organization desire such a presentation.

risk assessment, proactive   An assessment that examines a process in detail including sequencing of events; assesses actual and potential risk, failure, or points of vulnerability; and, through a logical process, prioritizes areas for improvement based on the actual or potential resident care impact (criticality).

risk-management activities   Clinical and administrative activities that organizations undertake to identify, evaluate, and reduce the risk of injury to residents, staff, and visitors and the risk of loss to the organization itself.

GL

root cause analysis A process for identifying the basic or causal factor(s) that underlie variation in performance, including the occurrence or possible occurrence of a sentinel event.

run chart A display of data in which data points are plotted as they occur over time (for example, observed weights over time) to detect trends or other patterns and variation occurring over time. Run charts, as opposed to tabular frequency displays, are capable of time-order analytic studies.

safety The degree to which the risk of an intervention (for example, use of a drug or a procedure) and risk in the care environment are reduced for a resident and other persons, including health care practitioners.

safety management Activities selected and implemented by the organization to assess and control the impact of environmental risk, and to improve general environmental safety.

scope of care or services The activities performed by governance, managerial, clinical, or support staff.

secure In locked containers, in a locked room, or under constant surveillance.

security *See* information management.

security management A component of an organization's management of the environment of care program that maintains and improves the general security of the care environment.

self-administration *See* medication management, administration.

sentinel event An unexpected occurrence involving death or serious physical or psychological injury, or the risk thereof. Serious injury specifically includes loss of limb or function. The phrase *or the risk thereof* includes any process variation for which a recurrence carries a significant chance of a serious adverse outcome.

sexual abuse *See* abuse.

Shared Visions–New Pathways® An initiative to progressively sharpen the focus of the accreditation process on care systems critical to the safety and quality of resident care.

social work services Services to assist clients and their families in addressing social, emotional, and economic stresses associated with illness or injury. Such services are provided by a qualified social worker or a social work assistant under the supervision of a qualified social worker. These services can be provided directly or through contract with another organization or individual.

staff Individuals, such as employees, contractors, or temporary agency personnel, who provide services in an organization.

staffing effectiveness The number, competence, and skill mix of staff as related to the provision of needed services.

standard A statement that defines the performance expectations, structures, or processes that must be in place for an organization to provide safe, high-quality care, treatment, and services.

Statement of Conditions™ (SOC) A proactive document that helps an organization to do a critical self-assessment of its current level of compliance and describe how to resolve any *Life Safety Code®* (*LSC*) deficiencies. The SOC was created to

GL

be a "living, ongoing" management tool that should be used in a management process that continually identifies, assesses, and resolves *LSC* deficiencies.

sterilization   The use of a physical or chemical procedure to destroy all microbial life, including highly resistant bacterial endospores.

subacute care   Care that is rendered immediately after, or instead of, acute hospitalization to treat one or more specific, active, complex medical conditions or to administer one or more technically complex treatments in the context of an individual's underlying long-term conditions and overall situation. Subacute care requires the coordinated services of an interdisciplinary team.

Subacute care is generally more intensive than traditional nursing facility care and less intensive than acute inpatient care. It requires frequent (daily to weekly) resident assessment and review of the clinical course and treatment plan for a limited time period (several days to several months), until a condition is stabilized or a predetermined treatment course is completed.

This definition addresses the following seven factors the Joint Commission considers integral to the provision of subacute care:

Time: Subacute care is rendered immediately after, or instead of, acute hospitalization.

Reason: It treats one or more specific, active, complex, or unstable medical conditions or administers one or more technically complex treatments in the context of a person's underlying long-term condition and overall situation.

Caregivers: It requires the services of an interdisciplinary team who is trained and knowledgeable to assess and manage the specific conditions and to perform the necessary procedures.

Site: It is provided as an inpatient program.

Frequency: It requires frequent resident assessment and review of the clinical course and treatment plan.

Intensity: It provides care at a level generally more intensive than provided in a traditional nursing facility and less intensive than provided in acute inpatient care.

Duration: It lasts for a limited time or until a condition is stabilized or a predetermined treatment course is completed.

supplemental finding   A recommendation that is not required to be addressed in an organization's Evidence of Standards Compliance (ESC) report (*see* definition), but should be addressed by the organization internally. A supplemental finding is also factored into an organization's Priority Focus Process (PFP) at its next survey.

surrogate decision maker   Someone appointed to act on behalf of another. Surrogates make decisions only when an individual is without capacity or has given permission to involve others. *See also* advocate; family.

survey   A key component in the accreditation process, whereby a surveyor(s) conducts an on-site evaluation of an organization's compliance with Joint Commission standards.

full survey   A survey that assesses an organization's compliance with

GL

all applicable Joint Commission standards.

initial survey   A survey of a health care organization not previously accredited by the Joint Commission, or a survey of an organization performed without reference to any prior survey findings.

surveyor   For purposes of Joint Commission accreditation, a physician, nurse, administrator, laboratorian, or any other health care professional who meets the Joint Commission's surveyor selection criteria, evaluates standards compliance, and provides education and consultation regarding standards compliance to surveyed organizations or networks.

system   A set of interrelated parts that work together toward a common goal.

system tracer   A session during an on-site survey devoted to evaluating high-priority safety and quality-of-care issues on a systemwide basis throughout the organization. Examples of such issues may include infection control, medication management, staffing effectiveness, and the use of data.

systems analysis   The evaluation of how well a health care organization's systems function.

threshold for Conditional Accreditation   At least two but not more than three standard deviations above the mean number of not compliant standards; the threshold for Conditional Accreditation is one rule for receiving Conditional Accreditation.

threshold for Preliminary Denial of Accreditation   At least three standard deviations above the mean number of not compliant standards; the threshold for Preliminary Denial of

Accreditation is one rule for receiving Preliminary Denial of Accreditation.

timeliness   *See* information management.

titrating orders   Orders in which the dose is either progressively increased or decreased in response to the individual's status.

total parenteral nutrition   *See* nutrition, parenteral nutrition.

tracer methodology   A tool used by a process surveyor(s) during an on-site survey to analyze an organization's systems, with particular attention to identified priority focus areas (PFAs), by following individual residents, residents, or clients through the organization's health care process in the sequence experienced by the patients, residents, or clients. Depending on the health care setting, this may require surveyors to visit multiple care units, departments, or areas within an organization or a single care unit to trace the care rendered to a patient, resident, or client.

transfer   The formal shifting of responsibility for the care of an individual (1) from one care unit to another, (2) from one clinical service to another, (3) from one licensed independent practitioner to another, or (4) from one organization to another.

transfer agreement   A written understanding that provides for the reciprocal transfer of individuals between health care organizations.

transmission   *See* information management.

urgent/immediate care services   Those services sought for conditions that are considered less critical than those that need to be seen in an

GL

emergency center, but are not scheduled with the individual's primary care provider or the provider's designee.

utilities management   Activities selected and implemented by the organization to assess and control the risks of utility systems of buildings that support the provision of care, treatment, or services. Included are those activities that ensure the operational reliability of such systems and those activities for responding to a failure of such systems.

utility systems   Building systems for life support; surveillance, prevention, and control of infection; environment support; and equipment support. These can include electrical distribution; emergency power; vertical and horizontal transport; heating, ventilating, and air conditioning; plumbing, boiler, and steam; piped gases; vacuum systems; or communication systems including data-exchange systems.

utilization management   The examination and evaluation of the appropriateness of the utilization of an organization's resources. Also referred to as a utilization review.

waived testing   Tests that meet the Clinical Laboratory Improvement Amendments of 1988 (CLIA '88) requirements for waived tests; are cleared by the Food and Drug Administration for home use; employ methodologies that are so simple and accurate as to render the likelihood of erroneous results negligible; or pose no risk of harm to a resident if the test is performed incorrectly.

GL

Index

IX

IX

IX

IX

IX

IX

IX

IX

IX

IX

IX

IX